Managing Mad Mast Cells

A Practical Guide to Living with Mast Cell Activation Syndrome (MCAS)

Joy A. Schweizer

ISBN (Paperback): 978-3-9526273-0-3
ISBN (Hardcover): 978-3-9526273-1-0
ISBN (eBook): 978-3-9526273-2-7

First edition, January 2026
Published by Greener Pastures Books

Cover design by Jennifer Federico Stimson
Edited by Michael Tizzano
Typesetting by Arjan van Woensel

Copies are available through Amazon and other major retailers.

Dedicated to the Mast Cell Community

Table of Contents

SECTION III — MANAGING YOUR DIAGNOSIS

SECTION IV — DAILY SURVIVAL TACTICS

SECTION V — DIET & NUTRITION

RESOURCES & REFERENCES

Foreword

I am a medical doctor specializing in general internal medicine. I earned my degree in human medicine from the University of Zurich in Switzerland in 2011 and completed my Doctor of Medicine (MD) at the same university in 2021. Over the years, I have built a broad skill set with extensive hands-on experience in cardiology, pulmonology, neurology, pathology, rehabilitation, and sleep medicine. I am also active in academic research, with three first-authored and four co-authored publications. Since 2019, my main focus has been on myalgic encephalomyelitis/chronic fatigue syndrome (ME/CFS), which is classified in ICD-10 under code G93.3.

This unusual career choice was primarily driven by personal reasons: I developed ME/CFS at age fourteen, and it took another seventeen years to receive a formal diagnosis. It was an incredibly tough and sanity-testing journey, to say the least. After seeing countless specialists from various backgrounds and enduring debilitating frustration with the generally prevalent misunderstanding of the condition, I felt it was necessary to cultivate and apply the often-overlooked knowledge to help others in similar distress. For clinicians, one of the main challenges in ME/CFS is the vast number of different conditions they must be able to recognize. Mast cell disorders (e.g., MCAD/MCAS) and their activities come up much earlier in the diagnostic process.

When Joy introduced herself in 2019, I had only a vague understanding of mast cell disorders. However, I was intrigued—she reminded me of myself: dead-set on finding the source of her suffering and effective treatments. Initially, I listened. Then I spent countless hours researching and reading. Finally, we devised a diagnostic testing plan, which at that time was a novelty in Switzerland. The rest is history. Word spread quickly, and I soon began receiving more referrals for patients with allergy-like symptoms but no clear diagnosis.

Screening for and differentiating mast cell disorders and other immunological disorders has meanwhile become part of my daily routine. There turned out to be a substantial grey area of obvious immunological anomalies orphaned by regular specialties that remain focused on a pre-selected variety of more sharply definable conditions. One of my primary purposes in my work is identifying these overlooked cases for further referrals. Regardless of whether a clearly defined condition is present, many of my patients require practical models and tangible, hands-on approaches to manage their daily lives. Ultimately, clinicians, therapists, and coaches may offer information and guidance, but even the most seasoned specialists should not confuse their long-term experience with the individual experiences of those suffering from a given disease.

This is where self-help and experience books become invaluable. They consolidate knowledge across physical, psychological, financial, and personal domains, translating complex information into accessible language and presenting it in a more personal way than scientific papers. People with mast cell disorders often face similar issues and benefit greatly from shared experiences. Joy's book offers a unique approach: it presents academic fundamentals in a clear, relatable way, is grounded in her story, and gathers all the practical information in one place. Identifying triggers, finding useful dietary modifications, supplements, or medications can be tricky—even more so learning how to manage everyday situations with MCAS since relevant information is scattered and hard to find.

While books, articles, and online resources can't replace specialists, they do offer understanding and serve as vital companions in the trial-and-error journey of recovery. They benefit patients, caregivers, and families alike. As a clinician, I'm grateful for such works—they fill a gap beyond what medicine alone can reach. Joy's book may well become an essential part of many personal journeys.

If you suffer—or believe you suffer—from a mast cell-associated disorder, don't give up. Please seek help from a medical professional experienced with mast cell-associated disorders beyond the clinically well-defined entities. Although this remains uncommon as of now, the future seems brighter—with increasing demand, increased supply must follow.

— **Protazy Rejmer, MD**

Preface

When I was diagnosed with mastocytosis, my doctors told me my health would likely only deteriorate over time. They suggested I just come to terms with the fact that I was now living with a chronic, lifelong condition that would never go away.

I really wasn't cool with that! I was incredibly sick and wanted nothing more than to return to at least some semblance of normal. Hearing this bleak prognosis, I instantly resolved to learn everything about mast cell disease and find a way to improve. After that meeting, I headed straight to the town's top bookstore to buy every book on mast cell disease I could find—only to discover that there weren't any!

With no books available, I had to wrap my head around this pernicious disease by studying research papers, consulting with other patients, and experimenting on myself—alongside countless doctor visits. A few years later, my initial diagnosis turned out to be wrong: I was actually dealing with mast cell activation syndrome (MCAS), Ehlers–Danlos syndrome (EDS), and Hereditary Alpha Tryptasemia (HαT).

Over the course of those years, I went through phases of debilitating pain, hopelessness, and fear, along with countless nerve-wracking attempts to convey my experience to others. Despite the challenges, I found ways to improve. Bit by bit, I began to feel better. Knowing what I know now, I am certain I could have felt better faster. Because of that, I felt it was finally on me to provide others with the book I wished to find at the beginning of my journey. I hope my insights will benefit others with MCAS and will contribute to a greater understanding of this disease; for those affected and for anyone interested in learning about it.

Managing Mad Mast Cells offers insights on the key topics I personally needed to understand in order to make sense of the condition and begin managing it effectively. Organized into five sections, it features bite-sized subchapters, allowing you to jump straight to the topics that interest you most.

- *Section I recounts my personal journey, highlighting what may have contributed to MCAS, the challenges of diagnosis, the difficulties that followed, and how I overcame them.*
- *Section II offers explanations of the fundamental medical aspects.*
- *Section III addresses psychological hurdles that can arise with MCAS.*
- *Section IV discusses methods for mitigating the impact of various triggers in daily life.*
- *Section V looks at diet and nutrition in the context of MCAS.*

Keep in mind that MCAS is complex and varies from person to person. My insights likely won't cover all the challenges you personally face, and some patients are worse off than I am. This book offers a good overview and starting point, but responses differ; what suits me might not suit you, or could even be harmful. Always consult your doctor and use your own best judgment when trying new approaches.

Also, let me state this clearly: I am not a doctor, and this book is not a substitute for actual medical treatment. I have no medical degree of any kind, so I am in no way suggesting that you should forego professional medical care. This book doesn't claim to be a way to heal MCAS. It's intended as more of a general guidebook and map of the territory, providing insights and strategies to assist you on your own path toward the effective management of this disease.

I am simply sharing a thorough summary of my own research as someone living with MCAS, drawn from sources like PubMed, JAMA Network, and other reputable platforms. The facts presented are backed by scientific references, which I encourage you to explore for deeper insight. Throughout the chapters, I indicate whether the information comes from scientific studies, my personal experience, or the collective knowledge of self-help communities.

I offer this book in the hope it may help ease any fears that come with your diagnosis, support you in learning how to manage your condition, and help your loved ones better understand your struggles with MCAS.

Good luck on your journey, and don't ever give up!

With love,
Joy

What Is MCAS?

Before we even start, let's get the big question out of the way: What the heck is MCAS? MCAS stands for mast cell activation syndrome, a relatively newly discovered chronic health condition that affects multiple organ systems in an inflammatory manner. It can present with or without allergic-type symptoms and the abnormal or dysfunctional growth of tissues, known as dystrophy.

Symptoms vary greatly from patient to patient and fluctuate in intensity over time. They tend to migrate across different body systems and range from mild to severe. The most dangerous manifestation is anaphylaxis, a severe, life-threatening allergic reaction that can be fatal in rare cases.[1]

To better understand MCAS, it helps to first have an idea of what mast cells are and what they do:

The roles of mast cells in our body

Without mast cells, we wouldn't be able to survive. As part of the immune system, these cells serve as a first line of defense against various threats such as parasites, bacteria, and venoms. They also aid in wound healing and tissue repair, help maintain vascular and bronchial homeostasis, and play a role in forming new blood vessels. Furthermore, they regulate bone growth and turnover and support mineral balance in bones.[2,3]

Characteristics of MCAS

In MCAS, mast cells are inappropriately active and release excessive mediators in response to various triggers. These triggers can vary widely from patient to patient and may also change for individuals over time. Furthermore, patients with MCAS may be triggered by substances and factors that are typically harmless to healthy individuals.

Examples include physical and emotional stress, infections, certain medications and excipients, specific foods, temperature changes, hormonal fluctuations, smells, vibrations, environmental toxins, and chemical components in body care products, furniture, fabrics, and building materials. Simply put, if you're affected by MCAS, you may experience allergic-type reactions to everyday substances and situations, which can be severe and, in the worst-case scenario, potentially life-threatening.[1,4-6]

As mentioned earlier, mast cells can activate in less than a second. This rapid response can be immediate and serious. For instance, if the scent of someone's perfume triggers an MCAS patient, they may experience symptoms such as facial flushing, difficulty breathing, or, in extreme cases, fainting within seconds to minutes due to the sudden release of mast cell mediators.

In the simplest terms, you could say that mast cells (in MCAS) are like overprotective bodyguards

If you've seen the movie *Iron Man*, think of "Happy" Hogan as played by Jon Favreau—exceedingly loyal and well-meaning, but honestly a bit over-concerned. They react to everyone and everything, and before long, you have to look after them more than they protect you.

Snobs

This is my favorite way to describe them. Mast cells act like a bunch of self-entitled snobs who take reign in your body. They are incredibly picky, very particular, and radically irritated if they don't get their way. Their way of wanting things might have very little to do with your preferences, but these little snobs are in charge right now. For now, they must be accommodated and appeased because they'll make life a living hell for you if you don't.

Symptoms

Symptoms of MCAS may be chronic or acute and are characterized by inflammation. Since virtually every organ or body system can be affected, the clinical signs can be constitutional, gastrointestinal, dermatologic, respiratory, immunologic, hematologic, neurological, psychiatric, ocular/ophthalmologic, and/or oral.[1,4-6]

The difficulty of diagnosis

It is not uncommon for MCAS patients to be repeatedly misdiagnosed and labeled as hypochondriacs by their families and doctors before ultimately receiving the correct diagnosis. MCAS often goes unrecognized because routine testing isn't effective in detecting mast cell involvement, and symptoms frequently overlap with other conditions. The high variability of disease manifestations and its episodic nature complicates diagnosis even more.[6]

Additionally, patients often appear much healthier than one might expect, given their extensive list of complaints. Dr. Lawrence B. Afrin, a leading expert in the field of mast cell activation disorders, has noted that many patients come to regard their symptoms—including daily episodes of anaphylaxis—as "normal," simply because they have never found clear explanations for their experiences.

Diagnostic frameworks

MCAS is both underdiagnosed and overdiagnosed. An additional challenge is the existence of several diagnostic proposals, with the two major classification frameworks being Consensus-1, which takes a stricter approach that relies on specific biomarkers, and Consensus-2, which is broader and more symptom-based. Neither has been established as superior or more accurate, and both are considered valid approaches for diagnosing MCAS, each with its pros and cons.

To compare the two proposals, refer to the following key papers:

1. "Definitions, Criteria and Global Classification of Mast Cell Disorders with Special Reference to Mast Cell Activation Syndromes: A Consensus Proposal," published in *International Archives of Allergy and Immunology* in 2012 (Consensus-1).[7]

2. "Diagnosis of mast cell activation syndrome: a global 'consensus-2'" published in *Diagnosis* in 2021(Consensus-2).[1]

The key similarities in both approaches include:

1. clinical signs and symptoms of mast cell activation

2. evidence of abnormal levels of mast cell mediators

3. favorable response to mast cell-targeting medications

The primary difference lies in how strictly they define the condition and, thus, in the number of patients eligible for an MCAS diagnosis, which can significantly affect treatment strategies and patient management.[1,5,7,8]

Prevalence

Estimates of MCAS prevalence also vary greatly. While many experts suggest that 17–20 percent of the population may be affected, others contend that MCAS is rare.[1,5]

Treatment and management strategies

Although MCAS is considered a chronic condition that poses significant challenges in a patient's daily life, life expectancy is typically not compromised. Many individuals eventually find effective treatment strategies tailored to their unique needs. These treatment plans usually include antihistaminic medications, mast cell stabilizing agents, and lifestyle changes, such as strict avoidance of triggers.[1]

The Irony of MCAS

"Oh, you look fine to me!"

Ironically, people will often say, "Oh wow, you look so healthy! What do you do to look so good?" Alternatively, I'm also told, "Oh, you look fine to me! I don't think it can be that bad." And other times, I've heard, "You look fantastic; you must be feeling better now!" Some have even said outright that they think that it's all just in my head, while others have suggested that I may be anorexic.

Sure, I might look pretty good when I feel reasonably well. I'm likely still in pain even on such days, but pain is often not visible. I guess I do look pretty healthy, because there is simply no way for me to live an unhealthy lifestyle. I cannot eat unhealthy foods, drink alcohol, go over my limits, or deprive myself of sleep. I've got to avoid everything toxic because I would react to it so severely that it would just hurt too much.

The invisible reality of bad days

The thing is, nobody sees me on a bad day, because I am not going outside. There are days when I cannot stand on my feet because they hurt so much. In fact, on some days, everything from the bottom of my feet to the top of my head is in agony.

On such days, I must avoid further triggers to prevent things from worsening—bright lights (even sunlight), harsh noises, certain foods, perfumes, smells, excessive heat or cold, and any physically or emotionally taxing situation can all intensify the reaction.

Dealing with doubters and setting boundaries

Dealing with those who don't believe me can be incredibly frustrating. On one hand, it's emotionally draining; if you're seriously sick, you'd hope that those who say they love you would take the initiative to learn about your disease instead of questioning your experience. On the other hand, I hate arguing about my limitations, because it contradicts my decision to focus on the positive.

What I'd hope for is constructive compassion—that those around me would at least try to learn about my condition and take steps to ensure I won't get sicker when we visit, such as forgoing perfumes, for example. Unfortunately, the reality for many MCAS patients is that we are often not understood and are sometimes even labeled as hypochondriacs. People with the flu or someone who burned a hand on a hot stove usually receive more sympathy and support than those with MCAS, because their pain is visible and familiar—something others can easily relate to.

What hurts the most is knowing that, unlike the flu or a burn, MCAS doesn't simply go away. It's chronic. Those affected must live with the constant awareness that every day requires careful management to avoid making things worse.

So, over time, I've learned to set boundaries. If I sense that someone isn't genuinely interested, I keep conversations about my illness brief. If someone says, "Oh, you look so healthy!" I simply say, "Thank you." If they remark, "I don't think it's so bad," I tell them that it's complicated—and if they genuinely wanted to understand, they'd need to set aside an entire afternoon to listen. This is a good example of where I've learned to set boundaries by choosing carefully where and how I spend my limited energy.

A helpful metaphor

The following story is a good example of the irony of MCAS. A member of a self-help group broke her arm and arrived at the hospital wearing a sling. A gentleman noticed and quickly jumped up to open the heavy door for her. She said she was, of course, grateful—but admitted that on any ordinary day she wouldn't have had the strength to push that same door open, simply because of the weakness her mast cell issues caused. She even joked that wearing a sling might be a clever way to signal she could use a little help.

Helping others understand

Of course, there are some people in our lives who we want to know what is going on and who definitely *should* know. If we share the same household, for example, they must understand what triggers us and take steps to avoid these substances just as we do, so that we can stay as well as possible.

Thanks to the Mast Cell Disease Society, you can access a host of infographics to print and share with your friends and relatives. These resources, designed to help explain your condition, are available on their website at tmsforacure.org.

Stay true to yourself

Whatever others say about you doesn't really matter. You have to stay true to yourself. Believe your body when it tells you something, and take care of it.

People cannot see what they cannot see. They are often at a loss for understanding when they face situations they've never experienced and therefore struggle to relate. Forgive their lack, and don't be afraid to move on… lovingly. I know this can hurt, but I think it's part of living with this disease that real friends will show up, while sunny-day friends will go their separate ways. In the end, we're better off that way.

Sharing this book

Writing this book has enabled me to share what it means to be in such a situation with friends and family. Equally, you, dear reader, can pass this book on to those who want to learn about your life with MCAS.

SECTION I

My Story

CHAPTER 1

From My Childhood Through My Twenties

I was born in Switzerland in the summer of 1982. My family lived in a small, picturesque village in the northern wine country, so I got to spend the majority of my childhood surrounded by nature. I loved to roam through the forests, fields, and vineyards, ride my bike around the region, and swim in one of the many nearby lakes.

The youngest of four, my siblings are ten, eight, and three years older than me. My mom had been married once before, so my two older siblings have another dad. My father worked as a teacher in the city, so, I only got to see him in the evenings and on the weekends, but my mom stayed home with us while we were still young. Besides being a fantastic mother, she is a teacher and a very talented artist as well. During these years, she also managed a pottery studio, where she created her artwork and taught classes.

My extended family is composed of entirely contrasting characters. As the youngest, naturally I observed a lot, and this rather chaotic potpourri of personalities was indeed fascinating to behold. Among my relatives, we had an artist, a teacher, a drug addict, a housewife, an alcoholic, a scholar, a craftsman, a punk rocker, and, I'd say, a status seeker. Angry, happy, unhappy, eager, desperate, arrogant, fulfilled, caring, and uncaring—I got to observe all this. I sincerely appreciate the diverse range of lifestyles and viewpoints I could learn from, as it has undoubtedly contributed to my self-understanding and helped me to identify my own preferences in life more precisely. It has kept me from repeating some of their biggest mistakes, yet it has also, perhaps inevitably, led me to make my own set of major missteps later on in life.

Compared to my siblings, I was the only kid who had so many health issues. Not that I was sick and miserable all the time—quite the contrary. I was actually very active, lively, and happy. I enjoyed many sports and physical activities, including Judo, ice and inline skating, running, biking, swimming, soccer, handball, basketball, and horseback riding. Besides all that, I have also loved making music for as long as I can remember. I started playing the violin at age five. Yet, despite a deep admiration for classical music, I wanted nothing to do with note-reading. This made it so difficult to deal with my music teachers that, unfortunately, I quit before long. By age seven, I had already determined that I wouldn't continue with these hidebound lessons anymore because I truly feared losing my love for music if I did. Instead, I just proceeded with the actual playing itself and taught myself the piano, drums, and later the guitar.

I had a good childhood. I had good friends with whom I could play, was out in nature every day, and had a nice home with a lovely family. In truth, I enjoyed my life overall; but some health issues were present from the beginning.

EARLY SYMPTOMS IN CHILDHOOD

From ages one to three, I suffered from chronic colic. To my parents, this surely seemed somewhat out of the ordinary, but apparently not unusual enough to take me to a doctor. Around age two, just starting to be able to string words together, I repeatedly tried to tell my family that my back hurt. Unfortunately, to no avail. I guess everyone around me thought I was way too young to have backaches, because my complaints were always dismissed out of hand as something I might have just picked up from a complaining adult. It took no less than three years of my unwavering insistence until I finally got taken to a doctor for a checkup. This physician found no explanation for my complaints other than a slight curvature of my spine, and the only help offered was a few ultimately useless strengthening exercises.

I also frequently exhibited both excessive bruising and recurrent, prolonged nosebleeds. Yet, besides the people who happened to see some of the bruises asking me whether I'd been beaten at home, which I definitely hadn't, no further questions were ever raised about it. The adults around me often told me that I was just that way, and by hearing this repeatedly from a young age, I really had come to believe that it was all somehow normal for me.

Besides all this, there were allergies. I was always sensitive to dust and cat hair. Not extremely sensitive, but they made me awfully itchy! And I've also always had somewhat of a round, swollen belly. I often wondered why this was so, but once again, whenever I'd asked, I was told that this was probably just the way I was. For a long time, I didn't even realize that I might be allergic to some foods, but my symptoms started to get significantly worse around age sixteen, so I finally had to start considering the possibility that I might have some food intolerances after all.

My parents got divorced when I was seven. After that, my dad moved to the city, and my brother and I visited him every other weekend and during school vacations. Going back and forth between these two worlds was quite challenging for me. My parents have rather contrasting personalities, along with very different lifestyles and perspectives. They also have wild discrepancies between their ultimate expectations, ideas, and hopes for their kids. Naturally, due to my love for both of these people and wanting to please them both, my repeatedly bouncing back and forth between them wasn't easy at all. Quite often, I ended up getting sick with fevers and nosebleeds on the first day of these visitation weekends—or I was grumpy or homesick, and later felt guilty about that, too.

EARLY TEENS

I started suffering from depression around age twelve. It's plausible that the shared custody was a major contributing factor, because I felt like I could never just be myself at home due to people around me trying to push me in very different directions simultaneously. On the other hand, it's also possible that the constant back pain, with no clear explanation as to why it kept hurting all the time, had something to do with it, too. Additionally, based on my perpetually swollen belly back then, it's likely that I was already allergic to some foods. Allergies can trigger inflammation, which in turn will often trigger depression all on its own. Most likely, it was the combination of all of these things that led me to entertain a death wish at such an early age, seriously enough to act on it.

After my second suicide attempt, this time at age thirteen, my mom decided we would move to the city. She wanted to be able to spend more time with us, which would be much easier if we lived closer to her work. My two older siblings were already old enough to live independently, so they both moved out and got their own apartments at the same time. Now it was just my mom, my brother, and me. I was eventually taken to sit down with a psychologist, but after talking to him once, I knew only two things for sure: first, I really didn't like the guy, and second, I never wanted to see him again. Consequently, this was both our first and last meeting. Instead of going back to therapy, I ventured on to find ways to distract myself from the depression.

Since I was still here and alive, I decided to give life a chance. And as I felt I had absolutely nothing to lose, I quite boldly went out exploring to see what else life had to offer. Depression would come crashing in time and time again, but I somehow always found a way to climb back out of it.

Our apartment in Zurich had been newly renovated, and it took us quite some time to detect that a pretty large mold spot had formed behind my brother's wardrobe. The walls had most likely not been allowed to dry properly before being painted. Our landlord had it fixed right away, but in retrospect, I can't shake the thought that this toxic mold exposure might have played a role in the subsequent decline in my health.

A BODY IN CRISIS

Around age fourteen, my back pain started to get so intense that I couldn't properly move, sit, or even sleep anymore. My doctor ordered me to go for weekly massage therapy, and my parents got me a good mattress. Both measures brought about some slight relief, but I had to get a massage every week without fail to remain even remotely functional. Aside from the minor reduction in pain, no real progress was made. If I didn't make it back for another session by the seventh day, my back would lock up all over again. I was certainly thankful for the massages, but I just really wanted to know why I had this pain in the first place and what, if anything, I could do to make it go away—not just for a few days, but for good! I kept pestering both my doctor and my massage therapist about it, but time and time again, I was told to hold better posture. I genuinely tried that, but I couldn't do it! Maintain my posture? I couldn't even figure out how to keep my back upright for a moment—it just didn't work!

At fifteen, I began experiencing nonstop finger, wrist, and hand pain. Doctors couldn't find a clear cause, with no swelling or visible signs, but they suspected joint inflammation based on how I described my pain. I was told to take cortisone thrice daily and avoid using my hands whenever they hurt. For the following three years, I had to wear wrist splints most of the time. I also remember reacting badly to my mom's citrus-scented body cream, feeling nauseous whenever she used it, even from two rooms down with closed doors. Looking back, I still wonder if the previous mold exposure might have caused these reactions.

My digestive system began to deteriorate when I was about sixteen years old. I experienced a range of symptoms, including stomach pain and acid reflux, along with alternating constipation and diarrhea. Thinking at the time that it must be an intolerance to either wheat or milk, I eventually checked for allergies, but all the tests came back negative. Over and over, I was told everything was fine and was encouraged to keep eating everything. So I did, despite the pain, but I kept on searching for answers and eventually started learning about and actively experimenting with alternative diets and various medicinal plants.

Around age seventeen, I started fainting time and time again. Whenever I asked doctors why this happened, they said it was most likely due to low blood sugar. They told me to eat more and see if it helped. My backache was still ongoing, and the underlying issues hadn't been resolved in any lasting way despite all the massage therapy, so I kept asking healthcare providers what the cause was or at least what I could do to ameliorate the symptoms. Most of them said that I'd have to hold better posture and continue doing strengthening exercises. One physician even told me to *find my inner balance.* Well … I tried all that, but nothing worked, so my search for answers continued.

One day, a school friend suggested that one of my legs might be shorter than the other after noticing how I walk. Initially I dismissed it as preposterous, but since I'd never found an explanation for my pain, I decided to ask my doctor. He laughed, shook his head, and dismissed it—but after I literally begged him to check, he finally agreed to measure anyway. Turns out, my left leg was, in fact, about half an inch shorter. He apologized and prescribed orthopedic insoles, which also supported my flat feet. They helped while I was wearing them, but barefoot, I was back to being off-balance.

MY FIRST ATTEMPT TO WORK

Reaching the age of eighteen, I took up an apprenticeship in hospitality. The first part of the training consisted mainly of maintenance and cleaning, with an interim month of fieldwork in an industrial laundry facility. My hands got so inflamed after working amidst all those chemicals that I couldn't even bend a finger anymore. It eventually became so bad—in the doctors' views, completely hopeless—that I got put on disability. I had to quit my apprenticeship and was told never to work with my hands again. The doctors stressed that even office work, such as typing on a keyboard, would be too much strain on my hands! Furthermore, I was urged to stop playing music if I wanted to make it to thirty and still be able to move my fingers at all.

Of course, it was altogether discouraging, and even downright demoralizing, to be told that I probably shouldn't ever even think about working with my hands again! It felt awful to be put on disability, having only just recently turned eighteen, and I was already getting pretty exasperated by the complete lack of progress with my condition—but the moment I was told to stop playing music, I was fed up. There had to be a way to fix this! The wrist splints and medications certainly helped soothe the pain to some extent, but they hadn't done a thing to solve the problem, so I decided I needed to go down another route.

It had been over three years since I was advised to rest my hands whenever they hurt. Unfortunately, this pain never really went away, so I almost always had at least one hand in a splint at any given time. My wrists had meanwhile become awfully frail, so I figured strengthening exercises might be worth a try. It would be painful to begin with because it hurt even to bend a finger at this stage, but I was determined to fix this. I was going to work through the pain and try to build up some muscle to help stabilize the joints. I started very cautiously, at first only gently kneading playdough, and then slowly and gradually working my way up to more challenging exercises.

A naturopath eventually suggested that quark and cabbage wraps can help soothe inflammation. Initially, this sounded quite absurd, but with nothing to lose, I ended up giving it a try. Much to my surprise and delight, it worked so well that it quickly became my first go-to remedy. After doing the strengthening exercises for over a year and a half, I successfully built enough muscle to support my joints and regain the use of my hands. Finally, I could discontinue the cortisone pills entirely. As of writing this book, I'm forty years old, my hands are strong, and I can still play my instruments. Inflammation still crops up, but now I know how to treat these flare-ups naturally. I have also come to know my body well enough to be much more careful in my movements, and I've learned to recognize when it's time to rest!

RISING JUST TO FALL

By age twenty, I had strengthened my hands enough to work again and started a sales apprenticeship at an organic bakery with a café and health food store. Though my hands felt better, my digestive issues and back pain kept getting worse. On top of that, depression hit me hard that year, especially after the breakup with my first love, who I had lived with for over two years. It left me feeling suicidal. It eventually became so severe that I sought help. This turned out to be quite a journey: After consulting seventeen psychiatrists and psychologists, I finally found a polarity therapy practitioner, which ultimately felt like the right approach.

Most of the other therapists were out of the question because I was absolutely averse to taking medication. I'd witnessed people becoming entirely numb to their feelings while on antidepressants, and I didn't want to mask this pain with any pharmaceutical crutch—I wanted to get to the bottom of it. I wanted to learn why my mind worked the way it did, why I tended to see things as dark as I did sometimes, and what I could do to truly free myself from this horrendous pain. It was my aim to master and overcome this grueling depression once and for all.

Polarity therapy proved to be the right choice for me. It helped me feel calmer, but the most significant benefit I got was realizing the value and power of staying present. I learned to pay attention to how my body feels and discovered that I usually have the means to make myself feel at least a bit more comfortable. Regardless of how I feel at any moment, if I recognize the need, I can make myself feel better, both physically and emotionally. I also learned techniques to prevent myself from going even deeper into negative thinking and to take charge and engage in activities that make me happier. I eventually felt stable enough to discontinue the therapy.

However, my back pain was still ongoing. Despite weekly physiotherapy sessions, massages, and continuous strength training, my back would still often lock up so badly that I simply couldn't move anymore. A couple of times when that happened, my doctor decided to inject cortisone into the joints to help restore the mobility, but I didn't tolerate these shots well at all. Within less than a minute of receiving the injection, I was drenched in sweat, my heart racing, and feeling so weak and dizzy that the nurses had to prop me up to prevent me from falling off the bed. Cortisone was clearly not going to be the answer for me—but continuing with the training was.

OUT OF AIR

At age twenty-one, my lungs collapsed twice; in medical terminology this is referred to as a spontaneous pneumothorax. I was sitting in school when I suddenly noticed an especially nasty sting in my back and all around my ribs. Attempting to stretch, which had often helped to alleviate such pain, only spiked it further this time. Even just trying to take another breath hurt! I felt a little light-headed, but still dismissed it as the usual pain and just sat with it. At some point, my teacher called upon me to answer a question. I couldn't speak up, so I waved him closer to me and asked him, now just in a frail whisper, to please not call me up because I couldn't breathe properly. He jolted into action right away, and I was rushed to the hospital.

At the emergency room, I was put on an oxygen mask and a chest X-ray was ordered, stat. When results came back, the doctors really sprang into high gear. My right lung had shrunk to less than half its size, risking collapse and wrapping around the heart. To prevent this, they quickly inserted a chest drain to remove the trapped air, allowing the lung to expand. A pneumothorax occurs when air leaks into the space between the lung and chest wall, increasing pressure and causing collapse. Draining the air relieves the pressure, letting the lung expand again.

I had to stay in the hospital for about a week. The doctors couldn't identify an apparent cause and casually mentioned that it could have something to do with my connective tissue. Yet they rushed right past that and dismissively said that, after all, it wasn't all that unusual for young, skinny women to have their lungs collapse. They also told me that this could happen again any time, and I should get myself to the nearest hospital immediately if it did. No kidding!

About four weeks later, it really did happen again. Now it was decided that I needed a surgical intervention to prevent yet another collapse as soon as possible. They would remove the pulmonary alveoli—those tiny, delicate air sacs—from the upper part of my lung and fix the right wing of the lung to my ribcage to reduce the likelihood of it happening again.

During the surgery, they discovered that my blood platelet count was alarmingly low, so shortly after that, I was sent to a hematologist. The hematologist couldn't pinpoint the underlying cause, so I was referred to an oncologist.

After weeks of testing, even the oncologist was still puzzled. She was able to rule out serious diseases like cancer, HIV, and hepatitis, and also to determine that my platelet count drops significantly during infections or fever. However, she couldn't tell why this was happening. So, without knowing the underlying cause, she diagnosed me with ITP (idiopathic thrombocytopenia) and explained that "idiopathic" simply means the cause is unknown. A bone marrow test could have revealed more, but she advised against it unless my levels became dangerously low. She recommended regular checkups, warned me to avoid blood thinners, and cautioned me to prevent serious injuries, as bleeding could be life-threatening. Although I hadn't worried about any of this before, I was relieved not to have cancer, HIV, or hepatitis—and I was glad to finally have an explanation for my lifelong bruises.

FINALLY ON MY OWN TERMS

I graduated from my apprenticeship when I was twenty-two. Psyched to finally finish my education, I couldn't wait to travel! In fact, I was so ready to get away that I found myself on an airplane bound for San Francisco the very first morning after graduation. I had booked a three-week stay, but thanks to my newfound freedom, I never boarded that return flight and ended up living in the Bay Area for the next five years instead.

I initially did a work trade at a yoga center, exchanging help for room, board, free classes, and sauna access. There, I learned about yoga, raw food, and detox, and through client connections I discovered meditation, Tai Chi, various massage styles, and osteopathy. My interest in bodywork grew, leading me to complete a Shiatsu program at the San Francisco School of Massage. To make ends meet, I took various jobs: cleaning, interior design consultations, apartment refurbishing, working as both a personal chef and a café barista, and occasional babysitting or dog walking gigs. I explored the city's neighborhoods by bike, made many new friends, and often enjoyed music jams and open mics. After a few years in, I decided to study travel and tourism, with a year at City College followed by practical training as a front desk clerk in a youth hostel near Fisherman's Wharf. My visa finally expired after graduation, so I decided to return to Switzerland.

Luckily, I found a super cute apartment right away, situated in the old center of Zurich. The rent for this place was so incredibly low that I could juggle a bunch of part-time positions instead of taking on a regular full-time job. This way, I could take time off whenever I had enough money to get by and use this extra time to delve into creative projects like music, art, and writing.

I eventually had as many as eleven different part-time positions that would hire me as needed. Some were vacation fill-ins or just temporary gigs, while others were sporadic. This was perfect for me because I love variety, and it's much easier on my body than repeating the same motions all day. I did some sales and market research, freelanced on events, and cared for a disabled woman for some time. I assisted an elderly artist and architect with his household affairs and occasionally helped out in a forest kindergarten. Besides all that, along with a few other random odd jobs, I built up my own clientele for house cleaning gigs and massages.

Shortly after I turned twenty-seven, I noticed a rash on my arms. I went to see a dermatologist who examined it carefully and finally took a punch biopsy to send it to a lab. When the results came back, he told me they couldn't find anything and not to worry about it. He really did conclude his analysis by saying it was nothing. Really! That's precisely what he said: "It's nothing." It still strikes me as remarkable that he could take a sample of nothing, examine it carefully, send it to a lab, and then tell me there wasn't anything at all!

CHAPTER 2

Turbulent Times

Two years into living this beautiful life—with plenty of room for creativity, steady work opportunities, and the immense luxury to choose when and what to work—a dear friend came to visit me. I felt incredibly honored that, of all the people I knew from California, he was coming to see me. When I had lived there, this man had helped me with my back issues more than anyone I'd ever met. I had great admiration and respect for this guy, and because he's helped me so much, I felt as if I would be forever grateful to him.

Like so many in the Bay Area, he called himself a healer. His work blended massage, acupuncture, and a kind of counseling that touched on life, love, and everything in between. During my last two years there, I regularly received treatments from him and achieved remarkable progress with my back issues. He inevitably noticed that my back was quite a mess, so he asked me if I'd be open to letting him try an acupuncture treatment on me. He said I was the perfect candidate, as the treatment would aim to realign the spine over time. My back was so locked up by then that I agreed to give it a try.

By then, seven of my thoracic vertebrae were essentially fused, and the rest misaligned, hardly any of them even facing the same direction. His experiment involved inserting acupuncture needles between each vertebra and on both sides, as well as at release points across my legs, feet, arms, hands, and head—about 180 needles per session in total. He treated my back every two weeks and alternated to the front of the body in the weeks in between. The pain was intense, but the results were amazing. I persisted because I felt I had nothing to lose and was hopeful it might help. Two years into this treatment, I was about one and a half inches taller. My vertebrae aligned, my spinal discs began to heal, and my posture, breathing, and focus improved significantly. I truly felt like I could think clearly for the first time in my life. Naturally, all of these changes made me feel happier and more at ease, and because of that, this man became very special to me. So, when he visited, I wanted to give him the best vacation ever. I took him to restaurants, introduced him to friends, and showed him around the country. He seemed moved by seeing the way I managed my life, and a week later, we fell in love. We married a year later, and he moved to Switzerland to be with me. Looking back, that might have been the dumbest decision I've ever made. This marriage turned my life upside down.

MOVING TO THE COUNTRYSIDE

My brother had just signed the lease for a beautiful farmhouse we could share. So, I gave up my sweet little apartment, and we moved to the countryside. The property was situated in a surprisingly pristine valley about three miles from the next town. The main house had two separate apartments and an adjacent barn with a stable for my brother's horses. A large pasture stretched alongside the house on the northern side, and a big garden was situated to the west. On the southern side, we had an apple orchard, and across the driveway there was even a little pond. Getting to live in such an idyllic place was a dream come true!

It was clear that my husband wouldn't be able to earn income right away, so to cover our bills, I had to work much more than before. At first, I did so very eagerly. I valued the fact that I could provide. I wanted to give him time to settle in, learn the language, and maybe explore the area for a while. Building up his massage business would also take some time. In California, he used to rely on word of mouth to get new clients and rarely needed to advertise. In Switzerland, he had no reputation yet, so establishing himself proved much more difficult than we'd initially expected. It definitely didn't help that he didn't speak German, and living in a relatively remote area without nearby public transportation was another hurdle. Plus, Switzerland isn't California. If you go around claiming to be a healer, most people will probably think you're just a quack.

For half a year, I managed to keep a work schedule of nine to twelve hours a day, with about three hours of commuting daily, while working five to six days a week. Our total expenses were three times my previous earnings, so I had to work that much more to make ends meet. Of course, this left me with no time for anything else—no time for music, art, or friends. No time to rest. The weekends were filled with cleaning, farm work, and attempts to set up a garden that never really came to fruition.

After six months of this with no real help from him, I started to worry.

I finally told him I couldn't keep this up much longer without getting sick. Unfortunately, instead of working together on a solution, we ended up in a nasty fight. I knew we needed to change things quickly, so I brainstormed and suggested everything I could think of, but I might as well have been talking to a wall. My husband was as flexible as granite. Instead of arriving at any real collaboration, I just faced tons of criticism.

WORSENING SYMPTOMS AND EMERGING INSIGHTS

The following summer, my digestive issues got so bad that I finally decided to see a doctor. At this point, it was clear that something was off, but my husband kept insisting, "Don't go to the doctor! Doctors kill. It's probably candida because you eat too much sugar. Do a cleanse instead!" And because I'd had so many futile interactions with doctors by then, I put my faith in him as a healer and started doing his cleanses and diets. Yet nothing helped! The symptoms persisted, the pain kept getting worse, and even the rash on my arms flared up more and more.

While working at the health food store one day, a customer told me about a long-term allergy test requiring just one blood sample to assess reactions to two hundred foods. He told me that he'd had skin problems and digestive issues for years. The doctors could never find the cause despite doing multiple allergy tests and trying different treatments. Finally, this particular test revealed the culprit: an allergy to carrots, of all things! He said he had been fine since removing the carrots from his diet.

Truthfully, I had never heard about long-term allergies before. These, as opposed to immediate allergic reactions, can trigger symptoms that don't appear for hours, or even up to fourteen days! Of course, I immediately ordered the test. The results I got back turned out to be very helpful. The most important finding was that I had an extreme allergy to gliadin, which is a component of gluten. This was such a crucial insight because I had long felt that I reacted unfavorably to grains. Over the past thirteen years, I had done quite a few allergy tests for gluten, wheat, rye, and spelt, but nothing ever came back positive. Funnily enough, these tests were both right and wrong. I am not allergic to any of these grains or to gluten per se, but rather to a protein that is contained inside all of them. Furthermore, the findings also revealed allergies to sunflower, basil, saffron, and milk.

I immediately removed these foods from my diet and experienced tangible improvement within as little as two weeks! It certainly wasn't easy to find foods that didn't contain at least one of these ingredients. Many packaged foods and milk substitutes contain sunflower oil, and many gluten-free products are made with sunflower seeds or dairy, so it was pretty frustrating initially. Nevertheless, these adjustments were well worth it because the pain in my gut started to diminish, and my ability to focus improved yet again. I was happier and more balanced, and I had more energy. Even so, my digestion still didn't feel right, but I had no clue which foods were causing it.

NEW PLANS AND UNEXPECTED DETOURS

Since my husband hadn't managed to build up his business on the farm, toward the spring of the following year we resolved to move back to the city. I was so glad about this decision that I immediately wrote an application and addressed over three hundred copies to property owners in Zurich. I also signed up for a sound-engineering school because I wanted to eventually work in a profession where I could use some of my actual talents. I was super excited about these upcoming changes, but then, the next day, before I even had time to send the letters out, my husband got a job offer in California! A friend of his needed help to develop some land. He offered us a pretty good salary, and what's more, he said he'd pay for us to build our own house on that land! We could design it, build it, and then keep it for good. Alas, our plans changed yet again, and instead of moving back to Zurich, we ended up moving back to America.

His friend wanted to start work immediately, so my husband left ahead of me. I still had to organize all of our paperwork, pack everything, and ship our belongings overseas. I canceled my course at the school and, determined to achieve at least something with my music, used my remaining time in Switzerland to record an album. I celebrated its release with a small show, loved seeing family and friends, and partied till dawn. Just like when I finished my apprenticeship, the very next day I traveled to San Francisco. On the trip, I had time to reflect on everything ahead of me: building a house, playing shows, and getting a green card. I dreamed of working at hot springs or opening an allergy-friendly restaurant, and I couldn't wait to reconnect with my California friends.

However, the reality turned out to be not quite what I'd expected. The land was a remote forest in Northern California, about a three-hour drive from San Francisco. Located at the lower part of a hillside with limited farmland, we had to cut trees and forge trails through the dense thickets, most of them overgrown with poison oak. There was a spring for water, but it hadn't been developed yet. With only one car essential for work, we rarely had a chance to leave, spending most of our time there working.

The house I was so excited about building turned out to be nothing but an empty promise. In short, it didn't happen. We lived in a tent. Working under the scorching heat of the Californian summer sun, with no place to cool off, was brutal. And yet, as soon as fall came along, it got extremely cold. I was bitten by fleas and spiders every day and got continuously reinfected by poison oak. My backache kept worsening because there was no level area where I could sleep properly, or at least do yoga or exercise. At this point, I felt an awful tiredness setting in, the likes of which I had never experienced before. Trying to make sense of it at the time, I attributed it to the extreme weather conditions and the fact that I probably wasn't getting enough aerobic exercise. Back home, riding my bike had always boosted my energy—now I was either doing hard work in the sun or getting around in a car.

Besides all this, there was something else that constantly worried me. We had never gotten a written contract. I kept bringing this up, which seemed to irritate my husband greatly. We had quite a few arguments about it, and after a particularly heated one in late June, he decided to send me back to Switzerland. This was the very same day I finally had the complete stack of paperwork for the green card ready to send in. Despite that, he said I could not stay with him anymore—he would not sign the papers. With the hope of getting a regular job and thus a somewhat independent social life suddenly slipping right through my fingers, I literally fell to my knees and begged him to let me stay. Yet my words seemed to fall on deaf ears because, in the end, he denied me.

BACK HOME

My friends and family welcomed me back to Switzerland wholeheartedly, and not one of them seemed unhappy to hear that this undertaking hadn't worked out for me. They were all glad to have me back. I honestly thought this was the end of my marriage, and, based on everything that had gone down so far, part of me was relieved to let it go.

Yet, another part of me was now suffering an enormous heartache, so heavy it began to echo through my body. Every single day, I woke up to a sensation akin to being struck by lightning, followed by a gnawing pain that pierced my heart and got my head spinning with questions that I couldn't seem to solve. It just didn't make sense to me that someone who had once chosen to marry me would suddenly become so incredibly cold and cruel. He had sent me off like a postal parcel right on the day I would have started to have an actual chance of a bit of independence. I tried to let it go and leave it all behind me, but this heartache was eating me up inside. I finally tried to reach out to him, hoping to find a way to understand it all and restore at least some semblance of inner peace. He never seemed available to talk, though, responding to my emails only occasionally by saying he was busy and needed time.

Fall of that year brought what was later found to be one of the most devastating wildfires in California's history. Raging through and ravaging large parts of the region, the fire couldn't be contained and eventually reached our home. It didn't spare our land. Within less than a week, all our efforts and hard work were reduced to nothing but coal and ashes. That's when I finally heard back from my man. When he initially called, I understood that he intended to visit me for only two weeks so that we could talk. Yet when I arrived to pick him up at the airport, this guy stood there with four suitcases and his ukulele, saying he had finally decided to give our relationship another chance and was ready to live with me again!

I've only shared a brief outline of what happened between us, but you can imagine this was a shock. To me, trying again without first clarifying our issues was a terrible idea, especially since I didn't have an apartment yet, and housing in Zurich had meanwhile become extremely scarce. However, since he was already there without a place to go back to in California, I finally agreed. After all the back and forth, I just wanted a normal life—home, stability, security—and in all honesty, I still hoped to restore our love. I wanted my beautiful life back; a life of love, peace, and happiness.

Despite still feeling uneasy, I resolved to proceed as efficiently as possible. Setting up my husband's massage business and finding a home were the top priorities, as without these, our relationship would certainly not stand a chance. Sorting out my own career had to wait. To get him started, I set up bookkeeping, compiled advertising addresses, and created a website, business cards, gift certificates, and flyers. My husband only needed to send the flyers.

Finding a home was tough, especially since we were completely out of money. Neither of us had valuable credentials for finding work, and our business partner from California hadn't secured insurance, so we had truly lost everything and our work wouldn't get compensated. It took months to sign a lease, and the place we finally found was only temporary since the house was scheduled for a complete renovation, requiring all tenants to move out nine months later. So we did have a stepping stone, but couldn't truly settle, still searching for our real home.

The delays made me increasingly eager to find work. My previous managers would have welcomed me back, but after what had happened in California, I wanted steady income. I didn't want to repeat running between jobs and barely making enough; I needed better pay and something suited to me. Sound technician school was no longer feasible due to costs, and I was uncertain about my next step, eager to find out.

Not long after my husband returned, I started to be unable to sleep properly. While we had been separated, I had been sleeping reasonably well, even with the tormenting heartache that woke me up each day. But now that he was back, still flatly opposed to reconciling in any concrete manner and rigidly insisting that it would be best to just forget about what had happened between us and simply move forward, I started to feel extremely uneasy. I honestly tried to put it all behind me and get past these feelings, but whenever I'd lie down to sleep, a sense of absolute terror would come crashing over me like a tsunami. Along with it, my digestive symptoms continually worsened, and the rash on my arms started to flare up more and more. It felt like thousands of needles were poking right through my flesh and out of my skin! I had no idea what the cause was and, consequently, no clue what to do about it. On top of that, I didn't even have time to consider these problems properly because finding an apartment and bringing in some money seemed much more urgent at the time.

I worked in a grocery shop and a dollar store, and occasionally picked up cleaning gigs, but I started to have such severe reactions to working in these places that it usually took me several days to recover after just one day of work. After a day at the dollar store, my skin would turn red like a lobster and I'd get unbearably itchy. My eyes would feel scratchy, and my throat often felt sore for a few days afterward. Working at the health food store, I reacted to the flour dust from the bread they sold, and some of the customers' perfumes closed up my throat to the point where, several times, I had to drop whatever I was doing and run outside to catch a breath—not ideal if you're working in sales. I eventually had to quit these jobs because I always got so sick working there. I muscled through the cleaning gigs as best I could, but my joints started to hurt so badly that sometimes I couldn't help but cry. Other times, I was literally left bleeding from underneath my fingernails. In short, this time of my life was just horrible.

SUCCESSES AND SETBACKS

A few months later, my husband visited California for three weeks, leaving me some room to focus on my professional path. During this alone time, I unexpectedly created a delicious gluten-free bread. Gluten-free baking is like secret alchemy; I'd often produce completely unappetizing baking failures, but this time I'd nailed it! When I opened the oven, I was honestly baffled to find something that actually looked like real bread. It also tasted delicious, so I repeated the recipe the next day, and it was just as good. Inspired, I decided to start a gluten-free bakery, turning my struggles into a positive venture to help others with food intolerances enjoy life more fully. For the first time in a long time, I felt excited again—like reconnecting with an old friend—which, I concluded, confirmed I was on the right path. Energized and motivated, I began developing new baked goods and planning my business.

In June, I finally found our place! I was so relieved to sign the lease, knowing that we could move in that September. But then, during that summer, I started getting seriously ill. My digestive symptoms became so severe that, usually within half an hour of eating, I'd be drenched in sweat and left writhing in excruciating pain! This wasn't anything like normal stomach cramps—it was a completely crushing pain that persisted for hours, draining me of my last bit of energy. The pain in my arms increased and started to spread throughout my body, and the skin rash flared up more and more. Sometimes it hurt so much that I couldn't help but scream, hoping to get at least some of it out. I was at my wits' end. I didn't know what was causing these horrible reactions, and to tell the truth, I started to fear eating anything at all. In August, right as we were getting ready to move, I collapsed a total of eight times in just three weeks. After that, I was done, finished, kaput. I just didn't function anymore. That's when I finally went to see a doctor.

CHAPTER 3

Finding the Cause of My Illness

My family doctor referred me to a gastroenterologist and issued a medical certificate for a month. He urged me to rest as much as possible and put everything else on hold. Of course, I knew it was crucial to rest, but I also knew we needed to bring in some money pronto. I needed to get back to work, or else we couldn't pay the rent! The certificate he'd provided didn't help, since not having a full-time position meant that no sick pay would be coming in, and my husband's nascent income wasn't nearly enough to pay for even half of our expenses. However, it was also an inescapable fact that I couldn't keep going anymore. Whatever the consequences might be, I needed rest. So, as contradictory as this might sound, I figured I needed to rest as efficiently as possible so that I could get back to work that much sooner.

If I had any hope of recuperating within a reasonable timeframe, I had no choice but to ask my husband for help. That didn't go over well. He got so upset that we ended up in a violent fight, during which he finally choked me out. I had already stopped fighting back when he had me pinned to the floor underneath him, but then his hands squeezed my throat so tightly that it was impossible to breathe, and within no time, my body went completely limp. My vision rapidly blurred, and it soon felt like my whole being was enveloped in flickering darkness. Only then did he finally release his vice-like grip from my throat and lift his bone-crushing weight off of me. After that, he left, and I didn't hear a peep from him until he finally came back four days later. As he walked out the door, he sarcastically tossed off one last remark: I could have the house to myself and enjoy the silence.

It was indeed very quiet after he was gone, but it wasn't restful at all. It was all extremely confusing and unsettling. I was lying there on the couch, staring at the ceiling, my thoughts swirling, and I had no idea what to make of this. I couldn't talk, could barely even swallow due to the pain in my throat, and my head was spinning—so much that I wouldn't have known what to say or whom to talk to, even if I could speak. This was the first time in my life that I had experienced such violence, so I didn't have a single clue how to handle it.

When he finally did come back four days later, he didn't want to talk about it. He only said that I had gone too far, but he offered me a hug as long as I didn't press further. Strangely enough, I did go for that hug. I truly needed one badly. Having reached such a desperately low point of being so sick, flat broke, stressed out, and seriously sleep-deprived, probably nobody would have been able to think clearly anymore. I guess I felt like I needed comfort and peace more than anything else. Just a pause, a break, a breather... I was yearning for a normal life. I wanted to feel good again, and I was desperate for some clarity over my health issues.

NO CLEAR ANSWERS

The gastroenterologist performed a gastroscopy and took biopsies from my stomach and duodenum. He couldn't find anything abnormal, so he suggested that I might have irritable bowel syndrome (IBS). He gave me some basic instructions for the FODMAP diet and strongly admonished me to stop following my husband's advice. During our first visit, my husband confidently asserted that candida was the problem, attributing it to the sugar I was eating. This doctor now told me that it most definitely was not candida overgrowth and that I certainly shouldn't substitute sugar with honey as my husband had advised, because that would just make matters worse.

Ironically, the negative results left me more disappointed than not, and if anything, even more concerned because I was sure that something was off and had hoped this doctor would find an answer. With no apparent indications, the FODMAP diet was my most promising path forward, so I gave it a try. Like when I learned about my long-term allergies, this diet brought some relief, but it didn't fully resolve the pain.

I was given a doctor's note to rest for yet another month. However, being entirely out of savings at this point, I just had to get some money coming in, or we'd be in even more serious trouble. My head was spinning in circles because my physical state didn't allow me to just buckle down and get back to work, so I finally had to apply for social aid. This might sound easy, but you can't just go there, say that you need money, and expect them to give it to you. You have to prove your case in writing and submit a mountain of evidence that you don't have any savings or any other options left. If you're self-employed, as my husband was, you must prove why this is your only option and explain why you can't take on another job. With no alternatives left, I had to attend to this mountain of paperwork instead of getting the rest I desperately needed.

After managing to submit all the documents, we had a few more meetings at their office before we were finally approved for aid. However, we weren't completely out of the woods yet. During the final round of this application gauntlet, we were told that our apartment was too expensive.

"What does this mean?" I asked, concerned.

"It means you'll have to find a cheaper apartment," the lady explained.

Now the whole world came crashing down around me again like a house of cards. We had only just moved in, and it had taken me so freaking long to even find a place at all! We'd been on the move for years, and I was relieved to have finally reached the end of this grueling ordeal—and now this journey was about to start all over again?! Inconceivable!

But rules are rules, and such were the rules. At least she gave us six months to find a cheaper place, with the additional requirement to apply for at least ten apartments per month and submit a copy of each application to their office. It sure was a huge relief to know we were financially taken care of for now, but learning that the search for a home wasn't over yet was crushing.

A DOCTOR WHO LISTENED

By October 2016, I began to feel so depleted that I got worried the depression might come back. I didn't have the strength to deal with depression on top of everything that was already going on, so I started to ponder it. Having been unable to eat properly for months by then, with my whole GI tract inflamed and afflicted by constant diarrhea, I was undoubtedly missing out on vital nutrients. I knew that some nutrient deficiencies could pose a risk for depression. And then, as well, serotonin, which is known as one of our happiness hormones, is also primarily created in the gut. My gut clearly wasn't working right, so I reckoned it was unlikely that anything good could be made in it at the time. Even if there were, it would have been flushed out long before having the chance to reach any other part of my body due to the constant diarrhea. I wondered if it might be possible to artificially replenish my serotonin levels, just until I could eat properly again, so I sought a clinic to inquire about this. That's how I came to meet Dr. Franziska Saissi.

During our first meeting at the beginning of November, I brought her up to speed with my medical history and shared with her that I had just gone through an incredibly challenging time after getting married. Bless her heart! She listened attentively for an hour and a half, and toward the end of the meeting, she finally told me something I'll never forget for the rest of my life. She paused and looked at me for a long moment, sincerely and with great concern, and said, "When I look at you, I see a brilliant young woman, but when I listen to you, you sound like an experienced psychiatrist with a degree. Note that I am saying psychiatrist, not psychologist. I see you are sick, and something is wrong, but I must admit I do not know what it is. Regarding your question about serotonin, some tests measure its concentration in the blood, but they aren't very reliable. Additionally, the medications used to increase serotonin levels always contain blood thinners, which means we can't use them on you due to your ITP. Let me tell you, I honestly don't know what you have, but if you are open to coming back, I'll do my very best to find out."

Never in my history of visiting doctors had I met one who openly admitted not knowing the answer but showed the willingness to investigate a matter they couldn't pinpoint yet. This in itself was already a huge blessing, and what she said about me sounding like a psychiatrist definitely perked me up a bit, this coming from a medical doctor who also has a degree in psychology. At any rate, I gratefully agreed to come back again. Over the next few months, I visited her office weekly and underwent extensive testing, but almost every test returned negative, like always. The only clear results were very low iron and vitamin B12 levels. While discussing this, I told her of a severe adverse reaction I had to an iron infusion years before, so she decided to start me on supplementation with drops, and later I could try chewable tablets. For the B12, I had to come back weekly for a series of eight shots.

TOGETHER BUT ALONE

The relationship with my husband was steadily deteriorating. He seemed downright disgusted by my state because, even though I now desperately needed his help, he started spending more and more time at my brother's ex-girlfriend's house. This woman offered to let him work from her home and helped him pick up new clients. So now he was often gone for days at a time to bring in a little bit of money while establishing his clientele at her place, about an hour's drive away from Zurich.

What also worried me was that he accepted all this help from the woman who had left my brother right after getting pregnant with his baby. I also believed she had been making things rather difficult for my brother over the upbringing of their child, so her closeness with my husband made me uncomfortable, but the two of them seemed to feel perfectly comfortable in their bond. They both stated they had found a *soulmate* in each other. In short, it was bizarre and certainly didn't help with our ongoing relationship issues one bit. When he did come home, we would often get into arguments, or he would retreat into his room and be about as responsive as a rock.

At the end of December, I finally asked for a divorce. For a long time, I clung to the notion that I never wanted to get divorced because I felt that saying yes to something meant that I should stick to it. I thought if things get tough, I have to find a way to work through it. But at this point, it had become undeniably clear that our relationship was a disaster beyond any hope. Since we'd gotten together, absolutely nothing had worked out. So, I just had to come to terms with the idea that it might never happen. I finally realized that it would be easier for me to handle my life alone than to keep feeling as if I was being pushed and pulled by this constant back and forth—waiting, hoping, arguing—while also doing all the housework, applying for apartments, and handling all our official paperwork. All that on top of being so miserably ill! It was clear to me that I couldn't possibly cope anymore, so I had to tell him that I wanted a divorce. When I finally did, he broke down crying, and this time he begged me on his knees to give us just one more chance. Believe it or not, I let compassion get the better of me once again and ultimately gave in to his entreaty.

DOWNWARD SPIRALING

To clear our heads and start fresh, we went to the mountains to visit my best friend's family at their vacation home. It felt so good to be away from the city and noise, but on the first morning, I woke with a high fever and a crushing headache. While everyone else went sledding, I stayed to rest, feeling soothed by the quiet, yet very sick, drifting in fever dreams and waking soaked. When they got back in the evening, they told me my husband had slipped on ice and fallen hard on his arm. They said it looked hilarious at first, but he was probably badly hurt. I returned to bed, too weak to stay up, missing out. The next day, we canceled our trip and went back home because I was still sick and he was in significant pain from his fall. At this point, it seemed things couldn't get worse—but the downward spiral continued.

When I woke up the next day, the house was absolutely quiet. I noticed that I'd slept much longer than I had in months. I hadn't woken up in the middle of the night; it was already morning! Delighted about this, I turned over and almost immediately fell back to sleep. It had been years since I'd slept through an entire night. Around noon, I woke up again. Still snug in my cozy bed, suddenly, it hit me like a thunderbolt—something was off. I hadn't yet heard a single sound from my husband, who was usually impossible to miss.

I got up and poked my head into his room. And there he was, lying in his bed, staring back at me with one hand covering the left side of his face and a panicked look in his right eye.

"What's up, baby?" I asked with rising concern.

"My face… can't move it," he mumbled desperately.

Panic shot through me like a lightning bolt. The left side of his face was frozen!

"Get dressed. We're going to the hospital!"

And gone was my sweet but all too brief moment of peace and relaxation.

He slowly got up while I dashed around the house to gather what we needed, but then he stopped me right in my tracks. He said he wanted to wait; maybe this would pass. Hearing that, I felt like he had just pulled the emergency brake on a freight train. I knew it was absolutely wrong to wait, and the thought made me nervous as hell, but what could I do if he didn't want to go? I couldn't carry him! This really seemed like an emergency to me—not something you should delay to see how it develops. So I got on the phone to call a few doctors I know personally and ask for their advice. All of them affirmed that it was urgent: He needed to go to the hospital immediately, if not sooner. I relayed to him precisely what they said, but he still refused. Instead, he asked me for a massage. You can guess how I felt about this; I was still seriously sick myself and felt a great urgency to take this man to the emergency unit, but he wanted a massage! I eventually gave in, but upon touching his face and feeling how cold and completely numb it was—I had to stop. I insisted he get dressed immediately, and we finally headed to the ER.

It turned out to be Bell's palsy, most likely caused by the same virus that I had gotten in the mountains—just that he was unlucky enough for the virus to have found its way into his facial nerves. The doctors explained that such paralysis usually heals on its own after some time, but they advised him to rest for a month and strictly avoid any cold air on his face. This last bit seemed practically impossible, as it was January in Switzerland, snowing, with temperatures well below zero. While at the hospital, he also showed them his injured arm. They determined that he had torn some of his tendons and that surgery would be necessary, but advised him to wait until the Bell's palsy had passed.

Now it was clear that he wouldn't be able to do anything for quite a while. He wouldn't be able to work, do the shopping, or help around the house. Once again, it was up to me to keep things going. At this point, I felt as though my own death was pretty much imminent, and yet now I had to shoulder an even heavier load somehow. Now I had to pamper and nurse my husband—the same man I'd asked for a divorce just a few days before!

I tried to pull myself together, but it was simply too much. After four days of doing all the cooking, shopping, caring, and trying to stay strong, I finally broke down in tears and asked him for a hug. Probably unsurprisingly by now, this sparked another ugly fight.

ONE LAST LEAD

It was February 2017 when Dr. Saissi finally told me, "Now I have reached my wits' end. Whatever I thought could be the cause of your illness has come back negative. There's one last thing I've found in the literature, which might be consistent with your symptoms, but it's a rare disease. And rare diseases, well… they're rare. We'll have to take another blood sample to measure your tryptase. If the results show normal levels, I'm sorry, but I'll have to let you go without an answer because I can't do anything else for you."

Hearing this felt quite dispiriting because I was desperate to feel better, and the prospect of just aborting our quest before having found the cause of my illness made me feel very uneasy. But then, a week later, the first abnormal test result finally did come back!

Dr. Saissi decided to repeat the test to ensure the result was accurate and that we were on the right track. A week later, it was confirmed: my tryptase levels were up to 17, while the normal serum tryptase range is between 0 and 11.4 μg/L. Finally, we had a hint!

Dr. Saissi told me then that I might have something called mastocytosis, and if it were so, she would have to refer me to a specialist at the university hospital. She also arranged for me to see a dermatologist who would perform a punch biopsy of my skin rash to check for mast cell involvement. Although we weren't entirely sure whether it was mastocytosis, she suggested I look it up online.

Walking out of her office that day, I was a bit amused at the irony of it being called *tryptase* because my situation was indeed quite trippy. At the same time, I was also glad to finally have an indication that something was off, since that unequivocally proved that it wasn't all just in my mind. I went home and eagerly looked it up on the internet.

I saw right away that avoiding foods high in histamine might well help. It certainly wasn't easy to figure out what all these foods were, and even less so to determine what I could still eat, given that I was already avoiding FODMAPs and all the things I was allergic to—but at least this was something I could implement right away to possibly feel better. However, it didn't take long for my initial elation to fade. Reading on about mast cell disease, I learned that some forms of mastocytosis are essentially benign, but others attack different organ systems to the point of possible organ failure, and there are even lethal forms, such as bone marrow cancer, where life expectancy could be only a couple of months. Now this was rather disturbing news, because I didn't know yet which of these versions I had. The sudden prospect of my illness being potentially terminal soon got me feeling, well, a bit edgy, to say the least.

Honestly, occasionally I wished I were dead already because I was in so much pain. My life was an unmitigated mess, my marriage a kind of living hell, and it seemed like absolutely nothing was going in the right direction. But then, getting the news that I might actually already be dying got me thinking. I wasn't cool with the idea of having my life end in such a tragic way. I've always had somewhat of a romantic notion about dying, and since I didn't manage to depart when I tried to kill myself during my early teenage years, I'd concluded that there must be a reason I still needed to be here. This couldn't be it. I always said that my aim in life would be to die happy and with a smile on my face. If I died now, that probably wouldn't happen.

The state I was in was just horrible. I had diarrhea up to sixteen times a day, was wracked with cramps for sometimes forty hours per week, barely ever got more than two hours of sleep per night, and was tormented by pretty scary heart palpitations where I never knew if these were my last moments alive. I needed to change my clothes up to eight times per day because they wound up soaking wet over and over due to incessant cold sweats. Quite frequently, I had sudden drops in energy, paired with debilitating dizzy spells that required me to immediately drop whatever I was doing and direct my entire focus on calming down to avoid passing out right on the spot. My joints hurt, my back hurt, and my kidneys hurt. I felt, quite simply, bloody awful.

SLOWLY FILLING IN THE BLANKS

A few days later, I had my appointment with the dermatologist. While he took the punch biopsy, I asked him whether he knew of any way to test for reactions to smells. By then, I'd realized that it was often merely the smell of certain odors that triggered tremendous discomfort in me. I wanted to know if there was some explanation, proof, and/or remedy for that. He told me that reactions to smells couldn't be measured, only the skin's reactions to certain substances could. He then proceeded to perform a patch test on my back. The patches had to stay on for two days—two perfectly miserable days of nonstop dizziness, excessive sweating, and nausea, during which I felt so ill that I couldn't sleep at all.

When he finally checked the results, he could only identify allergic reactions to nickel, cobalt, and benzophenone. He did say that he'd never seen such an intense reaction to nickel, and I should avoid it wherever possible. I was stunned that not everything was checked as *severely allergic*, because I had suffered enormously while having these substances on me. So, I couldn't get it confirmed through any medical test, but after this experience it seemed likely that it was really just the smell of these substances that caused this intense discomfort in me. At least I now had a bit more clarity and knew to steer clear of nickel, too. The punch biopsy revealed increased mast cells in the affected tissue, so with that, we had found another piece of the puzzle.

Back home, I started reading about nickel and quickly learned that it is found in many ordinary, everyday things, such as buttons, belt buckles, guitar strings, and jewelry. Now I finally understood why I could never wear jewelry; even as a kid, my skin would flare up whenever I tried to wear it. I also learned that nickel is found in varying amounts in different foods, and it's commonly used as a material in cooking utensils. So, I compiled a list of foods that potentially have high concentrations of nickel and added it to the ever-growing list of things I had to avoid.

MEETING THE FIRST SPECIALIST

Since the results of both the tryptase and the punch biopsy pointed to mast cell disease, Dr. Saissi then referred me to the specialist at the hospital. During my first consultation, the diagnosis of mastocytosis was confirmed. I was given an EpiPen and instructed to always carry it with me and not hesitate to use it whenever I felt I was going to faint. Now, this doctor explained to me that the reason for my repeated fainting was probably never low blood sugar, but more likely anaphylaxis, which in the worst case can be fatal.

Next, I got scheduled for several additional appointments. There were seemingly endless scans, more blood tests, prick tests, bone marrow density measurements, a colonoscopy, and a bone marrow puncture. Unfortunately, they couldn't schedule all the appointments at once because the results of the previous tests were always required to know how to proceed. I kept getting scheduled and rescheduled over the following five months, all the while unsure whether these were my last days on planet Earth because I didn't know yet whether I had, in fact, bone marrow cancer. Kind of a daunting feeling, to say the least.

PSYCHOLOGICAL SUPPORT

Before I got transferred to the hospital, Dr. Saissi urged me to contact Mrs. Pfleiderer, a psychologist friend of hers. By then, Dr. Saissi had been aware of my domestic situation for some time and had seen bruising on my arms. She had repeatedly tried to persuade me to get a divorce. Yet, since I had agreed to give the relationship another chance back in December, and now my husband was sick himself, I didn't have the heart or the energy to break up with him. Dr. Saissi was pregnant then and would soon be going on maternity leave. I knew she cared about me, and I didn't want her to worry. I knew I wasn't going to see her anymore, and she had become pretty much my only confidant. And so, because my situation was, in fact, extremely difficult, I finally agreed that I would at least meet this psychologist.

Mrs. Pfleiderer worked together with a psychiatrist, Mr. Kurz. He held the first session to assess my case, decide whether medication was necessary, and also to determine whether he or Mrs. Pfleiderer would work with me. I had initially been scheduled for ninety minutes, but he ended up greatly exceeding the allotted time. As I continued answering his questions, this man started sinking deeper and deeper into his seat while progressively leaning further to his left. He looked like he was going to fall right out of his chair at any moment, while his face started to turn a ghastly sort of green, and at some point, I thought he might vomit any second. Then, suddenly leaping out of his chair, he literally screamed at me, "But how many drugs does your husband take?"

A bit surprised at this unexpected outburst, I carefully replied that he liked to smoke weed, but I wouldn't say he was a drug addict. "He's just a bit arrogant," I suggested.

I'm still not sure what answer he was looking for, but I finally got accepted as their client. Medication was considered unnecessary, and Mrs. Pfleiderer would be working with me.

BREAKUP AND NEW BEGINNING

I am so glad I got this support, because what happened shortly after was so disturbing that I'm truly grateful I had someone to talk to who was paid to listen. I will spare you most of the details and share only this much: My husband left right before I got my diagnosis and moved in with my brother's ex. He genuinely seemed not to give a **** about me anymore. He never asked how I was doing and didn't even show any concern about whether I had bone marrow cancer or not. He disappeared the day before I had to go in for the colonoscopy.

Early that morning, I received yet another rejection for an apartment I had really hoped to get. I had filled out 140 separate applications during the previous six months, so I couldn't help but break down in tears when I read that letter. Nothing was working out, not between me and my husband, nor anything else in our lives. My health was down the drain, and I felt so wholly miserable, both physically and psychologically, that I had finally reached my absolute limit. At that point, I just had to tell my husband I needed to split up because I genuinely couldn't see any other way. Usually things had worked out for me, but since we'd gotten together, nothing ever did! Once I managed to get this through to him, we got into yet another nasty fight, after which he left again, but this time, it turned out to be for good.

Of course, it was tormenting to deal with this at the same time as the already agonizing scenarios concerning my health, but ultimately it was the best thing that could have happened. Why was it the best thing? There are a few reasons. One is that this breakup was so distressing that I completely lost my appetite. Before the colonoscopy, I was allowed to eat only white rice and meat. Thanks to the breakup, I didn't want to eat at all—neither before nor afterward. This complete loss of appetite lasted for another three weeks. You may think that it isn't good to go without food for such a long stretch, but in my case, it turned out to work wonders! This was the first time in years that my digestive system started to calm down. Since I'd been allowed to eat only white rice and meat before the colonoscopy, I figured these would be the first foods I'd reintroduce after this fast. This was the first time in more than a year that I didn't have a reaction to food.

Another positive effect of the breakup was that I finally had room to follow my own hunches instead of constantly arguing with my husband about his ideas on what I should do to feel better. The constant trying and worrying about our relationship was over. The back-and-forth of waiting, hoping, and trying had ended, and the certainty that the relationship was over allowed me to focus on myself, which was precisely what I needed. Besides that, my friends and family started coming back into my life. I was so delighted that they did. Most of them said it just wasn't feasible for them to be around both of us, and they all said they were glad to have me back.

A DIAGNOSIS AND A SAFE HAVEN

I was diagnosed specifically with cutaneous mastocytosis a few weeks later. It was a tremendous relief to know it wasn't bone marrow cancer! Also, with the tests complete, I could now finally take antihistamines. Initially, I was advised to take two pills daily, but that wasn't enough to get this horrible itching under control. My skin felt like it was on fire! Sleeping was nearly impossible, and I'd often wake up with bloody scratches. Doubling the dose on the doctor's recommendation slightly improved things, but it wasn't enough to calm the symptoms entirely.

Since my marriage was over and beyond all hope of reconciliation, I moved out of our old apartment; I couldn't stand being there anymore. My ex refused to return the keys, which freaked me out because I never knew if he would suddenly pop in. Sure, I could've changed the locks, but I desperately wanted to be somewhere he didn't even know. By a happy coincidence, during the first phone call I made after deciding to move out, I learned that a friend needed a place. As luck would have it, I was able to transfer the lease to her within two weeks. My next stepping stone was a dear friend's atelier, where I could crash for a while. I had helped him with household affairs for many years, and we shared a strong bond. The only catch was that he had dementia. It was much better than staying in the old place, but still demanding in different ways, so I couldn't completely unwind.

One day, I randomly called a friend I hadn't spoken to in years. When he heard about my situation, he instantly offered me his guest room and asked whether I'd be open to house-sitting while he went to Greece for a few weeks. Of course, I gladly accepted. This was perfect because no one in the whole wide world except my friend and his wife knew where I was. This gave me such a sense of safety that, at last, I started to be able to sleep again! Finally alone in a quiet, beautiful, and peaceful place, I slept like a bear for the first two weeks. On one occasion, I slept for thirty-five hours straight, got up only to pee and drink some water, and then crashed again for another seventeen hours!

When my friend and his wife returned, they generously offered to let me stay with them until I found my own place. After a few weeks of resting, I got back to applying for apartments. Unbelievably, I got my new place after writing only three applications! Things were starting to work out for me again.

CHAPTER 4

After the Diagnosis

Getting the diagnosis was such a relief! Not that it's nice to know that you're sick, but it was good to be able to put a name to the thing that had burdened me for so long. I was also glad to finally have some proof that I could use to counter the people who constantly insisted that it was all just in my head or any of their other silly interpretations. However, it didn't take long for reality to crash back in and shatter this initial rush of exhilaration.

During my next hospital visit, the doctors asked me how I'd been faring with the antihistamines. I reported that they helped reduce the itching to some extent, but they didn't completely stop it. Now I was prescribed ranitidine. Two pills per day, on top of the four doses of fexofenadine.

"What about the smells?" I asked, hoping for some helpful input.

They looked a bit puzzled. "It's not a common symptom," they replied.

"But I often feel awfully ill when exposed to certain smells. Is there any way you can test for that?"

One of the doctors responded brusquely, "No, there isn't anything we can do about it."

I considered this for a moment. If the doctors really couldn't help me with it, I would have to find a way to work around these smells. But how could I do that? Smells are all over the place; they're invisible—and they're everywhere! How can you work around something like that?

"Well, what should I do for work now?" I asked.

She quickly replied, "You can do an office job."

Starting to feel a little hopeless, I responded, "But I cannot sit in a chair for longer than twenty minutes because my back always goes out whenever I sit for too long. That's why I've always preferred jobs that involve lots of movement, like cleaning or sales. However, I've recently started reacting to dust, cleaning agents, and smells. And then there's the inflammation, which often makes it hard even just to hold something because my hands and joints hurt so much. I don't see how I could keep doing any of this without getting even sicker!"

Still, nothing I said seemed to get through to her. "You'll have to use ergonomic chairs or standing desks," she explained.

A bit frustrated, I finally replied, "Well, maybe this will all get better with time when I know how it all works."

I will probably never forget just how dispiriting it felt when both doctors looked at me with these sorry looks on their faces and asserted confidently, "If we were you, we would not plan on that. This is a chronic disease; it's for life. It won't get better. It usually gets progressively worse. We're sorry. If we were you, we'd try to come to terms with it."

I wasn't about to just be okay with it. I didn't want to keep getting worse! I felt really shitty already and wanted nothing more than to get back to normal, get healthy, and enjoy my life! I mean, if it can come, then it can go again, right? Determined to find a way out of this, the first thing I did after this meeting was head straight to the most renowned bookshop in Zurich to inquire about books on mastocytosis and mast cell disease—but they couldn't find anything!

"Nothing at all?" I asked, hoping for a little miracle.

The lady nodded and apologized, "No, I am sorry. It looks like there aren't any books on this topic. The only thing I can find are some references to scientific papers."

I had already read and reread everything I could dig up on the internet. Most of it just stated the same things in different words, but I hadn't yet found anything on how I could learn to live with this disease, let alone how to heal it. I was hoping to find a book that would provide some real insight and a few clues on how to move forward, but it increasingly seemed that I'd have to find my own way.

A SMALL SANCTUARY

Meanwhile, I had moved into my own apartment. It was a small studio, but luckily it was back in my old neighborhood. Returning to this familiar area where I felt a sense of belonging was balm to my soul. It also helped that I could keep my place exactly as I liked it: I got to decide which smells entered my home—body care products, detergents, and foods—and keep it as clean as I wanted. Yet, despite all these improvements, I still wound up getting hit by reactions all the time.

Whenever I got exposed to perfumes, noises, or harsh lights, for example,

I'd get hit by heart palpitations, my hands would start to shake uncontrollably, and my vision would get blurry. I'd usually get incredibly dizzy and often felt so sick to my stomach that it was just completely overwhelming. I mean, I frequently got close to passing out just trying to buy groceries! Even at home, I'd often get hit by the same reactions just from the residual smells on the packaging. I know this might sound exaggerated—it was hard for me to fathom, too—but it truly was the case.

I often experienced these sudden drops in energy, needing to sit down right away and breathe until this rollercoaster came to a halt. I had to do that regardless of where I was or how this might have looked to others, or else I'd run the risk of fainting yet again. All of this just became too much, so I started retreating inside my home and avoiding the outside world as best I could. As long as I stayed inside, I felt much better. I began journaling about my condition to better understand the dynamics of this illness and also to try to help my doctors understand my situation so that they could hopefully help me find better treatment. The social services urged me to apply for disability, so I filled out the paperwork and sent it at the end of September.

A few weeks later, my divorce finally took place. The certainty that I was now legally out of this contract and consequently no longer liable for anything that man would do was an unspeakable relief! I felt so liberated that, right after the divorce, I slept through the better part of the following two months. I simply needed the rest. I had just gone through a highly traumatic time and hadn't slept properly for more than two years, though the four doses of antihistamines may also have made me even more tired.

A CAUTIOUS RETURN

Toward the end of the year, I finally regained some energy. After being tucked away at home for a few months, I started feeling the urge to get out again. Having spent so much time alone, I wanted to meet some new people. Yet this wasn't easy, because I had truthfully become a little estranged from the world. Everything from getting so sick to my stormy marriage had been very challenging and time-consuming, and since then, I had spent almost all my time alone. The other hurdle was that I now had reactions to pretty much the entire world outside.

Wondering how I could reenter life, I decided to try yoga classes. This would allow me to be in a room with others gently focused on doing something good for themselves, and I wouldn't have to talk. After weeks of being alone and not speaking at all, I honestly didn't know whether I could still carry on a simple conversation. I just had to take it step by step. Luckily, I found a yoga studio within walking distance from my home. They had a good deal on unlimited classes, which I could afford even with my limited budget. The first step was to check out how it smelled to see whether I could even cope with being there. Fortunately, they used only natural cleaning products and didn't burn incense—and thankfully, none of the students wore perfume. I started going there almost religiously, immensely grateful to reconnect with life in such a gentle setting. I'd still get dizzy spells, heart palpitations, flushing, joint pain, and all that, but I informed the teacher about it, and we agreed that I would rest as needed.

My days now consisted of yoga, researching diet options and mast cell disease, and trying to understand how to calm my reactions. It took time to master simple tasks like shopping without severe reactions or passing out. Since I was almost always at home, with basically no social interactions besides the yoga classes, I used this time to write a children's book, which felt remarkably uplifting compared to just being sick. Despite all the yoga, my back still hurt; about once a month, my vertebrae dislocated, sometimes leaving me immobile for days. I'd just lie there on the floor, tears streaming, hoping it would pop back in. After nine dislocations in three months, I finally decided to find a doctor who could help. This physician determined that surgery wasn't necessary and referred me to a specialist in rehabilitation and physiotherapy. It took another few months to get an appointment.

A NEW TEAM OF DOCTORS

Early in 2018, I got a request from the university hospital to meet another team of doctors—a small group of physicians appointed to study the more complicated cases like mine. I was beyond thrilled about the prospect of working with a team of doctors who would help me improve my situation, so of course I gratefully agreed.

During the first meeting, I noticed a puzzled glance between the two doctors when they read that I was taking ranitidine. One even asked the other, "Why ranitidine?"

His colleague shook his head and mumbled, "Don't know."

I couldn't overlook this interaction, so I told them I had already been on fexofenadine, an H1 blocker, and I was given ranitidine, an H2 blocker, to help soothe the itching. They just nodded and skipped right ahead. Again, I told them about my reactions to smells, the digestive issues, shaky hands, heart palpitations, skin symptoms, joint inflammation, and the pain that shoots throughout my body whenever I'm exposed to a trigger—and finally, I gave them my journal. They couldn't give me a clear answer about any of it yet, but asked me to come back again in a few weeks. Before I left, they emphasized that they would do their best to help me and that I could contact them whenever I needed their support.

Back home, ready to take the next dose of medication, I looked at the ranitidine. Why were they so surprised that I was taking it? I had always been a little reluctant to read the package inserts, to reduce the chance of obsessing about something I didn't have, but now I wanted to know exactly what this stuff was for, because these two doctors were obviously surprised that I was taking it.

I also remembered the interaction between the other two doctors who prescribed it in the first place. One was still in training, which is often the case at a university hospital. When my lungs collapsed, for example, they let a student try to insert the chest tube. I vividly remember lying there, not sure if I was going to die any second, as I watched her try and fail about five times. I could see the senior physician mimicking the movements for her, with his hands nervously fumbling around in the air until he eventually just pushed her aside and jammed that thing into my chest himself so the machine could finally start to work.

As for the ranitidine, there seemed to be a moment of hesitation when they prescribed it in the first place. I could only imagine what their uncertainty meant. To me, it appeared to imply, "Well, we can't increase the dose of antihistamines, and other mast cell patients take ranitidine, too. So, let's give it a try?"

Anyway, I finally did read the insert and learned that ranitidine is typically prescribed for stomach acid reflux and heartburn. What the heck? They gave it to me to address my skin symptoms! As I kept reading through the list of side effects, I realized they included many of the very problems that I was already struggling with. So, I stopped taking it right then and there.

I only learned later that ranitidine, when combined with H1 blockers, is indeed known to help reduce itching.

MY FIRST ATTEMPT AT SOCIALIZING

In February, I went out for the first time since the previous summer. As a human being, you just have to connect with other people at some point, so I went to visit some good friends for dinner. We agreed that I would cook for everyone so nobody would accidentally make something that would make me sick. They had recently become vegan, and I was super excited to spoil them with a beautiful meal. I wouldn't be able to eat everything I made, but I decided on zucchini and eggplant appetizers with a tahini dip, followed by baked pumpkin served with vegan mashed potatoes and a colorful side salad for the main course. While stirring the tahini dip, which I make with sesame paste, salt, water, and lemon juice, I thought I should try a little drop to see if it had enough salt. I tried smelling it, but the thing is, you can't smell salt. So then, while stirring a little more to get the mix properly emulsified, I thought I might want to try just a tiny bit to be sure. I took another whiff, and—in a flash—I started to faint! I had just enough time to spin around and drop my ass down onto the floor.

My vision blurred into flickering black and gray, my heart and head pounding. Sweat soaked me as waves of nausea and heat surged through me like the ocean. I focused all my energy on not passing out completely, yet aware my friends saw this strange move; they were alarmed and asked if they could help. I couldn't talk, and their words sounded muffled like being underwater. Heavily relying on the kitchen cabinet for support, I tried to stay upright, feeling soothed by the cool floor but internally boiling. The room spun, and I felt the strong urge to lie down on the marble floor, but I fought to stay conscious. It took about ten minutes for the flickering to stop and the spinning to settle. My friends remained at my side, concerned and asking if I needed a hospital, but I insisted on staying for dinner, not letting this ruin my first outing in six months.

Yet this event did taint the mood, and I could feel their concern throughout the whole evening. They kept asking if I was okay and whether they should take me to the ER because, even hours later, my face was still as red as a tomato. Despite feeling extremely weak, I managed to make it through the rest of the night and finally leave under my own steam. The most curious thing was that my face had gotten red and hot, because whenever I had passed out before, I had turned pale and ghostly.

The next day, I visited my doctor, seeking an explanation. After recounting my experience, he said, "Well, I guess you should remember not to sniff sesame." *Gee, thanks, Doc!*

Not long after, I went to the university hospital, where I described the incident again. The doctors there explained sesame is a potent allergen and used an analogy about peanuts to illustrate the severity of reactions, explaining that simply smelling the sesame caused my anaphylactic shock. They did a skin prick test, which was negative, prompting questions about how I could pass out from smelling it. They said it was another indicator that I have mastocytosis, because reactions can occur even if tests are negative. *Well, great,* I thought—now my skin burned from the test, and the results were inconclusive. Hospital visits often leave me feeling like a guinea pig.

When I asked why my head was red, I was told it was due to excess histamine, and I should avoid sesame. I was genuinely shocked that such a tiny and seemingly harmless seed like sesame could affect me so strongly—especially since I love sesame: its taste, smell, and cooking with it. Yet now, that same beloved seed could send me into anaphylaxis! Alas, no sesame for me anymore.

In the following weeks, I was tormented by aches and pains throughout my body. I felt exhausted, weak, and jittery. My muscles were sore, and my joints were inflamed all over again. On top of all that, I couldn't even think clearly because my mind was veiled in a seemingly impenetrable, thick, dense brain fog. I could only conclude that all this was just an aftermath of my anaphylactic shock.

TOO WELL TO BE SICK

Ironically enough, it was precisely that same week that I received a letter from the disability agency. It stated that, based on my mention of feeling much better whenever I was at home, I wouldn't meet the eligibility criteria and could go back to work. And there I was, unable to move and in excruciating pain because, in addition to everything else, my back had gone out again. At least I was at home and thus protected from additional triggers for the moment, but reading that letter propelled me into enough of a panic that I contacted my psychologist, whom I hadn't seen for a few months.

After the divorce, I felt that I just needed to sleep, recuperate, and try coming to terms with having been diagnosed with a chronic disease—a condition that nobody seemed to understand completely or be able to help me with. I truly felt like it wouldn't be beneficial to keep talking about this dilemma with no positive prospects in sight. But now, I needed her help to figure out what I could do to get support from the disability agency, because I was dependent upon it.

But how do you prove something that is going on in your body that not even the doctors have a way of explaining, simply because it is not part of their literature? How do you explain something like that? Symptoms that are so strange that even you, who experiences this whole bewildering torment, think it sounds crazy and unbelievable.... And what can you do for work if you know you can't depend on your body? When you experience these reactions daily, to the point where even simple tasks like cooking or taking a shower become impossible, leaving you on the floor with cold sweats and muscle pain, as if you had a high fever? How would one approach this perplexing conundrum? Or even how could you explain something that you can't explain, even to yourself? I didn't know the answer to all these knotty questions. All I knew was that I needed support.

GETTING THE HELP I NEEDED

Returning to counseling seemed my best hope, but, as you can guess, my psychologist also doubted whether this was real or if I was making it up. But how can you make something up you don't even believe yourself? It was extremely difficult to prove that these reactions were really happening and not some attempt to fake illness to avoid work. I mean, I preferred having a job and not being sick, earning money and being self-sufficient. But I was genuinely very sick and needed support—financial, medical, and psychological. All these reactions were new to me, and I just didn't have a clue how to live with them. We finally decided to review my entire life to see whether disability was justified from a psychological point of view, because at this stage I still lacked enough scientific explanations for my physical ailments. She also helped organize information to contest the decision. Given my illness, it wasn't easy to attend these meetings on a weekly basis, but her support gave me a sense of security. It was also good to have someone unbiased to talk to—someone who didn't pretend to have all the answers. I liked this woman from the start, but over time, I came to value our relationship deeply. Since we met so often, she saw my ordeal firsthand and probably empathized more than friends or family.

People who've known you for a long time understandably think they know you. Yet they might not realize that such an illness changes everything in your life. It can become difficult to relate on both sides because, even though you still look pretty much the same, nothing in your life remains as it was before. We must alter so many things in our lives to deal with such a uniquely challenging situation. We have to develop various coping mechanisms and make countless adjustments to our surroundings just to be semi-well. We cannot continue as we used to, and this inevitably affects how we interact with others. The people around us—even and especially those who love us and think they know us—can often reach their limit in compassion and understanding.

THE SEARCH FOR ANSWERS CONTINUED

Since the doctors at the university hospital offered nothing beyond a load of antihistamines, I kept searching for answers. Suddenly remembering that one doctor mentioned a self-help group, I looked for their information and contacted them. This was a group of just four to six people who met quarterly to exchange their experiences on living with mastocytosis. The first meeting I attended was in May 2018.

The attendees informed me that there was also a self-help group on Facebook and gave me the address of a physician specializing in mastocytosis. He practiced in a town less than an hour from where I lived, so I soon scheduled an appointment with him. Just knowing that I would eventually get to meet a doctor who was truly invested in this disease gave me a great sense of hope, even though it was going to take another few months until he was available. Joining the Facebook group was amazingly helpful because the quick search option allowed me to find answers much faster than trying to find them online. Aside from that, it felt good to be part of a community of people who could truly relate to my experiences. One attendee mentioned that she had Dr. Afrin's book *Never Bet Against Occam* and offered to let me borrow it. I hadn't heard of it before and was eager to read it, so I met her the following week to pick it up.

I am not exactly what you would call a bookworm, but it took me only two weeks to devour those 470 pages! It was incredibly eye-opening to learn that the myriad symptoms I experienced, which the doctors said weren't common in mastocytosis, appeared to be quite prevalent in mast cell activation syndrome. Besides, it was comforting to read all these stories of others who had gone through experiences quite similar to mine. In a way, it made me feel less alone. Whenever I found a description that resembled my symptomatology, I marked the page. Two weeks later, I took the book to my psychologist—tagged with approximately 60 sticky notes—to tell her that I might have just found the direction in which to look.

I also brought the book to the next hospital session, where I was greeted by the two doctors I'd been working with, their students and, what I didn't realize at the time, their boss. Excitedly, I shared my discovery that my symptoms might stem from mast cell activation syndrome (MCAS) rather than mastocytosis. My primary doctor clearly disagreed and insisted that if I had mastocytosis, I also had MCAS. I countered that mastocytosis involves too many mast cells in specific tissues, which may not always cause symptoms, unlike MCAS, where mast cells may be overly active throughout the body.

Then I asked if they could measure mediators and do a brain MRI, as I had been suffering from a crushing and persistent headache for over seven weeks. One of the doctors sharply refused both requests and told me to stop relying on internet sources. The session ended with a medication change from fexofenadine to Aerius and a suggestion to send me to a mountain rehabilitation clinic where a team of doctors would help me understand my reactions and find the best treatments. They would contact me once insurance issues were resolved.

This idea sounded better than good to me! For one, I love the mountains, and of course it would be beneficial, because there are far fewer triggers up there compared to the city. What's more, I couldn't wait to learn how to get a handle on the reactions to smells. Having a whole team of doctors attend to my needs and at the same time be up in the mountains seemed like the perfect setting to make some real progress and hopefully feel better soon! I gladly accepted and was greatly looking forward to this retreat. In retrospect, my doctor was actually right that mast cell activation is fundamental to all mast cell-related diseases. However, without access to mast cell stabilizers in my treatment, I was still left struggling with a myriad of symptoms.

After the meeting, I went home and emailed Dr. Afrin. I described my situation and asked for his advice on how to progress with my doctors, who still maintained their opinion that my reactions to smells had absolutely nothing to do with mast cells. I couldn't believe that within only thirty minutes, he'd written a whole page-long reply! He reaffirmed that, with all due respect to my doctors, unusual reactivity to odors is indeed a common problem in patients with mast cell disease. He also stated that if I did have mastocytosis, my doctors were right that it wouldn't be necessary to measure the mediators, but that there are a great many drugs that help control mast cell activation. He kindly invited them to contact him if they wanted to discuss the disease in general or my case in particular. What an absolute angel!

I immediately informed my doctors that they were welcome to contact Dr. Afrin, but I doubt they ever did. As for myself, I certainly never got a reply from them. Amusingly enough, after this meeting, I never saw this particular doctor again. I've been to the hospital many times since, but he always seems to disappear, much to the confusion of his colleagues.

AN UNEXPECTED LIFELINE

A bit of serendipity came one day out of the blue. I randomly met a guy while bringing my compost to the community garden, and we subsequently became friends. After hearing about my situation, he quickly established that a friend of his, who lived in England, had pretty much the same ailments as me. He connected the two of us, and I soon emailed this lady. It turned out that she, too, had been diagnosed with cutaneous mastocytosis and suffered from nearly the same symptoms. On top of that, she'd been through a relationship very similar to the one I had just recently escaped and was still struggling to recover from. It was such a relief to finally have someone to talk to who could fully grasp the situation I was in!

When she heard about my incessant headache, she asked me to send her a comprehensive list of everything I ate—finally, an easy task: I was down to twenty foods. She soon replied that olive and coconut oils are high in salicylates, suggesting that this could be the culprit for my headache. I hadn't ever heard of salicylates, but, of course, I decided to cut them out. I removed these two oils from my diet and switched to canola oil instead. This helped so quickly, I almost couldn't believe it—my headache was completely gone after only four days! This rapid improvement left no room for doubt, so from then on, I began avoiding salicylates as well.

CHAPTER 5

My Stay at the Rehabilitation Clinic

WEEK 1 — A ROCKY START

In mid-June, I got admitted to the clinic in the mountains. I traveled up there by train, a somewhat grueling three-hour journey, such that I was utterly exhausted when I finally arrived. Trains, you see, are just chock-full of triggers, and there's not much you can do about that, except to a limited extent by wearing a mask. Not having a mask yet, I covered my face with a scarf, but I still arrived jittery and sweating, with a flushed face and watery eyes that blurred my vision.

Once I finally managed to drag myself into the facility, it didn't take more than a few seconds to be hit by the next set of triggers. The smells of carpeted floors, ham and cheese, baked croissants, aftershave, and soup saturating the air spiked my already present nausea only further. With my heart pounding wildly, I had to practically fight through the next fifteen yards to reach the reception desk, where I almost fainted when the staff's perfumes hit me full-on. Barely able to remain standing, I desperately clung to the reception desk and did my best to answer their questions to check in. More than ready to lie down and settle in, I was so glad when a nurse finally arrived to escort me to my room.

The room was nice and clean … too clean, in fact. As soon as we crossed the threshold, the nausea increased and I started to tremble. I instantly knew the room was freshly renovated—the fumes from the fresh glue and new flooring stinging in my eyes, skin, and lungs.

The nurse immediately grabbed the phone and called, "Strong allergic reaction in room 101! Request a transfer!"

I was glad this was obvious, so I didn't have to explain. We gathered my bags, and en route to the next floor, the nurse apologized and explained that the section had just recently been renovated and even he had mild reactions to the flooring. The next two rooms weren't any better, so I was finally placed on the top floor in an older room away from the renovation, laundry, and cafeteria. Now I could finally lie down!

I was more than a bit shaken by all this, but I kept reminding myself of what my doctor had said: *A team of physicians here will use their mutual knowledge to help me get better.* A nurse came by a little later to give me the next day's schedule and inform me about dinner time and location. I told her straight up that there was no way I would go down to a dining hall and expose myself to even more triggers. After I explained to her that I react to smells of certain foods, as well as perfumes, deodorants, shampoos, and so forth, it was decided that I'd get room service instead.

SO MUCH FOR THE REST

I had submitted a list of my tolerated foods weeks in advance, but one glimpse of my dinner plate made it frustratingly clear that this rather crucial information somehow hadn't made it to the kitchen. I looked at the plate, utterly dejected, and just felt so bummed. I was very hungry after all the turmoil of the day, but there wasn't a single thing I could eat! When the nurse returned to collect the dishes, she looked at me quite surprised and asked if I didn't like it. I told her that, unfortunately, I was allergic to everything on that plate. She profusely apologized and called the kitchen to make sure they'd consider my list from then on. I went to bed hungry and completely exhausted. By then, I was honestly a bit skeptical whether this whole affair would work out for me, but at this point, I was just thankful to settle in for some much-needed rest.

But then, like a waking nightmare, even sleeping wasn't possible! Lying in bed, dead tired, and so ready to sleep, I got awfully itchy and quickly started to sweat so profusely that my pajamas and the sheets were soaked within no time. I eventually got up to shower, and after that succeeded in perking me up a bit, I investigated that stupid bed. When I discovered that the mattress had a plastic lining, it was immediately apparent why I had this response. Argh! Alright, I do understand that hospital beds need to be clean, and plastic covers are a valid solution as a sanitary measure, but they're not a good idea for hypersensitive folks with mast cell disease. Thankfully, I found a wool blanket to cover the mattress. Yet, even though this did help make it more comfortable, I was still so riled up by then that I couldn't wind down anymore. In the end, I didn't sleep a wink that first night.

A FACILITY FULL OF TRIGGERS

I wish I could say that at least a brighter day awaited, but, sadly, breakfast was just as disappointing as that depressing dinner the night before. Orange juice, bread, butter, and jam were immediately out of the question. Coffee was the only option that I sometimes tolerated, but I felt a reaction to this one after the first sip. Feeling the need to get at least something in me, I decided to try my luck with the coffee vending machine down the hallway.

As soon as I hit the corridor, my eyes and skin started to sting and burn again. Spotting the cleaning bucket and floor mop next to the elevator, I couldn't help but feel a twinge of hopelessness. It became increasingly clear that the entire facility was full of triggers, just like most public places are. How could I work around all that during the entire length of my stay?

Unfortunately, I didn't tolerate the coffee from the vending machine either. Minutes after drinking it, my face was flushed and my stomach hurt. Trying to put this breakfast ordeal behind me, I headed to the first doctor's consultation.

I got into the elevator and pressed the button. Within seconds—before the doors could even close—my heart was racing again. The air inside this tiny, enclosed space was permeated with the smells of shampoo and aftershave. All I could do was hold my breath, hoping the doors opened again before I passed out. Unfortunately, that next breath knocked me right off my feet, because the little whiff of air I took in once the doors opened was saturated with the fumes of cleaning agents. I literally fell over because my legs just gave out beneath me. I shuffled over to the nearest chair and plopped down. Hardly even capable of sitting upright, I did my best to calm down while waiting for my appointment.

The doctor reassured me that they would do their best to help me. After hearing about my ongoing dilemma with the food, she called the kitchen to ensure they'd start serving me only the foods on my list. Concerning my insomnia, she suggested I take a sleep aid, at least for the first few days, until I'd be properly settled in. Then she took my weight and vitals and read through the information she'd received from my doctors. Finally, she asked me about my expectations for the retreat.

I answered that my main problem at the time was my reactions to smells—and I was greatly looking forward to finally getting to the bottom of it all.

"Well, reactions to smells are a known symptom in mast cell disease," she replied, seeming slightly abashed, "and unfortunately, we won't be able to do anything about that ... I mean, we cannot change the air or control what other patients here use."

Well, goodness me, hadn't I said this all along?! Reactions to smells are part and parcel of this whole mast cell madness! Why on earth was I up here, getting hammered by precisely that—in a facility flooded with smells and triggers—after my doctors had explicitly told me they were going to help me solve this problem? These people here knew that such reactions are common in mast cell disease, but they couldn't do anything about it. Honestly, by that point, I was starting to get upset.

"Let's just take it step by step," she suggested, adding, "I am sure there are things we can do for you."

I sat there wondering exactly how she thought they could help me.

SMALL WINS AND STALE CHICKEN

The first thing I did after this massively disappointing meeting was go to the village to buy some food, because I was starving by that point. I got corn waffles, safflower oil, Himalayan salt, hard-boiled eggs, and apples. I just needed to be sure I had something to eat. During the last year, I had already lost four sizes, and I wanted to avoid losing any more weight. Walking to the village, I got to take a breather. The surroundings of this hospital were just gorgeous! The air was clean and crisp, and a small lake sparkled nearby beneath the majestic beauty of the mountains. The comforting silence surrounding me and the sweet, slightly invigorating smell of pine trees wafting in on the warm breeze felt like a worthy counterbalance to the ordeal I had just gone through. I gathered my courage and decided to remain hopeful that something good would come out of this stay.

The next meal I got served was somewhat better, but still didn't quite do it. A dried-out puck of baked chicken breast accompanied by a sad little side salad and corn niblets from a can. Aside from being disgusting, canned vegetables are a no-go if you react to histamine and nickel, and there's no telling what preservatives were used. One look at the chicken breast made me wonder how long ago it had been prepared and whether it was still safe to eat, as it might have turned into a histamine bomb since then. I complained once again. There was no way I would put this stuff in my mouth without knowing the answers to these questions. It just felt like too much of a risk, so I asked if I could please talk to the chefs. Alright, I admit that I do love good food and could even be called somewhat of a food snob, but at this point, I really would have eaten whatever they served if I just felt confident that it wouldn't make me even sicker. This complaint turned out to be worth it in the end, because after that I did get scheduled for a meeting with the nutritionist. Finally, I could leave him with some simple ideas about what they could prepare for me.

In the afternoon, my heart health was assessed while I pedaled on a stationary bike. I got so dizzy that I could barely stand afterward, but neither did I pass out, nor did my heart stop. It was concluded that my heart appeared to function normally, and I was cleared for the rest of the day. After resting for a bit, I took another stroll outside.

Returning for dinner, I was so happy to find the first warm meal I could eat! Meat, rice, and steamed vegetables. Not that difficult after all, was it?

PARADOXICAL REACTIONS

Even though I'm not a fan of sleeping pills, that day I figured I'd make an exception. I truly needed some rest, so I took the dose they had so neatly prepared for me in a little plastic dish beside my bed. I lay down and closed my eyes. I was starting to relax, ready to drift off to dreamland, when suddenly my heart began to beat very fast. It quickly became so overpowering that I started to feel incredibly agitated. I remember thinking it might be a reaction to the bed material again, but I just turned over, trying to ignore it and relax. Yet the agitation kept increasing until I eventually jumped out of bed, so riled up I felt like I could run up the walls! Then it slowly dawned on me that it might be an adverse reaction to the sleeping pills. Years before, I'd been given a dose of Valium to help me sleep, but it ended up keeping me awake for two days straight. Like back then, I didn't get to sleep at all that night.

The following day, now suffering from just about complete exhaustion, I noticed my schedule was basically empty—one exercise class in the late morning, but no doctor's consultation at all! I lay there wondering when this team of genius doctors would arrive and how exactly they planned to apply their collective knowledge, experience, and great wisdom to help me get better! How were we supposed to make any progress like that? I wanted more clarity on my condition and to get into a better state, but the reality of this affair was that I just kept getting worse through being hit by all these triggers, day in and day out! When a nurse came by my room, I asked her whether she had any idea why my schedule was empty for the day. She said she didn't know either, but I could talk to Mrs. Huggins, who was available for patients to address problems concerning their stay.

I did that immediately. I told her how difficult it was for me to be inside the facility because of all the triggers, that I hadn't slept properly since I got there, and that I was getting ridiculously hungry by this point. I expressed my worries about having been sent up there to figure out my dilemma with the reactions to smells, yet it now seemed pretty clear that I couldn't expect any solution to that problem. I felt much worse than before I came! My entire body was in pain. My joints hurt, my eyes never stopped burning, my voice had gotten hoarse, and it was getting increasingly difficult to breathe. With a lack of clarity about the goals for my stay and, consequently, no idea why precisely I needed to be up here amidst all these triggers, I truly wanted to be done with this unfruitful undertaking and go home.

ESCAPE FROM THE RETREAT

Thankfully, she understood my concerns and asked me what I wanted to do. I replied that I would love to go home, at least just for the weekend, so I could catch up on sleep, eat right for a few solid meals, and nourish myself back up. I could then bring my own bedding, some extra food, and my coffee maker when I returned, so that I'd be more comfortable and better able to hopefully make actual progress. This sweet woman said she would make an exception for me, even though they usually wouldn't allow people to leave the clinic, especially at the beginning of a stay. She told me to go home and take good care of myself but be sure to make it back by Sunday evening. I was so relieved! I packed up quickly and dashed right over to the train station.

Upon arriving in Zurich, I went to buy a bunch of groceries, and as soon as I was home, I cooked up a massive pan of coconut chicken with vegetables and rice. After gobbling down the whole thing, I promptly dropped into my comfy bed and slept straight through the next sixteen hours! The next day, my best friend came by to visit. We played music, shared some good food, and just relaxed for the rest of the weekend.

WEEK 2 — TRYING ANEW

My dad offered to take me back on Sunday, a very kind gesture given the three-hour drive. I deeply appreciated it and felt relieved there wouldn't be triggers like on the train. Yet when they picked me up, I was instantly hit by the scent of a strong perfume. My throat closed, and my eyes burned. I asked, "Are you guys wearing perfume?" knowing they knew I react severely.

They had known for a while, yet they came drenched in it, not considering the impact. My dad said he wasn't wearing perfume, pointing at his wife, who admitted she had put it on before leaving and realized only afterward she probably shouldn't have. She then explained it's routine for her to wear perfume before going out, and added, "I mean, you wouldn't expect me to shower again just to wash it off, would you?"

I thought about just taking the train, but my dad insisted I stick with the plan. To cope, I rolled down the window to get as much fresh air as possible, but being immersed in the smell for the entire ride made me feel extremely ill.

As sick as I was, the truth is that this indifference felt even worse psychologically than my physical reaction. They clearly wanted to do me a favor, but either they didn't understand the gravity of my reactions, or they didn't believe me when I'd told them before. And if it were the case that they didn't believe me, what were they really thinking about me? Were they possibly thinking I was making all this stuff up, or what? Maybe they didn't realize just how important it was for me that they would at least try to adjust such routines around me so I could be more comfortable. Except comfortable isn't even the right word! It's not about me being comfortable, but rather about me being safe, not just from getting a little bit ill, but violently ill. I can be sick for days or weeks when these reactions hit. Such a fundamental lack of simple validation and understanding can really make you feel hopeless. Sometimes it seems like your only choice is to either resign yourself to being miserably ill whenever visiting with others, or you could retreat from life entirely and become a veritable hermit instead.

That day, riding in the car with them, encumbered by this awkward silence, I just felt like an absolute nuisance. I felt repelled by the idea of having to dictate to everyone around me what they would have to do, just so that I could even be around, but I also didn't want to keep getting sick over and over again. Silently weighing the pros and cons of these two choices, neither of them felt at all desirable.

More than anything, I was just sad. I had genuinely been looking forward to spending this time with my dad, to the conversations we might have during the ride, and the memories we'd make that day. Yet now, due to this pathetic condition, absolutely nothing about this day turned out to be enjoyable. All I felt was guilt now because I couldn't even be present! He had been so generous to spend an entire day on me; driving me all the way up to the mountains, and then he'd still have to return home afterward—and I couldn't give him anything in return. I hated this situation. All the nice things that could have happened on this day, but now I couldn't even have so much as a simple conversation with him because the whistling of the airstream was just too loud with the windows open. And sadly, it seemed that I was the only person there who fully understood the necessity of it, perhaps because I was the only one who actually felt the pain, which is hardly visible from the outside.

After arriving at the village, we decided to have a coffee together before they headed back home. I asked them if we could go to a place with a patio so I could get some fresh air and recover from the ride before going back inside the clinic. It was a bit cloudy, so my dad's wife insisted firmly that she wouldn't sit outside because she didn't want to get cold. I was reluctant to venture into a strange restaurant and possibly get hammered again by even more smells. So, sadly, we ended up skipping the coffee altogether. We finally pulled up in front of the clinic, I gathered up my bags, and they just drove off.

LITTLE VICTORIES

Bringing my own bedding really did make it more comfortable, and I slept considerably better that night. Bringing along my tiny fold-out camping stove, coffee maker, and some grounds was also a smart move. Life at the clinic had just improved tremendously! Happy about that, I was now eager for progress.

The following day, my lungs were thoroughly examined, and they appeared to be okay. Next, a dermatologist confirmed the diagnosis of cutaneous mastocytosis again. He advised me to keep up my regimen with the antihistamines and gave me some creams to help reduce the itching. He also ran a test for UVA and UVB light and discovered that I am highly allergic to UVB rays. I hadn't ever thought about that before. I guess I had always instinctively worn long-sleeved shirts in summer simply because having the sun directly on my skin felt uncomfortable. He also advised me to do this and strongly admonished me to always wear sunscreen when I'm in the sun.

STILL NOT SAFE

Despite better sleep, I kept getting sicker due to triggers at the clinic. My eyes burned so badly that it hurt to keep them open, and my sore throat made speaking painful. I was hoarse, with frequent heart palpitations, dizziness, and relentless full-body pain. I felt like being trapped in a trigger suit with electric stimulations firing randomly, frying me from the inside. My skin burned and my recent headache returned with a vengeance, pounding under the flickering fluorescent lights throughout the clinic.

Next, I was scheduled to meet with a psychologist. She suggested we have our conversations outside, which made it easier for me to focus and talk. Although I felt I wasn't there for counseling, I was actually grateful to have someone to talk to instead of lying in my room recovering from the latest reactions. I told her I felt uneasy about my stay because my doctors sent me there to figure out my reactions to smells, but it seemed nothing could be done. My well-being had steadily declined since I arrived, as there was no way to escape triggers inside the facility, even with a mask. Over five days, I had lost six pounds and truly felt safer at home. I was worried about losing the progress I had so painstakingly gained until then, and afraid of facing the aftermath of these reactions for a long time. I knew I was risking my health and couldn't endure this much longer, so I told her I wanted to go home. I also mentioned needing support from the disability agency because I didn't know what job I could do, given my reactions to almost everything outside. How could I responsibly accept a job, knowing I might collapse at any moment and likely wouldn't be physically stable? I still had the meeting with the specialist from the self-help group, leaving me with at least a sliver of hope.

THE LAST STRAW

The following day, my back went out. When that happens, when a vertebra dislocates, it often ends up pinching the nerves, and that pain can be completely debilitating. The best thing to do then is to get a massage or chiropractic work, or to get on a Pilates roller to try popping it back in. Sometimes it works, and sometimes it doesn't. Sometimes, I wind up lying around uselessly for days until it finally slips back in on its own. I suspect it went out this time because I was breathing rather shallowly to reduce the impact of the airborne triggers, at least to some extent.

When the nurses heard about my misfortune, they organized a massage for me. Yet, the first available slot wasn't until two days later, so I had to wait. With plenty of time to think about the pros and cons of my stay, it became blatantly clear that I'd only gotten worse since I had arrived. And now that my back had gone out again, my entire nervous system was completely fried. In Zurich, I had several good massage therapists who could have helped me by now.

So there I was, lying quietly in my room, contemplating the whole affair when suddenly, the gardener out front started up his leaf blower. The sound of this wretched machine came crashing in through my window, aggravating my headache to the point where it felt like my head would explode any second. Despite my locked-up back, I struggled to my feet and somehow schlepped myself over to the window. Yet, in my feeble attempt to close it, my shaky hand slipped right off the handle, and I sprained my thumb so badly that it turned blue within minutes. Now I'd had just about all I could take. I was done. I wanted to push the eject button and go home. I called the nurse and asked for an early checkout.

Unfortunately, it wasn't her call to allow me to leave—I had to wait for a doctor's approval. Since no doctor was available, I returned to Mrs. Huggins. She empathized with my situation but, not having the authority to allow me to leave either, all she could do was arrange a meeting with the senior physician as soon as possible.

SENT TO "CALM DOWN"

I visited him the following day to speak. In hindsight, meeting this doctor at the beginning of my stay would probably have been highly beneficial, as he appeared to be quite knowledgeable about mast cell issues. Perhaps meeting him earlier could have made a difference, but at this point, I just wanted to go home. I couldn't wait to get myself out of this danger zone! He empathized with my situation and expressed his regret about their inability to provide more help. He said that, had he known just how sensitive I was, he would have made it clear from the start that their facility wasn't appropriate for hypersensitive individuals like me. Glancing at my admission papers from Zurich, he said that the stated reason for my stay was to give me some time to rest and calm down, but he was aware that this wouldn't be possible for me in a setting where I had constant reactions.

"What did they say?" I sputtered in disbelief. "I was sent here to 'calm down'? They told me you would help me figure out my reactions to smells!" I was utterly dumbstruck and at a loss for words.

He confirmed that this was indeed what had been proposed in the papers.

Hearing that, I was absolutely livid. "It's not what they told me. I mean, how can I 'calm down' if I'm trying to figure out a physiological problem that causes havoc in my entire life, and still no doctor can assist me with it? Most don't even believe me, while others do, but they say nothing can be done about it. The worst thing is that I have to keep explaining myself, over and over, while feeling like I'm going to fall apart because I am in so much pain. My body just doesn't act right anymore. My problem is not that I need to calm down. My question is how to live life with this disease, because I can't do anything as I used to. The problem is that my body needs to calm down. I need to get support from the disability agency so that I can find ways to live without constantly getting sicker like I just did in this hospital."

He sympathetically replied, "I understand. How do you want to progress after leaving here?"

I told him my next hope was with the mastocytosis specialist from the self-help group. He seemed relieved I had an appointment. He nodded and agreed it was better for me to go home because my well-being truly couldn't be guaranteed there. I was discharged that day.

You can probably imagine my swirling thoughts all the way home. My doctors had actually lied to me! They had unceremoniously shoved me off to this clinic—certainly a beautiful place with a good reputation many would be grateful to be in—but I had been given misleading information, which led me to have unrealistic expectations about the retreat because I didn't know the instructions the doctors had received—and of course, this caused confusion on both ends. Now I finally understood why my schedule was so limited. If it was mainly for me to rest, not examine my case or find solutions, it made sense. I thought, *What a stupid move by my doctors*. How could I trust them now, knowing they withheld such vital information? After that, I lost all faith in them.

BACK HOME

I was so relieved to be back in my tiny, safe space. Sure, I regretted not having been able to get more out of this retreat, and I already missed the mountains, but it was good to be back inside my own walls. At least here I was protected from additional triggers and, thus, even more pain. It was clear that I had done nothing but get sicker at the hospital, but back home it became undeniably apparent just how urgent it had been for me to leave the clinic. I had lost close to eight pounds within a week, and my health had completely crashed. But now, like a dam waiting to burst, the aftermath of these reactions started to kick in—like when you take a vacation but end up getting sick on the first day precisely because you suddenly have the space for that to happen.

The next day, my entire body was sore; I couldn't stand due to pain in my feet, joints, and muscles, my skin burning and light sensitivity causing agony. I lay in bed, hoping to wait it out. Still unwell the following day, I called my house doctor, who advised Diclofenac, an NSAID. I confirmed this with my university hospital doctor, who agreed and urged me to go to the ER if my condition worsened.

I followed their advice to a T, but instead of relief, I got intense pain in my kidneys, and my hands and feet swelled up so much that they started looking like Mickey Mouse's gloves. I learned later that although most mast cell patients tolerate NSAIDs, they can strongly activate mast cells and are therefore contraindicated in a small subset of patients with mast cell activation disorder. Going to the ER seemed like a perfectly futile idea because, suffice to say, no medical institution had yet been able to help. Most of my recent hospital visits had made me feel even worse. Besides, I was in no condition to leave the house or even move at all.

However, I needed to get the inflammation down as soon as possible, or I felt I was going to smolder away. What I did then was use common sense. How to put out a fire? Water! I started drinking lots of water and chamomile tea. I also took *Boswellia serrata* extract multiple times a day—a powerful anti-inflammatory that had always helped with my GI symptoms. On top of this, I took arnica sugar pills and CBD oil that I'd once been given as a gift but had never used before. It took another six days of just lying in bed until I was able to move again, but this regimen seemed to help a lot.

After a week in bed and isolated, I finally managed to get on the computer briefly. It still hurt to move, and the bright screen pierced my eyes, but I wanted to make progress. At the clinic, I had asked the Facebook group how others manage reactions to smells. Some mentioned eye drops and nasal sprays with antihistaminic properties. I looked them up and called my doctor for prescriptions. I knew I had to stay home to avoid triggers for some time so I could get better, but I needed supplies for when I left the house again. Unfortunately, I couldn't tolerate either of these medicines because their taste caused further reactions.

For the next month, I was bedridden. It was a drag to spend the beginning of summer in bed while hearing the world outside my slightly open window wake up to the liveliness of warmer days. The chatter of people and the chirping of birds all sounded so happy and exuberant while I remained glued to my stupid bed. I felt frustrated about my upcoming birthday, knowing I wouldn't recover in time to celebrate it properly. I missed my life, my friends, my energy, and the sun. I missed those carefree, younger days when I could simply hop on my bike, ride off, and soak up life. I felt stuck and alone; aware of life around me but trapped in my own void where no one else could see me.

AN EPIPHANY!

After wallowing in this misery for several weeks, one day I got up and shuffled over to the kitchen to make myself some food. It still hurt so much, even just standing on my feet was pure torment. Not only did my feet hurt, but also my legs, knees, joints, arms, hands, head, and eyes. Simply said, everything hurt. I couldn't hold onto any thought except, *Ouch, it hurts!*

These words spun like a record in my head. *Ouch*. Every step I took. *Ouch. I am so sick!* It hurt so much, and this *ouch* was so continuous that at some point it finally made me laugh. It had become almost comical. The pain was downright excruciating and seemed never-ending! Usually, pain subsides at some point. Every cold comes to an end, most wounds heal after some time, and most headaches eventually taper off, but this shit was relentless! It had become so grueling that, at this point, it started to seem completely absurd!

In my attempt to drink a sip of water, the glass slipped right out of my shaky hand and fell crashing to the ground. *Ouch!* The sound of the glass shattering across the floor brought another shiver of pain rushing through my entire body. Crouching down to gather up the scattered pieces hurt immensely, but then lifting myself back up brought the pain to a whole new level. Again, it made me laugh—not to suggest that I enjoy pain, but this was just ridiculous. It was incredible! I couldn't believe just how bad this all was, so I guess laughing was the only thing I had left.

Taking the next step—*ouch!* That instant, something surged through me like a lightning bolt: I had an epiphany! My cells were listening! Somehow, I both consciously grasped and physically felt this insight at the same time. My cells were listening to me narrating my pain—my brain the commander, the cells dutifully following its orders. I froze in my tracks, allowing this insight to sink in fully.

Suddenly, an article I'd read some time before came back to mind; it said that no cancer patient had ever gone into remission without a positive mindset. Now, a cascade of thoughts rushed through my mind: *Mast cells. Cells. Cellular. Healing. Cancer cells. Cells. Healing. Brain. Commander. Positivity. Healing. Healing on a cellular level.* I needed to heal on a cellular level!

My doctors seemed to be at their wits' end, or maybe they just weren't as invested in my recovery as much as I was. Whatever the case, I wanted to feel better! I needed to take this into my own hands and do whatever I could to get better. The body is like an entire universe, intrinsically interconnected. Cells communicate with each other, period. I needed to keep my thoughts positive, no matter what! Right then and there, still standing in my kitchen with the dustpan of shattered glass in front of me, I decided to stay positive, come what may! I decided I'd start telling myself, and therefore also my cells, a different story. The one that had been going on for some years now, endlessly bemoaning how bad I felt and counting every one of my pains, had to go!

Right away, like a mad woman, I started saying out loud, "I'm healthy, I'm healthy, I'm healthy." My cells, or at least something inside of me, screamed back, *Are you fucking nuts? It hurts. It's painful. We're sick!* I countered, "I know it hurts, I'm here, I feel it, but fuck it. I ain't gonna go down that road anymore!

I am well, I am healthy, I am healthy, I am well."

I know, this sounds completely bonkers. Honestly, I thought so too. Yet, I decided to try it. I quickly found that saying, "It's getting better," was more believable than, "It's good," so I stuck with it. It wasn't easy—after years of chronic pain, I was used to constantly noticing it. But now, I realized I needed to reprogram these thoughts if I wanted any chance of improving, so I kept at it, going back and restarting whenever I lost focus, especially at first.

In retrospect, this was the best thing that came from my stay at the clinic. Maybe I needed to end up at such a desperately low point to find this insight. I can't claim that everything just magically turned good overnight. The journey ahead was still arduous, but things did indeed start to lighten up a bit. Even if not physically for a long time, energetically and mentally I began to feel better.

CHAPTER 6

Gradual Recovery

It ultimately took a bit more than a month until the pain started to subside, and at last I had my long-awaited appointment with the mastocytosis specialist. I was thrilled to finally meet this guy and went to the meeting with a bucketful of optimism. Yet, once again, I left a doctor's office rather perturbed. After scarcely an hour, he told me that, in his view, I didn't have mastocytosis at all! He said that the rash on my arms didn't look typical, and the various symptoms I displayed didn't fit the criteria in the books. He also said he wouldn't accept me as a patient because he only worked with people who had mastocytosis.

I was utterly perplexed by his statement and asked if it could be mast cell activation syndrome instead. He shortly replied that he didn't know. It was clear by then that he had shut the door on helping me. Trying to salvage at least something from the appointment, I brought up cromoglicic acid, since I'd read that it could help stabilize mast cells. He agreed I could give it a try, quickly scribbling a prescription and sliding it across the desk, perhaps just to get me out of his office. I grabbed the paper, thanked him, and left—still bewildered about the whole encounter but clinging to a bit of hope. I had asked for this drug multiple times, but no doctor had let me try it. Maybe this would finally help.

My psychologist looked at me with hesitation. "So, he thinks it's not mastocytosis? What do you think it is, then?"

"Well, what the heck do I know?" I said. Reading Dr. Afrin's book had left me fairly sure it was MCAS, but I had no proof. I'd been diagnosed with cutaneous mastocytosis by multiple doctors over the years and had only just started to feel like I might finally understand what was happening. And now this specialist just pulled the rug out from under me, throwing everything into doubt. Interestingly, though, in his letter to my house doctor, he noted that my symptoms might be consistent with MCAS.

FINALLY, A WAY FORWARD

The next stage of my odyssey took me to Dr. René Zenhäusern, the specialist I'd been referred to months earlier for my back. He confirmed I didn't need surgery and said physiotherapy and muscle balance training could help. According to him, my muscles weren't functioning properly despite my active lifestyle because my brain wasn't making the connection. The muscles supporting my spine, glutes, hips, and scapula were atrophied, and no matter how hard I tried, I couldn't consciously tense them. He reassured me that reestablishing this brain-muscle link was possible—it would just take about 100,000 repetitions of specific exercises.

Well, that was indeed exhilarating news! One hundred thousand isn't exactly a small number, but this was something I could do to feel better at some point. Besides, it was a bit perplexing to learn that some of the major muscle groups in my body weren't functioning properly, even though I've always been very active, doing all kinds of sports and yoga, not to mention all the cleaning, moving, and gardening jobs. After considering this for a moment, I concluded that I could feel tremendously proud of my body since it had done a pretty good job holding up all this time.

I was scheduled to come back weekly for physiotherapy and was flatly forbidden from practicing yoga, at least until these limp muscles were on par with the rest of my body. The prospect that these exercises could eventually help strengthen my back to the point that it wouldn't keep knocking me out was exciting. I also felt fairly certain it would help with the mast-cell reactions since the pain of a dislocated vertebra inevitably aggravated all the other symptoms.

I committed to daily exercises, which was tough, especially at first. Trying to do these isolated movements made me feel like a beginner again, because my stronger muscles would tend to kick in, preventing me from reaching the weaker ones that I actually needed to train. I had to stay laser-focused to target the right spots. New exercises often caused soreness, joint tenderness, and sometimes even vertebrae dislocations, and it was also crucial to find the right balance. Overdoing it triggered reactions that sidelined me, so I had to listen closely to my body's limits. It demanded patience and willpower to progress gradually within my body's capacity, but I stuck with it, knowing it would help.

SMARTER EVERY DAY

Meanwhile, I kept searching for solutions to the mast-cell reactions. I combed through the self-help groups again and again and exchanged many emails with my newfound MCAD-afflicted friend, Ellie, from England. I tried to observe my reactions closely enough to be able to gather as much additional data as possible, all in the hope of finding new ways to cope.

Day by day, I became a little smarter. I came up with some breathing techniques I could use while out in public to reduce the magnitude of my reactions to smells, at least to some degree. I also set up my house so it was easier to clean, which helped reduce my reactions to dust and facilitated the work, too. Eventually, I found cleaning agents and body-care products to which I didn't react, and I kept learning more about diet and nutrition.

All this took a great deal of time and effort, but I was determined to get better, so I didn't allow myself to shy away from it. I figured that every slight improvement might contribute to my overall well-being, and I was hoping that the cumulative effect of many minor improvements would eventually make all the difference. I stuck with my decision to stay positive and just kept trying whatever I thought might help.

By the end of August, it seemed as though I couldn't expect to achieve much more progress at the university hospital, so I decided to look further afield. Eventually, I remembered a pharmacist once mentioned a doctor who was supposedly remarkably good with complicated cases like mine. I went to look through the folder where I usually keep such notes, but I couldn't find it. Finally, I resorted to browsing the internet, hoping to recognize his name if I came across it. I did not see the name I was looking for, but during the search, another place popped up that immediately caught my attention.

The website's opening line said: "Learn about reasons for disease and experience cause-oriented healing." I honestly felt a rush of excitement reading their claim to seek the root cause of illness through a holistic approach, rather than just prescribing medication. Their nickname, *Last Chance Clinic*, made me chuckle, and while some might find it morbid, it actually motivated me to call and schedule an appointment. The receptionist, after hearing a brief outline of my case, booked me with the clinic's owner, Dr. John Van Limburg-Stirum, for a ninety-minute session. This sounded promising since such appointments usually last an hour, but complex cases need more time. I was delighted that they had set aside enough time—and that I would be speaking directly with the boss. This felt like a great start!

HELP WITH HURDLES

The meeting ultimately went well. It was the first time since I had left Dr. Saissi that I felt like a doctor really took the time to listen. Dr. Van Limburg-Stirum takes a thorough approach to assessing any case and is willing and able to think outside the box. Besides being a medical doctor, he also cherishes a holistic approach, which proved truly helpful. Over the next few months, we aimed to improve my well-being step by step. Some trial and error was definitely part of it, but I can say it was all worth it in the long run.

After discovering my iron count was still very low, he suggested an infusion. I was rather apprehensive about it because I had experienced a very intense reaction to such an infusion years before, so we agreed to first try a *baby dose* of just 50 mg. Despite the minimal amount, my body still didn't like it one bit. I shuffled out of the clinic twenty minutes later, feeling like I weighed a hundred tons. Trying to ride my bike home on a route that usually took fifteen minutes ended up taking me well over an hour because I'd gotten so weak that it felt virtually impossible to turn the pedals. I had to practically drag myself home while pushing the bike beside me and using it as a crutch to keep me upright.

It felt like one of those dreams where you desperately want to run, but all you can do is move in slow motion while the world around you keeps spinning at its normal pace. After finally making it home, I plopped into bed, overpowered by a profound lethargy, along with muscle cramps, waves of nausea, and cold sweats. On top of all that, an oppressively overwhelming sadness and hopelessness soon overcame me. Later that day, things got even weirder. I called someone on the phone, but the words I wanted to say just wouldn't come out right; some words were muddled up, and some just came out plain wrong—nothing like what I'd meant to say! This was so strange because I knew exactly what I intended to say, but I just couldn't talk properly. I finally had to give up and lie back down, hoping for a better day. Besides everything else, my skin rash flared up, the itching increased, and all my joints started hurting like hell! I still felt sad and hopeless, and now, as if all that wasn't enough, I started feeling agitated as I rarely ever had in my life. Thankfully, these symptoms lasted only two weeks, but since all this was pretty much the opposite of what an iron infusion should do, we stayed clear of trying another one and switched to oral supplements instead.

Regarding my skin reactions, Dr. John Van Limburg-Stirum (whom, for simplicity, I will refer to as Dr. John from now on) suggested I try some alkalizing bath salts. I didn't have a bathtub at home, so I had to arrange to use a friend's tub. This might sound easy, but it wasn't. If you are affected by MCAS, there's always the chance of having reactions to smells in other people's places. And if you bathe in water just a tad too hot, you might even end up passing out on their living room floor. All this has happened to me, but as I said, we learn step by step.

Next, Dr. John had me try a supplement he had developed to support mitochondrial health. It contained a little bit of lemon, so I broke out in a rash within minutes of trying it. Looking for other ways to improve my state, one day he asked me about the scars on my rib cage (from the surgery when my lungs collapsed). They were somewhat hardened, and since back in 2001, when the chest tube had been inserted, I had lost peripheral feeling in that area. The entire upper part of my right chest had been numb ever since. He then suggested trying neural therapy—a procedure in which a local anesthetic is injected into and under the scar tissue to help re-establish nerve pathways.

I was willing to give it a try, and it turned out to work wonders! First of all, the scar tissue softened remarkably, but most surprisingly, the sensation around my torso returned! After eighteen years of feeling absolutely nothing in that part of my body, I almost couldn't believe that such a simple treatment could produce such dramatic results.

INVISIBLE TRIGGERS

My mom came over for a visit one morning. I was still sleeping when the doorbell chimed, so I struggled out of bed to let her in and then went to the kitchen to make us some coffee. Standing beside me, she instantly noticed and said, "Your hands are shaking!"

I looked down at my hands and only then realized that they were shaking quite a bit. I paused and then replied, "Holy shit, you're right. They are shaking! I didn't even notice before because the dizziness gets me much more. Lately, I feel so light-headed in the mornings that sometimes I can't even lift myself out of bed. I often feel like I'm going to faint before I even manage to get up. Whenever I'm able to go out for a walk, this feeling dwindles, but it keeps coming back, and it's always at its worst when I wake up. Kinda strange, isn't it? After I sleep, I'm dizzier than before. Maybe I stop breathing when I sleep? I don't know."

She thought about it for a moment and then suggested we have coffee outside, which is what we did. As usual, I started to feel better after walking a bit, but the dizziness returned as soon as I was back home.

Suddenly I realized the gas heater might be causing my dizziness. Maybe it had a leak? I immediately called my landlord, who sent a technician to check the heater right away. No leaks were found, but he advised a hospital visit for carbon monoxide testing. Thankfully, the tests were normal, but the dizziness persisted. Eventually, I switched to an electric heater to see if it helped—and it turned out to do the trick. Burning gas likely used up too much oxygen in that small, enclosed space, but maybe it was merely the smell that triggered my reactions. Whatever it was, I felt remarkably better after I stopped using the gas heater: my dizziness subsided, and even my skin symptoms started to improve!

HIDDEN IN PLAIN SIGHT

In December of that year, I caught a horrible cold—a very rare occurrence for me. I have wondered if those overzealous, high-strung mast cells might be responsible for that, because even when everybody around me had the flu, I barely ever caught it. Maybe these mighty mast cells eradicate most invaders before they can cause any harm. If so, this mast cell madness has at least one potential upside.

Anyhow, this time I had a high fever and other common flu symptoms, so I decided to make some chicken soup. It turned out delicious, so I took a second helping. Yet, as soon as I had the first spoonful in my mouth, I spat it out, utterly disgusted. I tasted nothing but metal! Examining my spoon, I cautiously touched it to the tip of my tongue. It also tasted like metal—but of course it would, being made of stainless steel. I tried again with a plastic spoon, yet I still tasted nothing but metal. It was incredible! Even worse, soon thereafter, my entire mouth became saturated with the flavor of metal—my tongue, teeth, and throat! I finally just tossed the soup despite still being very hungry.

Waking up the following day, this disgusting taste lingered, as if my mouth was now entirely coated in steel. Everything I tried to eat or drink now tasted metallic. I checked my pans; they were all labeled as stainless steel. I had tested them for nickel with a test kit after the dermatologist advised me to avoid it wherever possible. The test showed that they weren't leaching nickel, but now I surmised they must be leaching something. When I looked it up online, I quickly discovered that cookware made of stainless steel is best avoided if you have a nickel allergy. Stainless steel is most often labeled 18/10, which means it's made of 18 percent chromium... and 10 percent nickel!

What an insight! At that moment, I could've kicked myself for not double-checking this before. I'd been blithely using these pans and potentially poisoning myself, bit by bit, each day. Despite diligently adhering to a diet free of milk, gluten, histamine, nickel, salicylate, and FODMAPs to stay as healthy as possible, the very utensils I'd been using to prepare these low-in-everything foods might have been exacerbating my symptoms all along! Having learned so much in the mast cell self-help groups, I instantly thought of joining a nickel forum. After gathering the few pieces of info I needed, I ditched all my stainless steel equipment for nickel-free options like glass, ceramic, or wood. This turned out to be a game-changer for me. It didn't take long for my skin reactions to diminish, and eventually my stomach started to feel better, too.

FRICTION POINTS

Only after my symptoms had already improved on several levels did I begin to notice other triggers. It soon became clear that the friction from the seams of my clothing was one of them. Trying to tackle this next step, I initially resorted to wearing my underwear inside out to prevent the seams from touching my skin directly. This did help somewhat, but it always felt a little strange knowing my undies were turned inside out, even if nobody would ever notice.

Looking for a less awkward solution, I soon found many seamless designs. Still, the fabrics are sometimes made of potentially irritating materials, or the waistbands contain plastics, which would certainly also aggravate my skin. Finally, I discovered a brand called Sloggi with a product line labeled "Zero Feel". The seams are glued, and the fabric is made of polyamide and elastane. Not knowing yet whether I would tolerate the fabric, I decided to buy just a couple to test them out. They were perfectly comfortable, so I replaced all my old ones. Before long, the skin around my hips started healing, and with that coup, my overall reactions went down yet another notch.

After that, I noticed just how much fabric in general contributed to these awful reactions. Sometimes, I'd feel flushed and utterly drained without an apparent cause. Yet, after showering and putting on fresh clothes, my energy returned. I soon realized I felt even better when wearing only pure cotton. So, I went through my closet and sorted out everything that felt less than comfortable, as well as anything even slightly tight. This turned out to be another game-changer for me. It made such a big difference that I honestly wondered how I hadn't noticed this sooner. Truthfully, I felt a bit embarrassed that it had taken me so long. But then again, after years of constant reactions throughout my body, it sometimes felt impossible to even hope to identify each trigger.

ALL-ONE

I spent Christmas that year alone. My family would gather at my mom's house, but I didn't want to go because I knew I would get sick even if I asked everyone to forgo perfumes. I would still get reactions to the smells of all the shampoos, body creams, deodorants, and laundry detergents. And I mean, how could I ask them not to use any of those? I knew that being in a room with even just two people would likely put me out for days or weeks to come, and there would be seventeen people present that night! I really didn't want to face another interminable stretch of time being confined to my bed again, and neither did I want to be that one sick person who always needs to be handled with kid gloves. Besides, I had barely enough money for groceries and couldn't possibly hope to afford gifts for everyone. It just didn't feel right to celebrate Christmas while bringing nothing except my sick self.

Spending Christmas alone for the first time in my life wasn't so bad after all. In fact, it turned out to be a wonderful night. I made myself a delicious candlelit dinner and listened to beautiful music. I had time and space to think about everyone I love, and I did this so thoroughly that at the end of the night, I was positively filled to the brim with love and gratitude. Even though I was alone and had been isolated from the world for quite some time by then—just thinking about all the beautiful experiences I'd had in my life and all the amazing friends and acquaintances I'd shared these beautiful moments with made me realize just how blessed I am, and just how much love I have in my life.

Giving myself this time was so deeply touching, completely lovely, and sensuous that I couldn't have dreamt of it. At some point, fat and sweet tears of gratitude and joy started streaming from my eyes until my whole shirt was soaking wet. I just sat there in my little apartment smiling, laughing, and crying all at the same time while feeling this oneness. I cherished myself, my life, and my path. Even though nobody else was physically there with me that night, it felt like I got to spend time with everyone I loved just by thinking of them. This may sound a bit odd, but up until now, this has been the most profound Christmas of my entire life.

CHAPTER 7

Greener Pastures

In January, Dr. John suggested trying sauna therapy. In his experience, it has sometimes helped to alleviate symptoms of chemical sensitivity (MCS), which he said matched some of what I was experiencing. He recommended a rigorous approach: three saunas weekly, staying in until my heart raced. Hearing his plan, I found it rather alarming and risky, given my history of heart palpitations and fear of exacerbating them, despite doctors dismissing these as common. In addition, both heat and sweating are known mast cell triggers, so—truth be told—I was afraid to submit to this experiment. Nevertheless, I decided to give it a try because I wanted to get better. I would just start cautiously, carrying my EpiPen and monitoring my response closely enough so I could quickly leave before it got too much.

The first time went pretty well, I'd say. I was able to stay in much longer than I'd anticipated, and the sweating didn't trigger a big reaction, probably because I took a shower immediately after leaving the sauna each time. The following few days, though, I was wiped out. On my second visit, I ended up passing out briefly at some point, but thankfully, I didn't become a public spectacle once again. It happened quite elegantly while I was safely lying on a deck chair and could easily have been mistaken for somebody just resting. I eventually recovered enough to return to the land of the living, but after that, I decided it really was too risky and didn't try again. Considering that heat, and therefore also saunas, can trigger a potentially deadly anaphylactic shock, I don't think that a hardcore approach to sauna therapy is a good idea if you have mast cell issues.

Trying was actually a stupidly brave idea, especially since I had nobody else with me who could have helped in case something went wrong. But suppose you've been sick for years, and most doctors told you there's not much they can do and that your condition will likely only get worse. In that case, you might be willing to try almost anything that could help, even potentially dangerous approaches.

In the end, whether it was a good idea or not didn't matter because I couldn't afford it. Going to the sauna even twice a month was already a stretch for my budget, let alone going twelve times. All that said, if someone had been with me in case I passed out and if I had taken a gentler approach by slowly adjusting to the heat, maybe it would have helped me get well faster. Sauna therapy has its benefits, but how we approach things also matters greatly.

Since sauna therapy clearly wasn't the answer for me, Dr. John suggested I try to fatten up a bit. He said that he didn't know of any fat people with MCS, so maybe it would help. I thought I was already eating plenty because I usually ate about twice as much as most other people I knew. However, my physiotherapist had also mentioned that I should eat more, and others kept nagging me about it, saying that they thought I was anorexic.

It was incredibly annoying, because I am definitely not anorexic. I am a real lover of food and rather something of an eating machine! The thing is, I am allergic to both gluten and milk, and the foods that I do tolerate just don't make you fat. So, I had to eat like a maniac to gain some weight. I managed to put on ten extra pounds over about five months by consuming around 4,000 calories per day. At first, this was actually quite entertaining, but after a while, I was literally fed up with eating that much every single day! In all fairness, being a bit *thicker-skinned* did help mitigate my reactions to some extent, but, unfortunately, my reactions to smells were still the same.

GETTING TO THE HEART

By the end of February, the ground beneath my feet shifted once again. My mom went to Italy over the weekend to visit a friend she hadn't seen in a few years. He was a doctor, so of course my illness came up in their conversation. When she showed him a picture of me, he suggested that I might have Marfan syndrome.

Coincidentally, I had just stumbled upon that term myself in my research. Learning that collapsed lungs, dislocating joints, elongated limbs and fingers, eye problems, a curved spine, a high-arched palate, crowded teeth, and even heart murmurs were all seen as defining features, I had to start considering the possibility that Marfan syndrome might explain just about all my inexplicable symptoms.

Reading on with increasing dismay, I learned that the most significant risk is a burst aorta, which can be fatal within as little as twenty minutes.

Additionally, if left undiagnosed, the average life expectancy is only around thirty-seven years—quite alarming, as I was then thirty-six and a half! So, when my mom returned and shared her friend's opinion, the alarm bells tripled. I didn't know how to proceed with that discovery yet, but figured I would ask my doctor about it during my next visit.

But then my back went out just a few days later. This time, I experienced a pain very similar to what was described in the Marfan syndrome literature, where it stated that you should have your aorta checked immediately because it may have just torn!

I had no clue which doctor to go to with this problem, so I called the Swiss Marfan Association and asked them for a recommendation. They sounded somewhat baffled by my call and appeared reluctant to give me any advice, but once I described the current pain and told them that my lungs had collapsed before, they became alarmed and promptly organized a meeting with a heart specialist knowledgeable about Marfan syndrome.

As soon as I arrived, these two doctors sprang into action and swiftly channeled me through their examination. They measured and scanned me top to bottom while texting back and forth with another specialist via instant messaging. After four hours of testing, they concluded that my heart was fine. Actually, it was more than just fine. They were genuinely baffled that my heart was, as they put it, about *27 percent stronger than average* for my age. They wanted to know whether I did elite sports and, if not, why was I so fit. This really made me laugh! I told them that I'd been mostly bedridden for the last two years and hadn't been doing anything except for yoga and physiotherapy until about a year ago.

It was such a relief to know my heart had been checked and was clearly in good shape. But, if not my heart, what else could it be? Both doctors found it outrageous that no one had ever considered Marfan syndrome, especially since I exhibited 9 of 20 points on the Marfan scale. They acknowledged that, given my heart's condition, it might be another connective tissue disorder, so they recommended a genetic test to identify the real cause. Additionally, I was scheduled for an MRI to ensure they hadn't overlooked anything.

The MRI confirmed that my heart was in excellent condition. This was so very good to know with absolute certainty. Now it became feasible to assume that the palpitations were probably linked to my triggers and possibly pure exhaustion. They still happened, and it was still very uncomfortable every time, but knowing that my heart was, in fact, as healthy as it could be, gave me such a sense of reassurance, that I could cope with these reactions more calmly from then on.

For the genetic evaluation, I was referred to a specialist who practiced at the Children's Hospital. I loved being sent to the Children's Hospital—at least it would be a refreshing change of scenery! This doctor repeated the same physical screening with identical results: something was clearly amiss with my connective tissue. She suggested it might be Ehlers-Danlos syndrome (EDS), and not Marfan. To confirm this, all the genes associated with connective tissue disorders needed to be checked. If none of these genes carried a mutation, it would be the hyper-mobility type of Ehlers-Danlos syndrome (hEDS), which she acknowledged can be linked to mast cell disease.

Since it would take a few months for the results to come back, I had time to read up on EDS. I soon learned that chronic fatigue is a common symptom. No wonder I was always so tired! Fatigue is indeed common with mast cell issues, EDS, and ITP. True, I didn't yet know whether I had EDS, but it seemed very likely at this point. This would also finally explain my endless joint pain, the dislocating joints, some of the digestive issues, and the chronic fatigue.

FATIGUE AND FOOD TRIALS

Meanwhile, my skin reactions had diminished appreciably, and I also had my GI symptoms largely under control. Now my reactions to smells, the inflammation of my joints, and my seemingly unconquerable fatigue had become the most taxing issues I faced. For the fatigue, Dr. John suggested doing another series of vitamin B12 shots. These shots did help reduce the fatigue to some degree, but they also hurt. Maybe they don't necessarily affect everyone this way, but they did hit me in a way that left my joints and spine feeling sore for a day or two after each injection. Once I was past that initial discomfort, I would indeed feel fresh and energized, but the fatigue would inevitably return to take me down again.

To give you an idea of just how tired I was, from February to June, I slept an average of fifteen hours per night. In the mornings, I could stay awake for only two to three hours until my energy crashed to the point where I couldn't possibly sit upright or even keep my eyes open. I needed to take a midday nap, often followed by another nap later in the afternoon, so I could be at least a little bit productive during the few waking hours I had left.

Sleeping so much might sound nice to some, but I can assure you it's not! You can take my word for it. Sleeping away three-quarters of your life yet never having the energy to do anything is not a nice feeling at all. Not being able to go out and do something you love because you don't have the energy for it really sucks! Having my energy crash after a ten-minute walk and then having to sit down for another ten minutes just to recover enough to make my way home always made me feel extremely old. When you're not even forty yet, that is a very unpleasant feeling!

Thankfully, I eventually found a vitamin B12 supplement that I tolerated. One of these chewables was even twice as effective as the shot, and I could buy two whole bottles for the price of just one shot. This was so much easier than going to the clinic for an injection: a wholly painless and cost-effective way to help keep my energy levels up.

At some point, Dr. John suggested I try reintroducing more foods into my diet. I agreed that if I tolerated the foods, it might indeed help boost my energy. Apart from that, I also liked the idea of having a wider range of foods to choose from, though I knew that if it backfired, the pain could be intense. Weighing up the pros and cons, I decided to give it a go. The first thing I tried was blueberries. It backfired badly. I only ate about a handful that evening, but was hit by severe cramps within the hour. My belly swelled up to the size of a basketball, and I got hit by cold sweats and agonizing pain in my limbs, stomach, and kidneys. This ordeal persisted until sometime the next afternoon, and now my entire GI tract was wrecked again!

This was so discouraging that I resigned from any more experimenting for a while. It took a few days to realize I'd made a big mistake when choosing the first food I would try. I had only looked at histamine content and completely missed considering nickel! Blueberries are pretty high in nickel, and I might have spared myself a great deal of misery had I been more thoughtful then. Regardless, as a result of this painful setback, I decided to continue sticking with the foods that I knew wouldn't hurt me for as long as it would take for my system to calm down sufficiently.

RESPITE, RECOVERY, REALITY

Early in 2019, my mom and stepdad went on vacation and asked me if I would be willing to house-sit for them. I welcomed this opportunity gladly because they live in a beautiful home with a balcony and a great view. Their house is full of plants, has a lovely kitchen, and a spacious bathroom with a tub. Above all, the air there is much cleaner than in the city. This respite resulted in a tangible improvement. I couldn't shake off the fatigue yet, but I started feeling much better otherwise!

It felt so refreshing to breathe clean air, sort of how I imagine it would feel to drink fresh spring water after being lost in a bleak and barren desert for days. It was incredibly soothing to be in a quiet place without the constant noise and bustling of the city. With less light pollution, I slept noticeably better, and it felt just heavenly to be so close to nature. All this made it crystal clear that I would unquestionably do much better living in the countryside.

One afternoon, I felt like going for a walk. Before I got so freaking sick, I would often go on walks. Sometimes, I would even walk all day. So, on one particularly sunny day, I decided to go up into the forest. I couldn't wait to roam under the shade of the trees and soak up the beauty, the stillness, and the scents of the forest. So excited to soon be amidst the lush greenery, I left the house and walked up the hill. The fresh, crisp air felt so invigorating, and the magnificent view over the lake to the mountains got my heart buzzing with joy, but the reality that I was still sick crashed in on me again after just ten minutes.

In a flash, exhaustion hit me like a lightning bolt, and I got knocked right on my ass. Instantly drenched in sweat, my heart pounding wildly, all I could see were those little floating cartoon stars swirling around above my head. I wasn't even anywhere near the forest yet, but I already had to wave the white flag! I was wrecked and had to pull myself together to make it back home, where I finally crashed out and couldn't even move for the next few days.

It was so upsetting to realize that my body had become so pathetically weak that, even without the triggers, I couldn't walk more than ten minutes! Incredibly annoyed by this, I became more determined than ever to find a way to overcome it all. I made up my mind that I was going to walk, and I was going to push myself as far as I possibly could. I wanted to be strong again! I wanted to have the freedom to walk as far as I pleased, and I needed to believe that I'd be doing these incredibly long walks again one day. What I really wanted to do was to run and exercise and go totally nuts with it, but I knew I had to take it one step at a time.

So, this is what I did. As soon as I could move again without excruciating pain, I made myself go on a walk every other day and gradually increased the distance that I could go—literally step by step. I remained very cautious not to overdo it, making sure I had enough strength to make it back home on my own, and to avoid ending up completely useless again the next day. By gently pushing myself to walk just a few steps more each time, I was able to increase my walking time from around ten minutes to half an hour within that one month. This might not sound like much, but in my situation, it felt like an absolute triumph, because I learned that I could get better!

MY FIRST VENTURE INTO SOCIETY

In June, my brother got married. I was, as they say, bound and determined not to miss this occasion. No way on earth would I allow myself to miss this special day! Having recently rediscovered my love for photography, I decided to bring my camera to see if I could capture the day's vibes. I had started to consider photography as a profession because a camera could serve as a kind of buffer between myself and the object I'm portraying. Maybe this little bit of distance would provide enough room for me to stay safe from certain triggers. At the wedding, the camera would also come in handy as a practical excuse to quickly escape a perfume cloud if I needed to.

I was incredibly nervous about attending this event. There would be lots of people, and some of them would surely be drenched in perfume like walking, reeking landmines. It was going to be incredibly busy and probably quite noisy as well, and I didn't want to ruin the day for anyone by fainting or having yet another stupid mast cell reaction. I was so anxious that I barely slept the night before. I had spent almost all my time alone for years. Every day and every night had been hushed, muted, and gentle to the senses. To go from this sheltered silence to a rather busy and perhaps loud and even hectic gathering such as this was quite a leap. The last time I'd mingled with people was over half a year before. After only four hours, I couldn't walk for the next four days. Thank goodness the wedding took place outside!

I held up pretty well, I'd say. Mainly focusing on taking pictures did indeed allow me to move around as needed, and whenever a smell got to be too much, I swiftly moved on without having to explain myself to anyone. However, my luck finally gave out a little later in the afternoon. At some point, exhaustion set in. When that happens, I have to get quiet as quickly as possible. If I don't, then any noises, lights, and smells will swiftly start to intensify, which can rapidly become overwhelming because, along with it, always come my tremors, palpitations, and dizziness. As soon as I noticed the scales beginning to tip, I looked for the quietest place I could find and sat down at an empty table to catch my breath.

Moments later, my stepmom approached and sat down beside me, heavily perfumed as usual. Not noticing the distress I was in, she started asking me a bunch of somewhat rhetorical questions, such as why people would want to ruin their beautiful bodies with tattoos. I tried to unravel her seemingly vexing conundrums, but she kept adding snide remarks about why someone would make themselves look so ugly and went on and on about how simply awful it was. I was able to pull myself together for a few minutes, but then my energy crashed to the point where my vision began to flicker, and I started to faint. With the last of my strength, I feebly mumbled back at her, "Sorry, gotta lie down, dizzy..." I got up, gestured to my mom what was happening, and luckily managed to retreat inside the house to collapse onto the couch—neatly out of sight from the wedding guests.

Since my family was already aware of the possibility of my fainting, it didn't scare anyone too much. My brother came in shortly to check on me and ask if there was anything he could do. By this point, I couldn't see anything but flickering dots in a gray haze, but I felt like I could probably keep conscious if I could lie there quietly and rest for a bit. I managed to murmur that I'd be fine. Resting up did the trick, and after about thirty minutes I was able to get back up.

Unfortunately, I had waited just a tad too long—the mast cells were already mad. Even though I had managed to keep conscious, I was now completely exhausted. Even so, I decided to stay. Some of the guests were clearly concerned now, but I told them this is just what happens sometimes, and did my best to reassure them I was fine. In all honesty, I wasn't even sure if I was fine myself. I didn't know how long the aftermath of this reaction would last, but I desperately wanted to avoid becoming the biggest topic of conversation of the day.

Fortunately, this one only took a day to heal. In the end, I am grateful I went, because I would have hated missing my brother's wedding. I am glad I took the pictures, because they came out great! I am pleased that I didn't cause a big fuss about my fainting, and I am proud that I stayed positive through it all.

MEETING MY DREAM DOCTOR

Toward summer, Dr. John informed me that he was about to hire a new doctor specializing in chronic fatigue syndrome. "Awesome! Yes! Of course, I wanna meet him!" I burst out in excitement. Meeting this guy was a stroke of luck. Dr. Protazy Rejmer had been affected by chronic fatigue since he was fourteen years old. He never found appropriate treatment despite having visited hundreds of different doctors. Consequently, he resolved to become an expert himself. He changed his initial plans to study physics and studied medicine instead. Probably because of that, he is truly dedicated to solving complicated cases like mine. So, I guess we were a perfect match, because he likes working on these unusually complex cases, and I desperately needed a doctor who was both willing and able to do precisely that.

During our first meeting, he wanted to hear my overall understanding of my situation before he would share his thoughts with me. I told him that I believed it would be crucial to diagnose mast cell activation syndrome because I wasn't sure whether it was mastocytosis or *just* MCAS. Also, retesting the biopsies from my stomach and duodenum was vital, because when they were initially taken, they weren't even screened for mast cells, and I was just told everything was fine. I speculated that my joint pain may be traced to loose connective tissues, a common symptom in EDS. Since mast cells are also located in these tissues, maybe their activation and the subsequent release of mediators within these tissues could explain why I was experiencing more joint pain than is usually observed in people with MCAS. Finally, I shared my presumption that the ITP must be related to the whole mast cell issue. Heparin is a known mast cell mediator and can, in certain cases, activate blood platelets. This could possibly explain my low blood platelet counts and their inexplicable fluctuations.

He wholeheartedly agreed with everything I said. He acknowledged that he wasn't specialized in mast cell diseases, but he had dedicated his entire weekend to studying my file and came to much the same conclusions. He even congratulated me on knowing so much and taking the time to learn about these issues. This was a dream come true! I finally had a doctor in front of me who was obviously very smart and willing to go the extra mile. On top of that, this guy certainly knew just how difficult it can be to be afflicted by health issues that profoundly affect your entire life, but are neither common nor at all simple to explain!

To ensure that nothing had been missed, Dr. Rejmer performed another physical examination before scheduling a twenty-four-hour urine test and sending in my old biopsies for additional mast cell screening. He also suggested testing DAO and HNMT, the main enzymes responsible for histamine breakdown. Regarding the fatigue, he suspected it might stem from sleep apnea, which, as he now told me, isn't uncommon in people with loose connective tissues. To find out, he gave me a device to take home and track my sleep cycle over the next few days.

A few days later, sleep apnea was already ruled out, making it clear that the reason for my fatigue would have to be found elsewhere. Once the biopsies were retested, they revealed an increased count of mast cells—three times the normal range. Finding a laboratory that could perform the twenty-four-hour urine test ultimately took a bit longer because, at that time, there weren't yet any labs in Switzerland equipped for it.

THE DISABILITY CONUNDRUM

In July, I finally heard back from the disability agency. They'd received my dossier more than two years before, and I was only now summoned for an interdisciplinary evaluation that would be performed by a rheumatologist, a psychiatrist, a general practitioner, and an allergist. The appointments were scheduled at a hospital in another town, about an hour's drive from Zurich. Maybe they do this to reduce the chances of patients and doctors knowing each other and therefore minimize the risk of bias or bribery.

This process was such an ordeal! The train ride was already a challenge, but then trying to find my way around an unfamiliar hospital while being put through a barrage of evaluations that all lasted between two and four hours was just grueling. At that point, I was already stable enough to pull myself together for a few hours, but, as you can probably imagine, I was done for after such a day. Luckily, they managed to schedule two meetings on the same day, so I only had to make the trip three times instead of four.

Most of the visits went pretty well, I'd say. The doctors seemed to be assiduously thorough and appeared to make an effort to understand my particular issues. My last stop was with the allergists. An assistant doctor interviewed me for nearly two hours, during which I had to relate the entire ongoing saga of my sickness for the fourth time in a row. Then she asked me to wait a minute while she called in the senior physician, a specialist in mastocytosis.

A few moments later, this doctor came in with a remarkably somber expression on his face. He quickly glanced at the rash on my skin, sighing heavily and giving me a terribly bleak look. Then, he said: "In my opinion, you don't have mastocytosis."

What? Just hearing that statement threw me for a loop. Still, I somehow managed to keep my composure and responded cautiously, "Well, I think it's mast cell activation syndrome, and maybe not mastocytosis."

To which he replied, "In my opinion, you neither have mastocytosis nor MCAS."

Now I was baffled. How could he know with such certainty after such a cursory examination? I wondered if he had even looked at the notes from the two-hour interview. Apparently, he had such confidence in himself that he could immediately conclude, with apodictic certainty, that I didn't have anything even related to mast cells. This struck me as beyond bizarre, so I asked him, "Well, how do you explain the increased amount of mast cells in my stomach and duodenum, my high tryptase levels, and all my reactions?"

He replied that he didn't know. There could be many reasons, but it wasn't anything related to mast cell disease. He then told me that a small group of doctors, whom he strongly agreed with, had concluded that there's only one way to diagnose MCAS. He said, "To diagnose mast cell activation disease, there is only one valid criterion: tryptase levels must be measured within two to four hours of an anaphylactic shock, and they must be at least twice as high as the baseline tryptase levels. There is no other valid marker."

Now I was stunned, because this was contrary to what I'd been told by other doctors and also what I'd read from other leading experts in the field. "Well…" I said, "if it's not mastocytosis, how come I've been diagnosed with it, over and over, by multiple physicians at various times? And what should I do with their opinions?"

What he said then was the strangest advice I've ever gotten from a medical professional. "If I were you," he said, "I would just not be sick so much. Accordingly, you won't have to visit doctors so often. Therefore, you'll have more time and energy to work—and that way, you'll be able to make some contributions to the world instead of just taking from everyone."

After hearing that, I immediately backed off, convinced that any further argument would be perfectly futile. I've encountered my share of startling opinions over the years, but this statement was truly beyond the pale. I figured the best I could do at that moment was to keep my composure and let it go. So, I exhaled fully, then took a long, slow breath and asked, "That's it?"

"Yes," he replied.

"Alright, bye!" I responded curtly, got up, and left.

It felt pointless to argue with someone who seemed to have made up his mind before he'd even met me. Making my way home with a somewhat heavy heart, I thought about it all. By then, I truly did feel much better than I had two years before. But that was most likely because I was living like a hermit. Only because of that was I able to dodge many of the triggers. I still felt dependent on at least a little bit of support so that I could take proper care of myself without deteriorating again as soon as I had to leave my safe haven.

Thankfully, my appointments with Dr. Rejmer were still ongoing. We were still waiting for the lab to get equipped for the twenty-four-hour urine test, and the results for EDS, DAO, and HNMT were underway. So, hopefully I would soon have conclusive scientific proof in my hands.

Having to constantly argue your limitations while being sick is such a drag, as if being sick was something you would want or would ever choose for yourself—it's freaking exhausting!

REAL ANSWERS

Fortunately, the process with Dr. Rejmer moved along fairly quickly. The tests soon came back with actual viable results. Huzzah! My DAO was indeed deficient, but HNMT levels tested fine. The urine test did reveal elevated levels of mast cell mediators, and my leukotriene levels were through the roof! Just a few weeks later, hEDS was also unanimously confirmed. Finally, I had my diagnosis!

Looking back, the first notion that I might be affected by mast cell disease came up in early 2017, but it took until October 2019 to complete the diagnosis. Finding these answers was a huge relief, both psychologically and practically, because now that we knew exactly what was happening, we could target treatment accordingly—and I finally didn't have to argue about my condition anymore!

Dr. Rejmer suggested I first try a DAO supplement to help break down the excess histamine. If I tolerated it, I could try reintroducing more foods into my diet. Luckily, I handled it well. This made it possible for me to reintroduce foods that I wouldn't have dreamt of ever being able to enjoy again. I can't put into words how much of a treat it was to finally savor these foods again after years of abstaining from them. Each new addition to my whitelist felt like a triumph, and before long, I was back in food heaven!

Of course, after my pitfall with the blueberries, I remained very cautious this time. I would try just a tiny amount, then wait at least two weeks before trying again to minimize the risk of triggering delayed reactions. If it seemed like I tolerated it, I would still only slowly and gradually increase the amount I ate. However, there were certain foods I continued to avoid, especially milk and gluten. They just felt too risky to try without another allergy test first. Even so, those small wins gave me the courage to keep trying new foods.

To target my leukotriene levels, Dr. Rejmer suggested a medication called Montelukast. Yet, given the extensive list of potentially intense side effects—suicidal thoughts among them—I was firmly opposed to trying it. Having recently learned that nettle leaf extract can help reduce leukotriene levels, we agreed I'd try that instead. Unfortunately, I didn't tolerate it. My skin-related symptoms immediately worsened after I started taking it, and because I'd also been experimenting with new foods, I couldn't be sure whether the supplement or something I ate caused the setback. My best bet then was to retreat to safer territory by cutting out everything new until the reactions subsided. Trying it again later confirmed that I didn't tolerate it well, so I stopped taking it. Even so, I kept getting better.

A HARD-WON VICTORY

The disability agency finally concluded that I was eligible for 30 percent support. Yet, since cash assistance is offered at 40 percent and above, their decision equated to no support at all. They demanded I perform a six-month work trial to reach a workload of 70 percent to ensure I'd hold up to it. The rather tricky part was that I had to work four days a week, but starting at only two hours per day and then slowly increasing the time to a full workday.

By sheer luck, I found a community farm nearby where I could embark on this task. The work was satisfying and fun, and because I was always outside, I was largely safe from my triggers. My coworkers were all super sweet and welcoming, and it felt really good to be part of a community again. Being needed and able to contribute in a meaningful way was truly gratifying. Yet, about halfway through, my health started to deteriorate again. I got so sick that the agency demanded that I stop at once, stating that it was too risky for me to keep working, because I was too sick.

Amazingly enough, they still held on to their decision not to support me financially. It took me over a year to recuperate from this setback, but I eventually did. The social service's legal department rechallenged the decision, this time adding the newest findings and confirmed diagnoses to my file. And finally, six years after I had filed my first request, my application was approved, granting me 100 percent disability.

Up until then, I had barely enough to cover food and rent, so the first thing I bought with that extra money was a really comfortable pillow—because now I could finally rest. And the second investment was a genetic test for hereditary alpha tryptasemia (HαT) that I couldn't possibly afford up until then. It came back positive. HαT is a genetic trait that causes elevated baseline tryptase levels and is increasingly recognized as a contributor to mast cell-related disorders like MCAS. Finally, I had an explanation for why I was predisposed to develop MCAS in the first place.

At long last, it all made sense.

STRONGER THAN BEFORE

A few years ago, I felt like I was dying. Compared to then, I feel strong now. It still takes a great deal of time and effort to maintain my equilibrium, but everything I've learned along the way helps tremendously in coping. The daily physiotherapy and muscle balance training have strengthened my back to the point where my vertebrae dislocate less frequently—and my joints hurt less because the muscles I've gained help stabilize them. This has undoubtedly helped reduce the magnitude of mast-cell reactions, because any kind of pain usually aggravates all the other symptoms.

The mast-cell reactions also happen less often than they used to because I now have the proper medications, including the mast cell stabilizing compounds—and I know my biggest triggers, so I am finally able to navigate around most of them. Because of that, my body and the mast cells have had time to calm down. These days, my reactions are significantly less intense than back when my entire system seemed to be stuck in a constant state of activation. Of course, by now I am used to these reactions and the associated pain, so maybe they just seem less intense because they don't scare me as much anymore. Who knows?

On the other hand, I now have the tools to get these symptoms under control. I know what I can do to get back on track comparatively quickly, and I've learned to live in a way that helps me stay relatively healthy in the first place. Last but not least, I have a team of brilliant doctors to turn to whenever I need their support.

Mentally, I am in a better place than ever before. Getting so very sick and my tumultuous marriage were definitely the biggest challenges I've faced in life, but now, looking back, I am so proud that I didn't ever give up. After going through all that, I feel unshakable, because I know I can count on myself. I did my best for myself and my health and stuck with it until I succeeded.

I am so thankful for each insight that helped bring me to a lighter place, because, in the end, it was all those tiny steps that added up to real change. I'm glad I did my research thoroughly and that I decided to stay positive no matter what. I'm grateful I've learned to listen to my body and gained the wisdom to always respect it. I've learned so much about health, nutrition, medicine, and psychology—and, along the way, I came closer to myself. So, despite all the torment this journey has put me through, I'm glad to be where I am.

SECTION II

Understanding MCAS

CHAPTER 8

Function and Purpose of Mast Cells

Mast cells are found throughout the body in tissues with blood vessels, especially where the body comes in contact with the outside world, such as the skin, respiratory system, and gastrointestinal tract. They are present in epithelial and mucosal tissues and also in connective tissues beneath the epithelium around structures such as blood vessels, smooth muscle, and hair follicles.[2] Epithelial tissues cover body surfaces like skin and organ linings—mucosal tissues are moist linings inside cavities, such as the respiratory and digestive tracts.

Mast cells originate from pluripotent progenitors in the bone marrow, acting as "starter" cells that develop into various cell types. They mature into mast cells at their tissue site. While mature mast cells are generally absent from the bloodstream, progenitors may circulate there to reach their destination. Once they arrive, these progenitors mature into mast cells under the influence of cytokines and stem cell factors. Their phenotype is mainly shaped by their tissue microenvironment.[2,9]

STRUCTURE & FUNCTIONS

Types of mast cells

According to current knowledge, we generally distinguish two major types of mast cells (MCs) based on the contents of the main enzymes, tryptase and chymase, and their location throughout the body.

- MC(T) produce tryptase and are associated with mucosal and epithelial tissues.
- MC(TC) produce tryptase, chymase, and carboxypeptidase and are associated with connective tissues.[2,3,10]

MC(TC) cells are located in the tissue layer beneath the mucosa and connective tissues near the conjunctiva and skin, frequently near blood and lymphatic vessels. Mucosa refers to the inner lining of hollow organs and cavities that communicate with the external environment, such as the mouth, lungs, and intestines. The conjunctiva is the thin, transparent tissue that covers the sclera and lines the inside of the eyelids. Connective tissue mast cells are essential for tissue repair.[10] Mast cell activation and degranulation result in varying impacts depending on their location.[2]

Mast cell structure

Mast cells are granule-containing immune cells[11] with a central nucleus, which is surrounded by a vast number of small granules that can be secreted into the surrounding tissues upon activation. These granules, often so densely packed around the nucleus to obscure it completely, contain potent inflammatory mediators such as histamine, heparin, and tryptase.[9,10]

Mast cell functions

Mast cells play a vital role in both innate and adaptive immunity; they eliminate parasites and bacteria, promote tissue repair, and form new blood vessels.[2,3]

They are also involved in several pathological functions, including allergic and inflammatory conditions such as Crohn's disease and asthma, autoimmune disorders like multiple sclerosis and rheumatoid arthritis, certain cancers—and mast cell activation diseases, in which dysregulated mast cells may have detrimental effects on the host.[3]

Mast cells are primarily known for their key role in inflammation, yet they also regulate numerous functions of other cell types. Due to their multi-potent mediators, mast cells can influence the functions of many tissues and organs. They maintain vascular and bronchial homeostasis, regulate bone growth and turnover, and help maintain bone mineral balance.[2]

ACTIVATION & MEDIATORS

Mast cell activation

Mast cell membranes express several surface receptors, enabling cells to interact with pathogens, antigens, and other stimuli. Stimulation of these receptors can activate the mast cells and prompt degranulation, releasing preformed, neoformed, and neosynthesized mediators.

Mediators

Mast cell mediators exert diverse effects depending on the tissue microenvironment and the specific triggers. They can induce vascular permeability (increased leakage in blood vessels), smooth muscle contraction (tightening of muscles), vasodilation (widening of blood vessels), bronchoconstriction (narrowing of airways), and enhanced peristalsis (increased movement in the gut). Some mediators recruit new mast cell progenitors to the sites of inflammation, while others modulate interactions between inflammatory cells. Mast cell mediators encompass cytokines, chemokines, growth factors, amines, neuropeptides, proteases, proteoglycans, and lipid derivatives. Mast cells bind to different surfaces, cells, and tissues via adhesive receptors and co-receptors, which are also expressed on their membranes.[3]

Degranulation

Degranulation, the most studied method by which mast cells release their mediators, occurs in distinct stages with the prompt release of preformed mediators upon activation. Neoformed mediators, such as leukotrienes and prostaglandins, are quickly generated and released in response to activation. Neosynthesized mediators, including cytokines and chemokines, are produced after transcriptional activation and are released hours later.[3,12] After degranulation, mast cells remain functional and regenerate their mediators. Their lifespan ranges from months to years.[3,13]

Triggers

Mast cell activation may be triggered through immunological pathways, such as antigens binding to IgE receptors, and non-immunological triggers, such as toxins, certain medications, fragrances, and physical stimuli like vibration, breezes, or temperature changes.[3,12,14] In immediate-type allergic reactions, for example, upon antigen detection, Fc receptors bind to the IgE antibodies attached to the antigen. Degranulation occurs if two Fc receptors cross-link, meaning they come into proximity and bind to the same antigen.[2,3]

CLINICAL IMPACT

Symptoms

Mast cell degranulation can lead to various symptoms, including swelling, itching, and redness of tissues, bronchoconstriction, increased mucus production, and enhanced peristalsis. In severe cases, it can result in potentially fatal anaphylaxis.[12] Continual mast cell degranulation resulting from repeated reactions to typically harmless substances can contribute to the development of allergies and asthma.[2] A more detailed explanation of these symptoms can be found in Chapter 12, "Symptoms of MCAS."

> **KEY TAKEAWAY**
>
> Mast cells are found throughout the body, especially where it interacts with the outside world. Originating in the bone marrow, they mature upon reaching their ultimate tissue location, where the local microenvironment shapes their mediator profile and function. Mast cells are involved in many healthy physiological functions, but when dysregulated, they can drive inflammatory diseases.
>
> They consist of a central nucleus surrounded by granules that store mediators like histamine. Surface receptors allow them to respond to stimuli; when triggered, they may degranulate and release mediators in a phasic fashion to alert other cells and prompt physical reactions to address perceived threats. Symptoms may include skin reactions, gastrointestinal issues, neurological effects, cardiovascular symptoms, and severe responses like anaphylaxis. Triggers include allergens, infections, medications, VOCs, scents, temperature shifts, and physical stimuli.

CHAPTER 9

Types of Mast Cell Diseases and Diagnoses

Mast cell activation disease (MCAD) refers to a group of conditions caused primarily by the inappropriate activation of dysfunctional mast cells and, to a lesser extent, by an abnormal increase in the number of these cells in the body.

Sometimes, these conditions do not occur in isolation. A notable number of people diagnosed with MCAS also present with what is commonly referred to as the *trifecta*: MCAS, Ehlers-Danlos syndrome (EDS), and postural orthostatic tachycardia syndrome (POTS). In addition, hereditary alpha tryptasemia (HαT)—a genetic trait associated with elevated baseline tryptase levels—may further complicate the diagnostic picture.

MCAD is categorized into two main subtypes: mastocytosis and mast cell activation syndrome (MCAS). Each condition has distinct characteristics and further subtypes, with mastocytosis considered rare and MCAS encountered much more frequently in clinical practice.

- Mastocytosis involves an excessive accumulation of mast cells in certain tissues, meaning that there are too many mast cells.
- MCAS is characterized by the inappropriate release of chemicals by mast cells, meaning that mast cells are overly active.

MCAS vs MCAD: Understanding the difference

It's important to understand that MCAS is not the same as MCAD. To simplify, MCAD is an umbrella term encompassing all mast cell diseases, just like *dairy* refers to all milk-based products. Just as yogurt is not the same as cheese, nor is it simply milk, MCAS is not the same as mastocytosis, nor is it correctly labeled as MCAD. While MCAS falls under the MCAD umbrella, it's important to refer to it accurately. Mislabeling it as MCAD would be like calling all dairy products *milk*—not quite accurate, is it?

TYPES OF MAST CELL DISEASES

Conditions marked with an asterisk (*) are associated with clonality.

Mast cell activation syndrome: 3 primary subtypes

- Primary MCAS* a.k.a. monoclonal MCAS (MMAS) or clonal MCAS (CMCAS)
- Secondary MCAS
- Idiopathic MCAS
- Additionally, a combined subtype is characterized by a primary disorder with allergy-triggered mast cell activation.

Mastocytosis: 4 subtypes

- Cutaneous mastocytosis* has three subtypes: diffuse cutaneous mastocytosis (DCM), maculopapular cutaneous mastocytosis (MPCM), also called urticaria pigmentosa (UP), and solitary cutaneous mastocytoma.
- Systemic mastocytosis* (SM) has two subtypes: indolent and smoldering systemic mastocytosis (SSM).
- Advanced systemic mastocytosis* has three subtypes: aggressive systemic mastocytosis (ASM), mastocytosis with associated hematologic neoplasia (SM-AHN), and mast cell leukemia.
- Mast cell sarcoma* has no subtypes. (Sources: [15-20])

Clonality

In some mast cell diseases, a genetic mutation leads to the development of clonal disease, meaning there is abnormal growth and proliferation of mast cells. One such mutation occurs in the KIT gene, which encodes a protein that controls how mast cells grow and function. This mutation changes one amino acid in the protein: Aspartic acid (D) is replaced with valine (V) at position 816 in exon 17 of the gene's blueprint.

Under normal conditions, the KIT protein acts like an "on switch," turning on only when it binds to a molecule called stem cell factor (SCF). However, the mutation makes the protein remain "on" all the time, even without SCF, leading to uncontrolled mast cell activity and growth. In some cases, clonality can also be determined by abnormal expression of CD25 or CD2 on neoplastic (abnormally grown) mast cells.[15]

MAST CELL ACTIVATION SYNDROME (MCAS)

In all forms of MCAS, mast cells may be highly reactive throughout the body, leading to symptoms in multiple organ systems, with anaphylaxis as the most significant risk.[1,15]

Primary mast cell activation syndrome (clonal/monoclonal)

- mast cells may or may not show signs associated with excessive proliferation
- considered by some to possibly be a very early form of SM or a pre-SM, though this is controversial[15,18,21]

Secondary mast cell activation syndrome (non-clonal)

- mast cells are present in normal numbers, with no signs of excessive proliferation[7,15,21]

Idiopathic mast cell activation syndrome

- mast cells may or may not show signs of excessive proliferation[1,7,15,16,21]

Diagnosis of MCAS

As of 2025, experts remain divided on the most accurate method for diagnosing MCAS. Two primary diagnostic proposals, Consensus-1 and Consensus-2, have emerged, along with three additional minor variations of Consensus-1. However, no scientific studies have yet compared the accuracy or effectiveness of these approaches, leaving it unclear which one is superior.[1,5,21]

While the two proposals share considerable overlap—requiring (a) clinical signs and symptoms of MCAD, (b) evidence of abnormal levels of mast cell mediators, and (c) a response to mast-cell-targeted treatment—they also differ significantly, as outlined below.

Consensus-1

Also known as the "Vienna consensus," this approach was initially published in 2010, updated in 2012, and refined in 2019. It adopts a strict, biomarker-based approach that requires a measurable increase in tryptase (typically defined as a 20% + 2 ng/mL rise from baseline) within 2–4 hours following symptom exacerbation. While Consensus-1 reduces the risk of false positives, its stringent criteria raise concerns about underdiagnosis.[7,18,21]

Consensus-2

First proposed in 2011 and revised in 2017, Consensus-2 adopts a more inclusive, symptom-based, and patient-centered approach. This method allows diagnosis based on clinical presentation, elevated biomarkers, and response to mast-cell-targeted treatment, even without a measurable increase in tryptase during an episode. While Consensus-2 is more accessible, it raises concerns about overdiagnosis and a higher risk of false positives.

For a more detailed comparison, I recommend readers refer to the following articles:

- "Diagnosis of Mast Cell Activation Syndrome: A Global 'Consensus-2'" (accessible via *PubMed*).[1]
- "Selecting the Right Criteria and Proper Classification to Diagnose Mast Cell Activation Syndromes: A Critical Review" (available at *Elsevier*).[21]

"Consensus-1" diagnostic criteria proposal

All three MCAS criteria (1+2+3) must be fulfilled to call a condition MCAS.

1. Typical clinical signs of severe, recurrent (episodic) systemic mast cell activation are present, often as anaphylaxis. (Systemic means involvement of at least two organ systems.)

2. Biochemical studies document the involvement of mast cells (MC). The preferred marker is an increased serum tryptase level from the individual's baseline to 20% + 2 ng/mL. Other MC-derived markers of MC activation, such as histamine and histamine metabolites, PGD_2 metabolites, and LTC4 metabolites, have also been proposed but are less specific than tryptase.

3. Response of symptoms to therapy with MC-stabilizing agents, drugs directed against MC mediator production, or drugs blocking mediator release or effects of MC-derived mediators (e.g., histamine receptor blockers or cromolyn).[7,18,21]

"Consensus-2" diagnostic criteria proposal

Proposed criteria to define MCAS after exclusion of all other diagnoses that could better explain the chronicity and full range of symptoms. The diagnosis is made upon fulfilling the major criterion and at least one minor criterion.

Major criterion:

1. Constellation of clinical complaints attributable to pathologically increased MC activity (MC mediator release syndrome).

Minor criteria:

1. Multifocal or disseminated infiltrates of MCs in marrow and/or extracutaneous organ(s) (e.g., gastrointestinal or genitourinary tract; >19 MCs/high-power field).
2. Abnormal spindle-shaped morphology in >25% of MCs in marrow or other extracutaneous organ(s).
3. Abnormal MC expression of CD2 and/or CD25 (i.e., co-expression of CD117/CD25 or CD117/CD2).
4. MC genetic changes (e.g., activating KIT codon 419, 509, or 560 mutations) shown to increase MC activity.
5. Evidence (typically from body fluids such as whole blood, serum, plasma, or urine) of above-normal levels of MC mediators, including:
    - tryptase
    - histamine or its metabolites (e.g., N-methylhistamine)
    - heparin
    - chromogranin A (note potential confounders of cardiac or renal failure, neuroendocrine tumors, or recent proton pump inhibitor use)
    - other relatively MC-specific mediators (e.g., eicosanoids including prostaglandin (PG)D2, its metabolite 11βPGF2α, or leukotriene E4)
6. Symptomatic response to inhibitors of MC activation, MC mediator production, or action.[1]

CUTANEOUS MASTOCYTOSIS

All forms of cutaneous mastocytosis involve excess mast cells in the skin. Mast cells may be highly reactive throughout the body, with anaphylaxis being the biggest risk.

Maculopapular cutaneous mastocytosis (MPCM), or urticaria pigmentosa (UP)

This form includes a subtype called telangiectasia macularis eruptiva perstans (TMEP).

- the most common presentation of mastocytosis
- red and brown spots
- spider veins associated with mast cells (TMEP), almost exclusively in adults[16]

Diffuse cutaneous mastocytosis (DCM)

- redness, blistering, and thickening of the skin
- almost exclusively in children
- can lead to skin damage

Solitary mastocytoma of the skin

- benign mast cell tumor on the skin
- redness and swelling when touched/scratched (Darier's sign)
- multiple mastocytomas may be present on the skin and in other parts of the body, including the GI tract[16]

Diagnosis is made based on the presence of typical skin lesions, a positive skin biopsy demonstrating characteristic clusters of mast cells, and a positive Darier's sign (although a negative Darier's sign does not exclude the possibility of CM).[19]

SYSTEMIC MASTOCYTOSIS (SM)

Systemic mastocytosis involves excess mast cells in organs other than the skin. SM is initiated in the bone marrow and may cause symptoms across multiple organ systems.[20] Mast cells may be highly reactive, and while anaphylaxis is a risk in all forms of SM, some subtypes are malignant and lead to organ damage.

Indolent systemic mastocytosis

- the most common form of systemic mastocytosis
- benign with a normal lifespan

Smoldering systemic mastocytosis

- signs of progression toward malignancy
- shortened lifespan
- major risks include progression to malignant forms of (ASM or MCL) and organ damage

Aggressive systemic mastocytosis (ASM)

- malignant
- rapid progression of organ damage
- shortened lifespan

Mast cell leukemia (MCL)

- malignant
- rapid progression of organ damage
- significantly shortened lifespan

Systemic mastocytosis with associated hematologic neoplasm (SM-AHN)

- can be benign or malignant
- lifespan depends on the subtype and other hematologic disorders
- risks include progression to malignant forms like ASM or MCL and organ damage[15,17,20]

Diagnosis is made primarily through a bone marrow biopsy. The World Health Organization (WHO) has established specific diagnostic criteria for SM, which are summarized below (adapted from Pardanani, 2023).

Major criterion:

- Multifocal dense infiltrates of mast cells (>15 MCs in aggregate) in bone marrow biopsies and/or in other extracutaneous organs.

Minor criteria:

- More than 25% of all mast cells are atypical cells (type I or type II) on bone marrow smears or are spindle-shaped in mast cell infiltrates detected in sections of bone marrow or other extracutaneous organs.
- Activating KIT point mutations at codon 816 (D816V) in other critical regions of KIT in bone marrow or other extracutaneous organs.
- Mast cells in bone marrow, blood, or another extracutaneous organ express one or more CD2 and/or CD25 and/or CD30.
- Baseline serum tryptase concentration >20 ng/ml (in the case of an unrelated myeloid neoplasm, an elevated tryptase does not count as an SM criterion. In the case of a known HαT (hereditary alpha tryptasemia), the tryptase level should be adjusted.

If at least one major criterion and one minor criterion, OR at least three minor criteria, are fulfilled, the diagnosis of systemic mastocytosis can be established.[20]

MAST CELL SARCOMA

- a highly malignant mast cell tumor
- symptoms in multiple organ systems
- rapidly developing mast cell leukemia (MCL)
- malignant
- significantly shortened lifespan
- mast cells may be highly reactive throughout the body
- major risks: progression to MCL, rapidly progressing organ damage, anaphylaxis[15,22]

Diagnosis is made through bone marrow biopsy, genetic testing, and immunophenotyping.[22]

HEREDITARY ALPHA TRYPTASEMIA (HαT)

HαT is estimated to affect 5–6% of the population. Although only about a third of individuals with HαT experience symptoms, those who do may present with highly variable manifestations, often including neuropsychiatric issues, gastrointestinal problems, musculoskeletal pain, and mast cell-mediated symptoms like itching, flushing, or anaphylaxis.[23]

Diagnosis is made via a blood or swab sample. Treatment generally follows the same routines used in MCAS, including antihistamines, mast cell stabilizers, and other mediator-blocking therapies.[23,24]

KEY TAKEAWAY

Mast Cell Activation Disease (MCAD) encompasses two main subtypes: mastocytosis and mast cell activation syndrome (MCAS), each with further subtypes. Inappropriate mast cell activation is the primary cause of MCAD, and to a lesser extent, an abnormal increase in mast cell numbers. Mastocytosis involves too many mast cells in certain tissues, whereas in MCAS, numbers may be normal, but they are overactive. In some cases, mast cell dysfunction is driven by clonality—genetic mutations (often in the KIT gene) that lead to abnormal mast cell proliferation.

Two main diagnostic proposals for MCAS exist: Consensus-1 and Consensus-2. Both require: 1) clinical signs and symptoms consistent with mast cell disease, 2) evidence of abnormal levels of mast cell mediators, and 3) a response to mast-cell-targeted treatment, but the criteria also differ. Consensus-1 requires a measurable rise in tryptase during a flare, making it more specific but less inclusive. Consensus-2 is based on symptoms, elevated biomarkers, and treatment response, making it more accessible but raising concerns about overdiagnosis.

MCAS sometimes presents alongside Ehlers-Danlos syndrome (EDS) and postural orthostatic tachycardia syndrome (POTS)—often referred to as the trifecta.

Hereditary alpha tryptasemia (HαT), a genetic trait marked by elevated baseline tryptase, is also closely related to MCAS. Though distinct, it often presents similarly and responds to the same treatments, such as antihistamines and mast cell stabilizers.

CHAPTER 10

Conditions That Can Mimic Mast Cell Disorders

(or May Sometimes Be Rooted in MCAD)

Mast cell activation disorders (MCAD) can be challenging to diagnose because their already complex symptom profile often overlaps with other conditions. A careful differential diagnosis is key to pinpointing the source of your symptoms and finding the best treatment.

MCAD is primarily characterized by abnormal mast cell activation and, in some cases, abnormal proliferation. However, mast cell activation (MCA) is not exclusive to MCAD and can occur in other conditions, further complicating the diagnosis. For both patients and clinicians, understanding the wide range of conditions that can mimic or be associated with MCAD is key to accurately diagnosing it and finding the most appropriate treatment.

The following section outlines examples of conditions that can mimic or sometimes stem from mast cell disorders, as described in a 2015 paper published in *The New England Journal of Medicine*[25] and a 2021 review by Gülen et al.[21]

Cardiovascular

- Arrhythmias
- Aortic stenosis with syncope
- Coronary hypersensitivity (Kounis syndrome)
- Endocarditis / endomyocarditis
- Myocardial infarction
- Pulmonary embolism
- Postural orthostatic tachycardia syndrome (POTS)

Cutaneous

- Atopic dermatitis
- Chronic urticaria
- Contact dermatitis
- Drug exanthema
- Hereditary or acquired angioedema
- Idiopathic flushing
- Rosacea
- Scleroderma

Endocrine

- Adrenal insufficiency
- Carcinoid syndrome
- Estrogen or testosterone deficiency
- Fibromyalgia
- Hypopituitarism
- Medullary thyroid carcinoma
- Parathyroid tumor
- Pheochromocytoma
- Thyroid disease

Gastrointestinal

- Adverse reactions to food
- Eosinophilic esophagitis
- Eosinophilic gastroenteritis
- Food intoxication
- Gastrointestinal motility disorders
- Gastroesophageal reflux disease
- Inflammatory bowel disease
- Irritable bowel syndrome
- Vasoactive intestinal peptide–secreting tumor

Immunologic

- Allergic episodes involving basophils but not mast cells
- Autoinflammatory disorders such as deficiency of IL-1 receptor antagonist
- Familial hyper-IgE syndrome

- Systemic capillary leak syndrome
- Vasculitis

Infectious

- Acute encephalitis/meningitis
- Acute gastrointestinal infections
- *Helicobacter pylori*–like organism–positive gastritis with urticaria; severe bacterial or viral infections (± septic shock)

Neuropsychiatric

- Anxiety
- Autonomic dysfunction / dysautonomia
- Chronic fatigue syndrome
- Depression
- Headaches
- Mixed organic brain syndrome
- Multiple sclerosis
- Panic attacks
- Seizures
- Somatization disorder
- Stroke
- Vasovagal syncope

> **KEY TAKEAWAY**
>
> Mast cell disorders have a wide range of symptoms that often overlap with other conditions, making diagnosis challenging. Since mast cell activation can also occur in other illnesses, testing for related conditions—a differential diagnosis—is important not only to identify MCAD but also to find effective treatments for the individual's symptoms.

CHAPTER 11

Comorbid Diseases in MCAS

MCAS patients may also have additional medical conditions independent of the primary disease. In medical terminology, this is referred to as "comorbidity," meaning an accompanying but unrelated pathological or disease process often used to describe the coexistence of multiple diseases.

While related conditions or those mimicking mast cell disorders require a differential diagnosis to confirm an MCAS diagnosis, comorbid diseases coexist with MCAS and require complementary treatment. Although not caused by or directly related to mast cell activation, these conditions can still significantly impact patients' lives. An overview of such conditions is provided below.[24]

Cardiovascular conditions

- Cardiovascular symptoms
- Dysautonomia
- Postural orthostatic tachycardia syndrome (POTS)

Dermatological

- Alopecia
- Eczema (atopic dermatitis)
- Urticaria (hives)
- Angioedema

Endocrine and metabolic conditions

- Diabetes (Types 1 and 2)
- Obesity

Gastrointestinal and genitourinary conditions

- Eosinophilic colitis
- Eosinophilic esophagitis
- Endometriosis, PMDD, and PCOS
- Food protein–induced enterocolitis syndrome (FPIES)
- Gastroparesis
- Interstitial cystitis
- Irritable bowel syndrome (IBS)

Musculoskeletal conditions and chronic pain

- Arthritis
- Ehlers–Danlos syndrome (EDS)
- Fibromyalgia
- Multiple sclerosis

Neurological and mental health conditions

- Alzheimer disease
- Anxiety/depression
- Attention deficit hyperactivity disorder (ADHD)
- Autism spectrum disorder
- Myalgic encephalomyelitis/chronic fatigue syndrome (ME/CFS)
- Post-traumatic stress disorder (PTSD)

Respiratory conditions

- Asthma
- Pulmonary fibrosis[24]

A 2017 paper in *The American Journal of the Medical Sciences* provides ranked data on the most common comorbidities in MCAS patients, which may help identify potential additional conditions. They are summarized here[6]:

Gastroesophageal reflux disease	35%
Hypertension	29%
Multiple/atypical drug reactions	23%
Abdominal pain, NOS	22%
Hysterectomy/oophorectomy	21%
Hyperlipidemia	20%
Cholecystectomy	20%

Environmental allergies	19%
Tobacco abuse	18%
Asthma	18%
Diabetes mellitus type 2	17%
Hypothyroidism	17%
Headaches	17%
Depression	16%
Sinusitis	16%
Fibromyalgia	16%
Anemia of chronic fatigue	15%
Sleep apnea	15%
Freq. upper respiratory infections	15%
Miscarriage	15%
Pharyngitis and/or tonsillitis	14%
Dysmenorrhea	14%
Thromboembolism	13%
Freq. and/or atypical infections	13%
Obesity	13%
Osteoarthritis	13%
Anxiety and/or panic	13%
Vertebral disease	12%
Cardiovascular malformations	12%
Dermatitides	11%
Presyncope and/or syncope	11%
Interstitial cystitis	11%
Chronic kidney disease	10%
POTS	10%

KEY TAKEAWAY

Comorbidity refers to a separate condition that exists alongside another disease. Comorbid conditions are not caused by mast cell activation, but may still significantly impact a patient's life and require additional treatment.

CHAPTER 12

Symptoms of Mast Cell Activation Syndrome

MCAS symptoms are highly variable: they range from mild to severe, manifest episodically or chronically, and can come on suddenly due to the rapid response of mast cells. Symptoms often migrate between organs and tissues, affecting nearly every system in the body, including the mouth, throat, respiratory system, digestive tract, skeletal system, immune system, cardiovascular system, blood system, skin, eyes, and central nervous system.[4]

The most common symptoms in MCAS include flushing, urticaria, hypotension, headache, angioedema, vomiting, and diarrhea.[26] To put it into perspective, a reaction that begins in the gastrointestinal tract may lead to respiratory issues, flushing, hives, a racing heart, palpitations, and, in the worst-case scenario, fainting due to anaphylaxis.

A study by Afrin et al. (2016)[6] identified the most common symptoms in MCAS patients, as shown below:

83%	fatigue
75%	fibromyalgia-type pain
71%	presyncope/syncope
63%	pruritus/urticaria, headache
50%–58%	paresthesias, chills, dyspnea, migratory edema, nausea ± vomiting, gastroesophageal reflux
40%–49%	abdominal pain, cognitive dysfunction, environmental allergies, fever, non-anginal chest pain, palpitation / dysrhythmias, rashes, throat irritation, sweats

30%–39%	alternating diarrhea/constipation, easy bleeding/bruising, flushing ± diaphoresis, insomnia, oral irritation/sores, proximal dysphagia, visual anomalies
23%–28%	adenopathy/adenitis, frequent or odd infections, diarrhea, poor healing, urinary symptoms
13%–17%	anxiety/panic, multiple/odd drug reactions, dental deterioration, weight gain/loss, alopecia, cough, dysmenorrhea, constipation, sinusitis, tremors, depression, onychodystrophy (abnormal nail growth), heat/cold intolerance, asthma

KEY TAKEAWAY

MCAS symptoms are highly variable. They may come on suddenly due to the rapid response of mast cells, range from mild to severe, manifest episodically or chronically, and often migrate between organs and tissues, affecting nearly every system in the body. Common symptoms include flushing, urticaria, hypotension, headache, angioedema, vomiting, and diarrhea.

CHAPTER 13

Mediator-Released Symptoms

Mast cells carry a vast array of mediators that can be released into surrounding tissues upon activation. These mediators act as messengers with diverse functions, enabling mast cells to influence immune responses and regulate physiological processes through interactions with other cells. They can, for example, increase blood vessel permeability, cause bronchoconstriction, and enhance peristalsis. They also play critical roles in inflammation, pain perception, tissue repair, and nerve signal regulation. The wide range of adverse reactions resulting from excessive mediator release is described in more detail in the preceding chapter, *Symptoms of Mast Cell Activation Syndrome.*

Human mast cells can produce at least 390 different mediators,[27] each triggering multiple responses from effector cells. These specialized immune cells (basophils, macrophages, B cells, T cells, and dendritic cells) carry out actions like attacking pathogens or coordinating immune reactions in response to mast cell signals. The large number of mast cell mediators and their varied effects help explain the complexity of symptoms in MCAS. Importantly, mast cells can selectively release mediators without completely degranulating. If this were not the case, every activation could result in an anaphylactic shock.

Mediators can be released through different mechanisms, such as complete degranulation, gradual release over time (piecemeal degranulation), or targeted mechanisms like synaptic interactions with neighboring cells and extracellular traps that immobilize pathogens. Mast cells survive degranulation and can repopulate their mediators.

Mediator composition in mast cells varies based on the tissue microenvironment in which they reside. It may also differ between specific organs and tissues due to various external and internal factors, including physical triggers. Moreover, following degranulation, mediator composition in mast cells may change, likely shaped by the stimulus that triggered degranulation.[27]

Below is a list of some of the more extensively studied mediators and their potentially associated symptoms, offering a clearer picture of the extensive range of effects they can cause.

MEDIATORS & SYMPTOMS

Chymase

cardiac arrhythmias, hypotension, myocardial infarction, syncope or near-syncope, tachycardia, and light-headedness

Cysteinyl leukotrienes (CysLT)

bronchoconstriction, mucus secretion, vascular instability, nasal pruritus, nasal congestion, shortness of breath, wheezing, and throat swelling

Cytokines and chemokines

inflammation, constitutional symptoms (fatigue), and osteoporosis

Corticotropin-releasing hormone (CRH)

syncope or near syncope, hypotension, tachycardia, light-headedness, pruritus, flushing, angioedema, urticaria, diarrhea, abdominal cramps, nausea and vomiting, esophageal reflux, depression, anxiety, insomnia, decreased concentration and memory, migraines, fatigue, weight loss, and generalized malaise

Histamine

migraines, hypotension, headaches, urticaria, pruritus, diarrhea, angioedema, anaphylaxis, syncope or near syncope, tachycardia, light-headedness, esophageal reflux, abdominal cramps, flushing, urticaria, pruritus, nasal pruritus, nasal congestion, throat swelling, shortness of breath, wheezing, fatigue, weight loss, insomnia, depression, anxiety, decreased concentration and memory, nausea and vomiting, and generalized malaise

Interleukin-6 (IL-6)

syncope or near syncope, hypotension, tachycardia, light-headedness, pruritus, flushing, angioedema, urticaria, diarrhea, abdominal cramps, nausea and vomiting, esophageal reflux, bone pain, aches, osteoporosis, osteopenia, depression, anxiety, migraines, insomnia, decreased concentration and memory, wheezing, shortness of breath, nasal pruritus, nasal congestion, throat swelling, weight loss, fatigue, and generalized malaise

Interleukin-8 (IL-8)

angioedema, pruritus, urticaria, and flushing

Interleukin-33

angioedema, pruritus, urticaria, and flushing

Neurotensin

nausea and vomiting, diarrhea, esophageal reflux, abdominal cramps, depression, anxiety, insomnia, decreased concentration and memory, and migraines

Proteoglycans

bleeding diathesis (increased susceptibility to bruising or bleeding)

Platelet activation factor (PAF)

abdominal cramping, urticaria, pulmonary edema, bronchoconstriction, arrhythmias, anaphylaxis, hypotension, headache, light-headedness, syncope or near syncope, tachycardia, pruritus, flushing, angioedema, nausea and vomiting, esophageal reflux, diarrhea, anxiety, depression, insomnia, decreased concentration and memory, migraines, nasal pruritus, nasal congestion, throat swelling, shortness of breath, and wheezing

Prostaglandin D2 (PGD2)

pruritus, flushing, angioedema, urticaria, diarrhea, abdominal cramps, nausea and vomiting, esophageal reflux, bone pain, aches, osteoporosis, osteopenia, depression, anxiety, insomnia, decreased concentration and memory, migraines, nasal pruritus, nasal congestion, throat swelling, shortness of breath, wheezing, weight loss, fatigue, and generalized malaise

Renin

cardiac arrhythmias, tachycardia, myocardial infarction, hypotension, light-headedness, and syncope or near syncope

Receptor activator of nuclear factor-κB ligand (RANKL)

bone pain, aches, osteoporosis, and osteopenia

Serotonin

nausea and vomiting, diarrhea, abdominal cramps, and esophageal reflux

Tryptase

inflammation, bleeding diathesis, light-headedness, syncope or near syncope, tachycardia, hypotension, pruritus, flushing, angioedema, urticaria, diarrhea, abdominal cramps, nausea and vomiting, esophageal reflux, bone pain, aches, osteoporosis, and osteopenia

Tumor necrosis factor (TNF)

light-headedness, syncope or near syncope, tachycardia, hypotension, pruritus, flushing, angioedema, urticaria, diarrhea, abdominal cramps, nausea and vomiting, esophageal reflux, bone pain, aches, osteoporosis, osteopenia, depression, anxiety, insomnia, decreased concentration and memory, migraines, weight loss, fatigue, and generalized malaise

Vasoactive intestinal peptide (VIP)

diarrhea, abdominal cramps, nausea and vomiting, and esophageal reflux[24,28]

> **KEY TAKEAWAY**
>
> Mediators are chemical messengers that enable mast cells to influence immune responses and regulate physiological processes by interacting with other cells. They play important roles in inflammation, pain perception, tissue repair, and nerve signaling. In MCAS, the excessive release of mediators can lead to a wide range of adverse reactions.
>
> Mast cells can carry hundreds of mediators, each capable of triggering multiple immune responses. They can also selectively release mediators without fully degranulating and repopulate them after degranulation. Mediator composition may change following degranulation, likely influenced by the stimulus that triggered the response. Common mediator-induced symptoms include itching, hives, digestive issues, swelling, low blood pressure, rapid heartbeat, reflux, fainting, and light-headedness.

CHAPTER 14

Triggers

Triggers refer to substances and factors that activate mast cells and lead to the onset of symptoms. To feel better, you'll need to identify your specific triggers as accurately as possible—and then avoid them as best you can. However, that's easier said than done, because triggers are incredibly diverse, they're often invisible, and they are everywhere!

They can include foods, medications, fragrances, physical factors such as cold or heat, and even emotional stressors like excitement or anxiety. Triggers also vary widely from person to person: I've met people with systemic mastocytosis who can eat just about anything and feel perfectly fine, while others with MCAS tolerate only three foods. Some can use scented products, while others may faint from just a trace of someone else's detergent.

To make matters worse, your triggers can even change over time! Something that has affected you in the past might suddenly not bother you anymore, while things you've always tolerated can unexpectedly cause reactions. The following list includes commonly reported triggers from MCAS self-help groups to help you identify your own.

Biological

- Animal hair
- Bee and wasp stings
- Dust
- Dust mites
- Insect bites
- Mold
- Pollen

Dietary

- Alcohol
- Certain foods
- Fructose in food
- Histamines in food
- Iodine
- Oxalates in food
- Salicylates in food
- Smells of certain foods
- Smells of overripe foods

Pharmacological

- Contrast agents
- Excipients
- Medications (some)

Physiological

- Dehydration
- Hormonal changes
- Menstruation

Psychological/Emotional

- Excitement
- Mental stress
- Strong emotions

Physical

- Barometric pressure changes
- Breezes
- Cold
- Exercise
- EMFs
- Fluorescent lights
- Friction
- Heat
- Noise
- Physical stress
- Smell of metal
- Sun
- Sweat
- Temperature changes
- Tight clothing
- Touching metal
- Vibration
- Weather changes
- Wind

Environmental / VOCs

- Aftershave
- Air fresheners
- Anything scented
- Bleach
- Body lotion
- Car exhaust
- Carpets
- Chemical fumes
- Chemical smells
- Cleaning products
- Conditioner
- Deodorant
- Disinfectant
- Dryer sheets
- Dyes
- Essential oils
- Fabric softener
- Fabrics
- Formaldehyde
- Gasoline
- Glue
- Hair dye
- Hairspray
- Hand sanitizer
- Incense
- Laundry detergent
- Linoleum floors
- Makeup
- Menstrual products (fragrances, plastics)
- Nail polish
- Nail polish remover
- Off-gassing of new furniture
- Off-gassing of plastics
- Paint
- Perfumes
- Pesticides
- Petroleum products
- Printer ink
- Scented candles
- Shampoo
- Smoke
- Soaps
- Toothpaste
- Wood finish

KEY TAKEAWAY

Triggers are substances and factors that activate mast cells, so they need to be avoided wherever possible. Triggers are tricky: they vary from person to person and may even change for an individual over time. They can include foods, fragrances, medications, excipients, or insect bites, as well as physical factors like temperature changes, barometric pressure shifts, or exercise, and even emotional stressors like excitement or fear.

CHAPTER 15

Medical Treatment Options

When it comes to medications, always consult your doctor to find the best treatment for you! Mast cell activation disease (MCAD) is generally considered incurable due to its genetic origin, but there are many medications that can help alleviate mast cell-related symptoms.

This chapter is primarily based on Molderings et al.'s article "Pharmacological treatment options for mast cell activation disease" (2016). While the text has been adapted for clarity and flow, the medical recommendations closely follow the original publication.

Molderings et al. (2016) stated, "Effective therapy often consists simply of antihistamines and MC stabilizing compounds supplemented with medications targeted at specific symptoms and complications."[29] However, treatment must be highly personalized. Every patient's genetic and epigenetic makeup is unique, affecting how cells send and receive signals and how we perceive and respond to sensations. As a result, these factors influence how mast cells develop and release mediators and how the disease manifests in each person.

Large-scale studies have yet to be conducted in MCAS and mastocytosis, so most available data on successful treatments comes from small clinical trials and individual case reports. Because inappropriate mast cell activation lies at the core of MCAD, first-line management focuses on identifying triggers as accurately as possible and avoiding them, along with taking medications that stabilize the mast cells and reduce their activity. If these measures don't provide sufficient relief, second- to fifth-line therapies can be considered.

TRYING NEW MEDICATIONS

Test with a small single dose

Testing medications in a single low dose is essential to lower the risk of adverse reactions. If tolerated, dosage should still be increased only gradually and with caution. In most cases, one to two months is enough time to determine whether a treatment is tolerated and effective. If a medication causes adverse effects or shows no benefit, it should be stopped immediately. However, it's best to discuss medication changes with your doctor, as some drugs should not be stopped abruptly.

Changing or adding several medications around the same time is not recommended, as this can make it challenging to know which one is responsible for any given effect. A therapy should only be continued if it demonstrably provides benefits. Otherwise, it's best to stop it to reduce the risk of taking too many unnecessary medications and of unfavorable drug interactions.

IMPROVING TREATMENT RESPONSE

Starting a new drug

Avoiding cow's milk protein, gluten, and yeast for three to four weeks when starting new medications may help improve treatment response. Therapies that strongly stimulate the immune system should be approached with caution, as they may significantly worsen MCAD symptoms, potentially even in the long term.

Adverse reactions

In MCAD patients, even drugs that are typically well-tolerated may trigger adverse reactions. Some individuals react to a broad range of medications, sometimes resulting in highly unusual and unexpected symptoms shortly after starting new medications. These patients may actually tolerate the active pharmaceutical ingredients, but react to the fillers, preservatives, dyes, and binders in these medicines—sometimes so strongly that only pure drug salts dissolved in water are tolerated. Trying alternative formulations with as few excipients as possible can be a solution for successful treatment.[30]

MEDICATIONS COMMONLY USED IN MCAD

The following medications are listed as described in the article by Molderings et al. (2016). While they reflect clinical experience, not all healthcare professionals may agree with their use or classification, and some carry black box warnings in certain countries.

Emergency & first-line treatments

- **Epinephrine** treats anaphylaxis.
- **H1 antihistamines** treat itching, flushing, abdominal discomfort, and allergic reactions.
- **H2 antihistamines** treat gastric reflux, abdominal pain, and nausea.
- **Cromoglicic acid (cromolyn)** stabilizes mast cell activity.
- **Preservative-free eyedrops with H1 antihistamine, cromolyn, ketotifen, or glucocorticoid** can be used short-term for conjunctivitis (secondary disease must be excluded).
- **Vitamin C** increases degradation of histamine and decreases histamine formation by inhibiting histidine decarboxylase.

Anti-inflammatory & immunomodulatory therapies

- **Corticosteroids** treat hives and wheezing, but are recommended only as a last resort.
- **Omalizumab** blocks binding of IgE to receptors and has been reported to reduce reactivity and sensitivity to activation, which can reduce anaphylactic episodes.
- **Budesonide and prednisone** treat colitis (should be used only for a few days).
- **COX-2 inhibitors**, such as etoricoxib or celecoxib, and paracetamol treat rheumatoid symptoms.
- **Aspirin** blocks the production of prostaglandin D2 and may reduce flushing.

GI & diarrhea management

- **Cholestyramine, nystatin, montelukast, ondansetron, and acetylsalicylic acid** treat diarrhea. (with extreme caution because of possible mast cell degranulation)
- **Proton-pump inhibitors** treat gastric complaints.
- **Metamizole and butylscopolamine** treat colicky abdominal pain due to distinct meteorism.
- **Additional H2 histamine receptor antagonists and proton-pump inhibitors** can be used for proven gastroesophageal reflux and non-cardiac chest pain.

Nausea management

- **Dimenhydrinate, lorazepam, 5-HT3 receptor inhibitors, and NK1 antagonists** treat nausea.

Dermatologic & topical therapies

- **Palmitoylethanolamide-containing** care products and **cromolyn-containing ointment** treat itching.

Anti-leukotrienes

- **Montelukast and zafirlukast** block the effects of leukotriene C4 (LTC4).
- **Zileuton** blocks LTC4 production, both of which are used to reduce wheezing and abdominal cramping.
- **Leukotriene receptor blockers** such as montelukast or zileuton treat respiratory problems.

Neurological & sleep support

- **Alpha-lipoic acid** treats neuropathic pain and paresthesia.
- **Triazolam** treats insomnia (sleep-onset and sleep maintenance).

Cardiovascular support

- **AT1-receptor antagonists** and **ivabradine** treat tachycardia.
- **Tranexamic acid** and **icatibant** treat angioedema.

Skeletal support

- **Bisphosphonates** treat osteoporosis, osteolysis, and bone pain.

Hematologic support

- **Iron supplementation** (oral or parenteral) treats anemia, but must be given cautiously due to the risk of potentially intense mast cell activation. Alternatively, red blood cell transfusion may be considered.

Other targeted treatments

- **Pentosan** and **amphetamines** treat interstitial cystitis.
- **HMG-CoA reductase inhibitor atorvastatin** may be trialed to treat hypercholesterolemia.

Targeted cancer/mutation-driven therapies

- **Imatinib** is a tyrosine kinase inhibitor used to treat cancer; it has shown efficacy against c-Kit-driven malignancies. One case report (Molderings et al., 2014) described success using imatinib alongside continuous diphenhydramine infusions to improve recurrent anaphylaxis in an MCAS patient who wasn't responsive to previous therapies.[29,31]

KEY TAKEAWAY

MCAS treatment typically starts with antihistamines and mast cell stabilizers, supplemented with drugs for specific symptoms—alongside avoiding triggers. However, because each patient's genetic and epigenetic makeup is unique, treatment must be highly personalized.

To reduce the risk of adverse drug reactions, always start with a small single dose, increase dosages gradually and with caution, and avoid changing multiple medications at once. If a drug causes adverse effects or provides no benefits, stop it immediately. To improve treatment response, consider avoiding cow's milk protein, gluten, and yeast for three to four weeks when starting a new medication.

CHAPTER 16

Histamine

Histamine is a biogenic amine, a small molecule that occurs naturally in various living organisms. Besides the human body, it's found in bacteria, plants, and food.[32,33] Histamine is synthesized by enzymatic decarboxylation of histidine, an amino acid present in various tissues of the human body and animals, as well as in plants and foods. Several lymphoid and myeloid cells can synthesize histamine, but only mast cells and basophils can store it in so-called vesicles, which are tiny organelles inside the cell.[32] Within these vesicles, histamine is inactive, but it can be readily released if necessary.[34]

HISTAMINE FUNCTIONS

Histamine is involved in many physiological and pathophysiological processes, such as the formation of new blood cells and the proliferation, differentiation, and regeneration of cells.[35] Histamine functions as a messenger substance and tissue hormone and plays a pivotal role in inflammatory responses, gastric acid secretion, neurotransmission, and immunomodulation.[33,36]

HISTAMINE RECEPTORS

Histamine exerts various effects by binding to histamine receptors, which are expressed on the surface of different cells.[32,35] There are four known histamine receptors, H1–H4, named according to the chronological order in which they were discovered. Each of these receptors triggers distinct signaling cascades:

- **H1 receptors** are present in numerous cell types throughout the body, and their activation leads to allergic responses, such as hypotension, tachycardia, bronchoconstriction, vasodilation, flushing, vascular permeability, increased pruritus, pain, and anaphylaxis. H1 receptors are furthermore involved in thermoregulation, locomotion, regulation of the circadian rhythm, memory, learning, and the regulation of appetite and emotions.[33]

- **H2 receptors** are expressed mainly in gastric parietal cells, the heart, and smooth muscle cells.[33] H2 receptor activation regulates gastric acid secretion, cardiac contraction, cell proliferation, and cell differentiation.[35]
- **H3 receptors** have been found in the central nervous system and in presynaptic and peripheral receptors, where they regulate the release of neurotransmitters and histamine.[35] It has been suggested that H3 receptors regulate leptin release, insulin resistance, and energy homeostasis.[35] H3 receptor expression has been linked to increased proinflammatory activity, bronchoconstriction, antigen-presentation capacity, and pruritus.[35]
- **H4 receptors** have been defined as immune system receptors due to their importance in inflammatory conditions and autoimmune diseases.[33] They are expressed in peripheral hematopoietic cells and the bone marrow, spleen, intestine, thymus, and immune cells.[35] Activation of H4 receptors triggers chemotaxis in basophils and mast cells, resulting in an amassment of inflammatory cells and reduced cytokine secretion.[35,37]

HISTAMINE DEGRADATION

Histamine is broken down via two main enzymatic pathways:

1. **Oxidative deamination** is catalyzed by an enzyme called **diamine oxidase (DAO)**, which acts as the first barrier that histamine encounters. DAO is mainly synthesized by intestinal cells that continuously release it from the intestinal mucosa into the gut lumen, where it combines with the food bolus and begins breaking down the histamine present.

2. **Cyclical methylation** through the action of an enzyme called **N-methyltransferase (HNMT)** is the second mechanism by which histamine is degraded. HNMT is found mainly in the liver and kidneys and, to a lesser extent, in the spleen, colon, ovary, prostate, cells of the spinal cord, and the respiratory system. HNMT breaks down histamine that gets absorbed through the intestinal mucosa and reaches the bloodstream.[34,38]

HISTAMINE INTOLERANCE

Allergens, immune reactions, tissue injury, and chemical, physical, and psychological stimuli can prompt the mast cells to release excessive amounts of histamine, leading to elevated histamine levels in the blood and consequent adverse reactions. Histamine intolerance often results from impaired histamine metabolism, that is, reduced levels or reduced activity of the enzymes that catabolize histamine.

> ### KEY TAKEAWAY
>
> Histamine is found in various organisms, including the human body and plants. It helps form and regenerate blood cells, acts as a messenger substance and tissue hormone, and is involved in inflammation, gastric acid secretion, neurotransmission, and immune responses.
>
> In the body, histamine binds to four different types of receptors (H1–H4), each triggering distinct effects. Breakdown occurs through two main enzymes: DAO in the intestines and HNMT in the liver. Mast cells can store and release large amounts of histamine. Impaired breakdown leads to histamine intolerance and adverse reactions.

CHAPTER 17

Antihistamines

Antihistamines—also known as histamine-receptor antagonists or receptor blockers—are used to treat allergy symptoms. Simply put, these drugs attach themselves to the histamine receptors in our body, thereby preventing the histamine from binding to its receptors, which then prevents the chemical reactions that lead to allergic symptoms. Antihistamines help prevent histamine actions, but they cannot reverse them.[39]

TYPES OF ANTIHISTAMINES

H1 and H2 receptor blockers

There are two main subtypes of antihistamines: H1 receptor blockers and H2 receptor blockers. There aren't any antihistamines that act on both receptors at the same time. H1 receptor blockers treat allergy symptoms like rhinitis, hay fever, and urticaria.[40,41] H2 receptor blockers treat conditions associated with gastric acid, such as GORD and peptic ulcers.[41]

H3 and H4 receptor antihistamines

The discovery of H3 receptors in the 1980s led to the understanding that "Histamine H3 receptors act as presynaptic autoreceptors that inhibit the synthesis and release of histamine in the histaminergic neurons in the central nervous system, and they also occur as hetero-receptors on nonhistaminergic neurons, modulating the release of other neurotransmitters."[41]

H3 antagonists, a promising area of research, could be therapeutically helpful in the treatment of obesity and various disorders of the central nervous system, such as Alzheimer disease, schizophrenia, sleep disturbances, learning deficits, and epilepsy.[41] The first approved H3 antagonist is pitolisant, which is used in the treatment of narcolepsy.[42]

H4 receptors are the most recently discovered histamine receptors. They are mainly found in immune cells in the bone marrow and peripheral tissues.[43] Potential pharmaceutical applications for H4 antagonists include treating various inflammatory disorders, such as asthma, allergies, autoimmune diseases, and pruritus.[43] As of 2024, there aren't any H4 blockers on the market, but clinical testing, trials, and research to develop such drugs are currently underway.[41,44]

HISTORY & DEVELOPMENT

Antihistamines were first developed in the 1930s, when regulatory authorities did not yet require randomized controlled trials or clinical pharmacology studies on the safety and efficacy of drugs.[40]

First-generation antihistamines

The earliest antihistamines, known as first-generation H1 blockers, were found to cross the blood-brain barrier. They are associated with a broad range of side effects—even at recommended doses—including fatigue, sedation, drowsiness, and headache, along with impaired cognition, psychomotor performance, and memory. According to the National Center for Biotechnology Information, first-generation antihistamines should be avoided because of their sedative properties and interference with REM sleep.[40]

Second-generation antihistamines

Second-generation antihistamines were introduced in the 1980s[41], and most of these drugs have been studied extensively. They cross the blood-brain barrier to a lesser extent, are unlikely to cause drowsiness, and do not increase the effects that co-administered CNS-active drugs or alcohol have on the central nervous system[40]. Since the withdrawal of terfenadine and astemizole from the market in the late 1990s, they are said to be devoid of cardiac side effects. However, interactions with other drugs or consumption of certain fruit juices can increase cytoplasmic levels and lead to cardiotoxic effects.[45]

Third-generation antihistamines

Third-generation antihistamines emerged in the 1990s with the aim of eliminating cardiotoxic effects.[46]

ANTIHISTAMINES ON THE MARKET

Currently available antihistamines include, but are not limited to, the following[40,47]:

First-generation H1 antihistamines

dimetindene, diphenhydramine, meclizine, doxylamine, promethazine, clemastine, dimenhydrinate, brompheniramine, hydroxyzine, chlorpheniramine, carbinoxamine

Second-generation H1 antihistamines

loratadine/desloratadine, cetirizine/levocetirizine, azelastine, ketotifen, mizolastine, ebastine, bilastine, bepotastine, quifenadine, nizatidine (astemizole and terfenadine have been removed from the market)

Third-generation H1 antihistamines

fexofenadine, levocetirizine, desloratadine

H2 antihistamines

ranitidine, cimetidine, famotidine

For topical use

azelastine, levocabastine, olopatadine, diphenhydramine

Eyedrops

azelastine, emedastine, ketotifen, olopatadine, pheniramine

Nasal sprays

azelastine, olopatadine

KEY TAKEAWAY

Antihistamines help prevent histamine actions but cannot reverse them. First developed in the 1930s, the earliest antihistamines (first-generation) were found to cross the blood-brain barrier and are associated with a broad range of side effects. Second- and third-generation antihistamines are considered safer.

H1 blockers treat allergy symptoms, H2 blockers target conditions related to gastric acid, H3 blockers may help with obesity and central nervous system disorders, and although H4 blockers are still in clinical trials, they may prove useful in treating inflammatory and autoimmune conditions. Antihistamines are available in the form of pills, ointments, eye drops, and nasal sprays.

CHAPTER 18

Mast Cell Stabilizers

Mast cell stabilizers are drugs that help prevent degranulation in mast cells. By stabilizing the cell's membranes, they inhibit the chemical reactions required for mediator release. They are therefore effective as a prophylactic measure prior to trigger exposure, but they cannot reverse reactions.

Mast cell stabilizing agents include both naturally occurring substances such as flavonoids, coumarins, phenols, terpenoids, and simple amino acids, and semi-synthetic and synthetic versions inspired by them.[48]

First-generation mast cell stabilizers like cromolyn sodium effectively prevent mast cell degranulation, while second-generation mast cell stabilizers like ketotifen also exhibit antihistaminic properties. Natural agents may offer additional benefits, such as the anti-allergic activity of flavonoids, which may ultimately enhance their efficacy in stabilizing mast cells.

Depending on where mast cells are located, they may react differently to different mast cell stabilizing agents. For example, both ketotifen and disodium cromoglycate (DSCG) are effective at blocking mediator release in mast cells located in the lungs and tonsillar tissues, but not in mast cells located in the skin.[48]

Billie Shellist, a Colorado-based nutrition practitioner and holistic health coach, had herself been affected by chronic Lyme disease, mold/biotoxin illness, and MCAS. She now specializes in treating people with MCAS, and emphasizes the importance of opting for pure formulations with as few extra ingredients as possible and trying each new agent separately.[49] Her advice aligns with the article "Pharmacological treatment options for mast cell activation disease" (2016) because often mast cell patients may actually tolerate the active ingredients of medications but experience adverse reactions to fillers, binders, preservatives, and dyes.[29]

SOURCES OF MAST CELL STABILIZERS

Flavonoids:	luteolin, diosmetin, apigenin, quercetin, fisetin, kaempferol, ginkgetin, EGCG, and silymarin
Coumarins:	scopoletin, scoparone, artekeiskeanol A, selinidin, 5-Methoxy-8-(2-hydroxy-3-butoxy-3-methylbutyloxy) psoralen, cinnamic acid, and ellagic acid
Phenols:	magnolol, honokiol, resveratrol, polydatin, curcumin, mangostin-alpha, beta, and gamma
Terpenoids:	parthenolide, sesquiterpene lactones (SQLTs), monoterpenes, sinomenine, indoline, and xestospongin C
Amino acids:	theanine[48]

PHARMACEUTICAL MAST CELL STABILIZERS

Examples

Cromolyn sodium (also known as sodium cromoglicate, disodium cromoglycate, or DSCG)

Often referred to as the gold standard mast cell stabilizer, cromolyn sodium effectively inhibits the release of histamine, PGD2, and leukotrienes.[50] However, according to a 2012 paper published in *PLoS One*, it is less effective in inhibiting pro-inflammatory cytokines.[51] Cromolyn sodium is indicated for treating mastocytosis and MCAS [50,52], allergic rhinitis, and the prophylaxis of mild to moderate cases of bronchial asthma. It can mitigate symptoms of headaches, flushing, vomiting, diarrhea, nausea, urticaria, itching, and abdominal pain.[50]

Ketotifen

Structurally related to H1 antihistamines, ketotifen functions as both a mast cell stabilizer and an H1 receptor antagonist, in addition to inhibiting the release of basophil mediators. It effectively inhibits the release of histamine, leukotrienes, tryptase, and prostaglandins from mast cells. Furthermore, it has been shown to reduce TNF-α, IL-8, and chemokines produced by macrophages, a type of white blood cell involved in the immune response. Ketotifen is used to treat bronchial asthma and allergic conditions such as chronic urticaria, allergic rhinitis, and atopic dermatitis.[53,54]

NATURAL MAST CELL STABILIZERS

Examples

Because herbal and natural agents can have side effects, interact with medications, or be contraindicated in some conditions, always discuss them with a knowledgeable healthcare professional before trying them.

Quercetin

A flavonoid in various foods (garlic, onions, ginger, apples, berries, grapes, citrus fruits, peppers, broccoli, herbs, wine, and tea), quercetin possesses powerful mast cell stabilizing properties, alongside antioxidant, anti-inflammatory, antibacterial, antiviral, and anticarcinogenic benefits. Quercetin effectively inhibits the release of histamine, PGD2, leukotrienes, IL-8, and TNF. It also helps prevent excessive calcium levels within cells and inhibits NF-kB activation, a process that causes inflammation in the body.[51]

Luteolin

A flavonoid found in various foods, such as olive fruit extract, tea, celery, and peppers, luteolin functions as an antioxidant, possesses mast cell–stabilizing properties, and exhibits anti-inflammatory activity. It effectively inhibits the release of IL-6, IL-8, and TNF, and because it crosses the blood-brain barrier, it offers neuroprotective effects as well. Luteolin inhibits the activation of T-cells and immune cells in people affected by multiple sclerosis. In animal studies, it has been shown to slow cognitive decline and improve spatial memory.[55–58]

Baikal skullcap *(Scutellaria baicalensis)*

A plant that offers anti-inflammatory, antioxidant, antibacterial, antiviral, and antitumor benefits, baikal skullcap is indicated in treating allergic diseases, respiratory tract infections, pneumonia, hepatitis, and colitis. The primary active substances, mainly flavonoids, inhibit pro-inflammatory cytokine production (IL-1β, IL-6, IL-8, and TNF-α), leukotrienes, prostaglandins, nitric oxide, and reactive oxygen species.[59,60] According to Billie Shellist, this herb can help reduce neurological inflammation, a claim supported in a 2018 paper published in *Pharmaceutical Biology*.[49,60]

Butterbur *(Petasites hybridus)*

Butterbur functions in a comparable manner to H1 antihistamines with less sedating effects. It contains petasines, compounds known to inhibit the synthesis of leukotrienes, which are involved in various inflammatory and allergic conditions. Butterbur is used to treat bronchial asthma, headaches, and smooth muscle spasms, and may be helpful in the treatment of seasonal allergies.[61–63] According to Shellist, it can also help mitigate anxiety and brain fog.[49]

Indian frankincense / olibanum *(Boswellia serrata)*

Long used in traditional medicine for arthritis, inflammatory conditions, and various other ailments, modern medicine now acknowledges its efficacy in treating arthritis, pain, and inflammation. It also offers mast cell–stabilizing, liver-protective, and blood lipid-regulating effects.[64,65]

Laboratory and animal studies have shown that Boswellic acids inhibit 5-lipoxygenase (a pro-inflammatory enzyme) and leukotriene B4—both of which contribute to increased vascular permeability, chemotaxis, and bronchoconstriction. Additionally, by inhibiting COX-2, *Boswellia serrata* may offer protection against Alzheimer disease and tumors.[64,65] In my personal experience, *Boswellia serrata* is extremely helpful in treating IBS symptoms.

Cannabis

Cannabis has been used since ancient times, with records dating back to 2700 BC. In therapeutic settings, it has been used as an analgesic and antiepileptic, and for its potential to relieve pain and anxiety. Modern research has additionally demonstrated anticancer, anti-inflammatory, and neuroprotective effects.

Of the three primary strains of cannabis, mainly *Cannabis sativa* has been employed for therapeutic purposes. Of over five hundred compounds in this plant, more than one hundred cannabinoids and over two hundred terpenoids have been identified—both of which help alleviate pain and inflammation.

Cannabinoid receptors are distributed throughout the body; they have the potential to reduce synaptic transmission and modulate nerve-related inflammation. Cannabinoids can decrease neuroinflammation by inhibiting nerve signaling and the subsequent release of inflammatory neuropeptides. Additionally, cannabinoids can suppress communication between mast cells, immunocytes, and nerves, resulting in diminished degranulation and release of inflammatory mediators.[66]

Evening primrose oil (*Oenothera biennis*)

Evening primrose oil contains a range of flavonoids and notable levels of linoleic acid and γ-linolenic acid. It may help treat chronic inflammation,[67] and offers antiproliferative, antimicrobial, and antiangiogenic benefits. In inconclusive studies, it has also shown potential in cancer therapy due to its ability to target A375 melanoma cells.[68,69] Shellist notes that it may also improve sleep, reduce anxiety, and alleviate pain.[49]

Feverfew (*Tanacetum parthenium*)

Feverfew has long been used in traditional medicine to treat fevers, migraines, rheumatoid arthritis, insect bites, stomach aches, infertility, and gynecological problems. It has also been used for allergies, psoriasis, asthma, nausea, vomiting, dizziness, and tinnitus. Feverfew offers a range of pharmacological benefits, including anti-inflammatory, anticancer, antispasmodic, and potentially cardiotonic effects, and it is known to stimulate menstruation.

Biologically active components of feverfew include sesquiterpene lactones, flavonoid glycosides, and pinenes. Chloroform leaf extracts of feverfew, abundant in sesquiterpene lactones, have been found to inhibit the production of pro-inflammatory prostaglandins in human leukocytes. Additionally, these extracts have been observed to inhibit the release of histamine in peritoneal (abdominal) mast cells from rats, even though the mechanism of action is not fully understood.[70] According to Shellist, feverfew can help treat headaches related to mast cell activation or histamine release.[49]

Holy basil / tulsi (*Ocimum sanctum L.*)

Despite limited scientific evidence on its effects on mast cells, *Ocimum sanctum* exhibits various therapeutic properties. Reports suggest it has the ability to inhibit IgE, suppress the release of inflammatory mediators, and stabilize mast cells.[71]

In Ayurveda, tulsi is revered as "the incomparable one," "the queen of herbs," or "mother medicine of nature," with a wide range of applications in the treatment of various disorders such as respiratory, gastrointestinal, dermatologic, and inflammatory conditions, as well as fevers, insect bites, eye problems, and anxiety. Experimental studies have confirmed tulsi's medicinal value, demonstrating antimicrobial, antioxidant, anti-inflammatory, neuroprotective, liver-protective, cardioprotective, antidiabetic, antiallergic, immunomodulatory, and anticoagulant effects. Furthermore, tulsi has been found to act as a central nervous system depressant, improve memory, and alleviate stress and anxiety.[72]

Licorice root (*Glycyrrhiza glabra*)

Licorice root is commonly used in traditional Chinese medicine to address respiratory and gastric conditions, support liver health, and aid in detoxification. Modern research has confirmed its broad spectrum of pharmacological benefits, including anti-inflammatory, antiviral, antimicrobial, antitumor, antidiabetic, immunoregulatory, liver-protective, and neuroprotective effects.

Licorice is considered pharmaceutically valuable due to its rich content of secondary metabolites such as triterpenes, flavonoids, and polysaccharides, many of which possess anti-inflammatory activity, primarily through decreasing oxidative stress and mediators such as PGD2, MMPs, and TNF-α. Studies have shown that glycyrrhizic acid (GA), the primary active ingredient in licorice, can balance Th1 and Th2 cytokines, promoting a regulated immune response. Additionally, GA has been found to inhibit degranulation in mast cells and reduce vascular permeability by downregulating the expression of calcium signaling proteins, thereby helping to prevent increased intracellular calcium levels.

Adverse effects of licorice are rare, with elevated blood pressure being the most frequently reported symptom. Sodium retention and hypokalemia have also been reported, but these symptoms typically diminish upon discontinuation. Those with salicylate intolerance should avoid licorice.[49,73-75]

Milk thistle (*Silybum marianum*)

Silybum marianum contains an active compound called silymarin, primarily used to treat liver diseases. Silibinin is silymarin's primary ingredient and has been shown to inhibit histamine release in peritoneal mast cells in rats. Additionally, it reduces the secretion of pro-inflammatory cytokines, including TNF-α and IL-6[76], and helps support gallbladder and liver detox.[49] Research indicates that milk thistle can interact with various medications, potentially affecting their metabolism and half-life. If you consider combining it with other medicines, it is best to consult a physician beforehand.

Nettle extract (*Urtica dioica*)

Nettle extract functions similarly to H1 antihistamines by blocking the histamine-1 receptors. Laboratory studies have also demonstrated that it inhibits tryptase (which hinders mast cell degranulation)[77], and the formation of prostaglandins by targeting PGD2 synthase, as well as the enzymes COX-1 and COX-2, which are involved in the production of pro-inflammatory molecules.[78,79]

Besides its anti-inflammatory benefits, nettle offers various pharmacological properties, including antioxidant, anti-proliferative, antibacterial, anti-rheumatic, antiviral, anticarcinogenic, and anti–Alzheimer effects. Additionally, it functions as a metabolic regulator and may be used to relieve pain.[77–79] Individuals who cannot tolerate nettle extract may find the whole plant tolerable.

Pycnogenol (*Pinus pinaster*)

Pycnogenol, an extract from French maritime pine bark, contains flavonoids that are potent free radical scavengers. It inhibits histamine release from mast cells in a similar manner to sodium cromoglycate. According to Shellist, pycnogenol can be a good alternative for people who do not tolerate luteolin or quercetin.[49,80]

Perilla extract (*Perilla frutescens*)

Perilla frutescens, also known as Chinese basil or shiso, is commonly used in Chinese medicine to treat headaches, colds, coughs, bloating, and seafood-related food poisoning.

Experimental studies have confirmed its diverse pharmacologic properties, including antioxidant, antibacterial, anti-inflammatory, anti-allergic, antidepressant, anticancer, neuroprotective, anti–ischemic, and liver-protective effects. Additionally, it offers anti-aging benefits on the skin.

Compounds derived from perilla—such as luteolin, glycoproteins, apigenin, and rosmarinic acids—exhibit notable anti-inflammatory, antiallergic, and antioxidant effects. A glycoprotein obtained from a water extract of perilla has been shown to markedly suppress the inflammatory reaction induced by mast cells. Perilla also reduces the production of pro-inflammatory cytokines and vascular permeability.[81] As Shellist states, it may help reduce hypersensitivity.[49]

Vitamin C

Vitamin C acts as an antioxidant and inhibits the production of free radicals, reduces bronchial hypersensitivity, and generally strengthens the immune system. While not a mast cell stabilizer per se, studies have linked low levels of vitamin C with increased levels of histamine.[82] Because of its ameliorative effects on systemic mast cell inflammation, vitamin C supplementation may be helpful as a complementary therapeutic measure in mast cell diseases.[83]

KEY TAKEAWAY

Mast cell stabilizers help stabilize the mast cell's membrane, preventing degranulation and mediator release. They are effective as a prophylactic before trigger exposure but cannot reverse ongoing reactions.

First-generation mast cell stabilizers, like cromolyn sodium, prevent degranulation alone, while second-generation options, such as ketotifen, also provide antihistaminic effects. Mast cells may respond differently to these agents depending on their location in the body—for example, some drugs work well in the lungs but not in the skin. Mast cell stabilizers include both pharmaceutical drugs and plant-based compounds, such as flavonoids, coumarins, phenols, and terpenoids.

SECTION III

Managing Your Diagnosis

CHAPTER 19

Finding a Doctor

Finding the right doctor is a crucial step, but unfortunately, it's not that easy. Doctors with a subspecialty in MCAS are still rare, and the few experts who can be found often have so much going on that they may not have the capacity to take on new patients.

Sadly, even some specialists aren't as proactive as many MCAS patients would hope. They might prescribe some medications and perform the necessary tests, but ultimately you're left out in the cold with the multitude of symptoms you have to manage.

WHERE TO START

Seek recommendations

To find a specialist, ask for referrals from different sources, including your primary care physician, pharmacist, and organizations like the Mast Cell Disease Society. You can also join a self-help community on Facebook and ask members for recommendations.

Work with your family doctor

If there aren't any specialists near you, see if your family doctor might be willing to learn about MCAS and help you experiment with possible treatments. Some doctors are open to working with a patient in this way. You could also ask your doctor to consult organizations like the Mast Cell Disease Society in the U.S. (tmsforacure.org) and Mast Cell Action in the UK (mastcellaction.org). They provide helpful guidance for healthcare professionals, including information about mast-cell diseases, signs and symptoms, testing, and treatment.

BUILDING A SUPPORT TEAM

Find specialists for your specific ailments

If no MCAS specialists are available, it can be helpful to find specialists for your specific ailments. This allows you to explore treatment options and improve your chances of effectively alleviating your symptoms.

I currently work with five doctors, all experts in their own fields. It took me three years to put this team together, and I surely wouldn't be where I am today without the support of each one of them.

My primary care physician, Dr. John Van Limburg-Stirum, always aims to help me improve my overall condition. This has been very helpful because maintaining equilibrium makes coping with the mast-cell reactions easier. Dr. Rejmer, a specialist in chronic fatigue syndrome and now also in MCAS, invested the time and effort to help establish mast-cell activation testing in Switzerland. I can turn to him with extra knotty questions. I do my physiotherapy and muscle-balance training under the supervision of Dr. Zenhäusern, who also helps me with spinal manipulation whenever my vertebrae dislocate. My dermatologist, Dr. Zepter, helps me manage my skin-related symptoms. And I see my psychologist, Mrs. Pfleiderer, about once a month. It's so good to have someone to talk with who's objective enough to provide constructive advice.

If you haven't found the right doctor yet, keep looking, and don't give up. It might take some time and patience, but it's worth the effort. Coping with this disease becomes so much easier if you can turn to experts with the knowledge and the means to help you.

> **KEY TAKEAWAY**
>
> To find a knowledgeable doctor, seek referrals from organizations like the Mast Cell Disease Society (US), Mast Cell Action (UK), Facebook support groups, your primary care physician, local hospitals, or pharmacists.

CHAPTER 20

Talking with Doctors

As strange as that might sound, simply knowing how to talk to a doctor is another important aspect of this experience. Many of us go through a nerve-wracking journey of being misdiagnosed over and over again. Eventually, we may be in such tremendous discomfort that having a calm, reasonable conversation becomes nearly impossible. Being in so much pain, it's perfectly understandable that we might end up crying out for help.

Unfortunately, doctors can be seriously offended by an overly demanding attitude—and might even feel insulted if they sense we know too much. Doctors are people, too. Unless they have an extraordinary bedside manner, they can quickly become disinterested in extending themselves to a patient who's difficult to communicate with, no matter how much that patient is suffering.

I've met doctors who shook their heads in disbelief and outright denied that all my symptoms could be connected, because most doctors specialize in one field of medicine. But mast cell issues simply aren't confined to one area of the body; it's truly a blessing to find a physician who can think outside the box or is at least willing to learn about MCAD and work collaboratively with you.

Until you find that gem of a doctor, try to remain as patient and calm as possible. Finding the right doctor is paramount, but until we do, it's important to stay on good terms with whoever we're able to work with in the meantime. The following are a few tips to help you get the most out of your doctor's appointments.

PREPARING FOR APPOINTMENTS

Keep your files organized

Always request your records and keep them well-organized, ideally in both paper and digital formats. This helps you stay on top of your information and simplifies sharing when consulting a new physician.

Make lists

Before your medical appointments, jot down everything you need to discuss. You can then either hand the list to your doctor or keep it handy to help ensure you cover all essential topics during the visit.

EFFECTIVE COMMUNICATION

Ask rather than demand

It can be helpful to frame your observations and concerns as questions for your doctor, so they feel validated too. If a doctor doesn't feel comfortable with you, it could seriously jeopardize your progress—and in the worst case, they may even withhold their help.

Give doctors some slack: no one knows everything

It helps to remember that nobody truly understands everything or has mastered every known skill, and the same applies to doctors. No single practitioner can be expected to understand every area of the body, so try to approach this with patience.

Each system of the body that a doctor might specialize in is like a little universe of its own—vast and complex. Only an exceptional diagnostician will connect the dots between these separate universes. Adding to the challenge are the differing diagnostic proposals for MCAS, along with the fact that mast cell disorders haven't been sufficiently researched. Even some experts acknowledge that medical science still has significant gaps to fill.

Balancing knowledge and experience

I guess in most cases, it's inevitable that individuals affected by mast cell disease will study and read whatever they can to try to understand what is happening to them. In doing so, we usually learn quite a bit, which can sometimes lead to a sort of power play between doctor and patient. We might even end up getting scolded for knowing too much.

Other patients and I have been told we shouldn't try to find information online. However, what we experience often seems so strange that it's only natural to look for explanations or validation of what we're going through.

Doctors have invested a lot of time, effort, and money into their education and training. Patients, on the other hand, haven't chosen to be ill—but they do have a lot of experience with their symptoms. It helps to see that both parties are human, each with their own knowledge and limitations. Approaching one another with respect and humility can significantly enhance the doctor–patient relationship—and may even transform it into a true partnership.

FINDING THE RIGHT DOCTOR

Don't settle for less

It's vital to find specialists who genuinely want to help you. If you sense that a doctor isn't truly interested in helping you, politely ask for a referral. Otherwise, as discussed in Chapter 19, "Finding a Doctor," ask for recommendations from self-help groups.

I've dealt with more than a hundred physicians during my life. From my observations, being a good doctor means more than being strong in medical knowledge and having the ability to diagnose correctly. It also means having good people skills, an agile mind, a thirst for learning, genuine compassion, and a true desire to help. Finding the right doctor might take some time, but don't give up—having one you can truly collaborate with is invaluable.

> **KEY TAKEAWAY**
>
> Get the most out of your medical appointments by keeping organized records and bringing a clear list of symptoms, questions, and concerns. Be patient and realistic—MCAS is complex and poorly understood. If a doctor isn't supportive, request a referral or keep searching until you find one who is genuinely committed to helping you.

CHAPTER 21

Alienation of Friends

It hurts to experience the loss of friends because your lifestyle becomes more limited with MCAS. It's a bitter pill to swallow, but it does happen. I've found it helps not to expect too much support from others and to realize that they might not understand the situation because they simply have no frame of reference. It's ultimately easier than trying to reason with them about this disease and why they should be there for you.

I know this is easier said than done because it's natural to want to be understood. At the same time, wanting to understand is normal. Usually, we learn these traits as we grow up. If we have an issue, we typically go to a friend or a loved one to talk it through. If we're sad, we get consoled, and if we're hurt or injured, we get pampered in some way. This is what we come to expect if that's what we experienced growing up. Yet once we're struggling with MCAS, it often feels as though no one understands, and we end up feeling utterly alone.

Try to see it this way: MCAS and its impact on the body are mind-boggling. As someone affected, you most likely long for support from your loved ones. But if even you—experiencing it all—are boggled by what's happening, try to imagine how hard it must be for others to grasp. No wonder they might not know how to respond to this new situation, even when they used to be there for you in the past.

They might feel helpless. They might be afraid of losing you—or of losing their own freedom if they decide to be available. Some may even become frustrated at not being able to understand everything or at not being able to be more helpful. In the worst-case scenario, friends and loved ones may distance themselves just when you need them the most.

Such alienation from people who used to be close to you hurts deeply. No one wants to be sick and in constant pain or to be so restricted. To be abandoned in such a state, on top of the agony of the disease itself, is indeed challenging. My take on this is to practice compassion. Once you get the hang of it, you'll probably take such things more lightly.

COMPASSION AS A RESPONSE

Compassion for yourself

Give yourself all the love and understanding you need to feel loved and understood. Give yourself time to rest and regain your energy. The body restores itself when it is resting; cells repair at night when you sleep—so the more quality rest you get, the better you'll feel.

Have compassion for yourself when you're out of strength. Energy will come time and time again, and it will leave time and time again. Just breathe through it and wait for the next burst of energy to follow through on what you need to get done.

Compassion for others

People who aren't affected by MCAS may struggle to understand both the nature of this condition and its impact on daily life for those who live with it. Exercise compassion for others where they lack empathy for you, because they simply might not have the capacity. So, have compassion for their lack; surrender and let it be what it is.

This might be the most thorough exercise in compassion you've gone through yet, but on a positive note, you'll be able to apply this technique in all areas of your life, and it might just make it all a little bit easier. Many of my friendships have ended, but others have grown even stronger bonds. Finally, I am happy to know who's with me—and I'm just as glad to know I've stopped giving my energy to people who weren't genuinely invested in me. In that sense, MCAS has provided invaluable lessons all around.

> **KEY TAKEAWAY**
>
> If friends pull away, remember that MCAS can lead to isolation for many reasons. Don't take it personally. Practice self-compassion and offer yourself the kindness and empathy you wish others would show.

CHAPTER 22

Hypersensitivity

Becoming ridiculously sensitive to all kinds of things seems to be a widespread issue with MCAS. For me, this certainly has been the case, and given that I've been quite sensitive to begin with, it's gone to levels that are difficult to comprehend. For people who weren't very sensitive before becoming ill, this may be even harder to grasp and cope with.

HEIGHTENED SENSITIVITY

How this feels for me

My perception of sound, light, scent, and touch has increased dramatically. Even ordinarily gentle sounds can now feel unbearably loud and distressing. For example, the simple trickling of water from the sink can trigger pain that reverberates throughout my entire nervous system like a current of electricity.

My sense of smell has become so intense that, at times, it's truly overwhelming. If I must take public transportation, I can usually distinguish who's wearing which shampoo, aftershave, or perfume just by my relative proximity to them. I've even been able to tell what kind of groceries people have in their shopping bags!

You might think this could be a valuable trait, but I can tell you it can be crushing! If you live in a populated area, you might perceive a cacophony of hundreds of overlapping smells, all assaulting you at once. It's like going to the movies with your olfactory system—but there's no pause button. It's on repeat, playing 24/7.

A real-life example

The moment I realized just how sensitive my sense of smell had become, I wasn't in a city but a mountain forest. I got up early that morning and went for a hike to enjoy the fresh, pristine mountain air. I had walked for about an hour, taking frequent stops to rest here and there, and began to tremendously enjoy the sensation of breathing deeply and fully.

In the city, I got used to shallow breathing; to avoid big reactions to triggers, I make my breathing cautious. But that day in the woods, I took deep, full breaths, filling my lungs completely and feeling downright ecstatic from this pure air. I immediately thought about moving to the mountains because it felt so invigorating.

Out of curiosity, I looked up how many times we breathe per day: about 17,000 to 30,000 breaths. So, I reckoned that living in a place with pure air might improve my quality of life by around 9,000, because these are roughly my conscious breaths while I'm awake. Then, while walking through the quiet forest, I suddenly felt a sensation akin to a punch in my stomach. I instantly knew it was a reaction to a smell.

Whenever this happens, it starts with a punch-like sensation in the stomach, followed by a mist of discomfort spreading through my stomach lining and respiratory tract. My heart rate speeds up, and I quickly feel nauseated, accompanied by a strange tingly feeling that spreads throughout my entire body, like an adrenaline rush that lingers for some time.

I knew someone was nearby despite seeing or hearing nothing. I paused, looked, and listened. Unable to detect any movement, I resumed walking. A few minutes later, I finally saw two people about two hundred feet ahead. The breeze might have carried their scent, but there wasn't much movement in the air that day—yet I felt a reaction from at least three hundred feet away! This moment made it crystal clear to me just how reactive mast cells really are.

THE OVERLOAD OF SENSORY INPUT

Now imagine that heightened sense of smell combined with an equally intense sensitivity to noise, temperature, movement, and light. There's a lot going on all at once, and it's quite a task to stay centered enough to take it all in without feeling overwhelmed.

COPING STRATEGIES

I say do anything in your power to reduce stress. Learn to quiet your mind, breathe through tension, and stay centered as much as possible. Give yourself permission to rest and make sure you sleep well. Create a home environment that feels safe and comfortable to you, so you have a space to truly recuperate.

Find mast cell stabilizers you tolerate, and try to keep your diet low in sugars and stimulants to support a calmer nervous system. Along with these, the tips throughout this book can help you cope more effectively.

The heightened sensitivity that comes with MCAS can be both physically and emotionally exhausting. On top of that, it often leaves you feeling lonely, as others may not fully grasp what you're going through. It's important to stay true to yourself and, if you will, become your own best friend. I'd say it's a good thing in life anyway, because we are the ones we must live with day in and day out, but I think it's especially valuable if you have a disease like this because the overwhelming sensory experience can leave you feeling rather isolated.

Without all the coping techniques I've developed over time, I think I would've gone nuts. I hope this description also highlights how anxiety can be a significant issue for many MCAS patients.

> **KEY TAKEAWAY**
>
> MCAS can cause extreme sensitivities to sound, light, scent, touch, and temperature—often even to trace amounts of triggers. This can be especially difficult in urban environments. Stress-reduction techniques such as mindfulness and breathwork can help manage sensory overwhelm and foster inner calm.

CHAPTER 23

Anxiety

Many patients with mast cell disorders encounter anxiety at some point, sometimes even progressing into full-blown panic attacks. These symptoms are closely tied to mast cell activation. Specific mast cell mediators, such as histamine, corticotropin-releasing hormone (CRH), and cytokines, have been linked to neuropsychiatric manifestations, including anxiety.

For instance, histamine can cross the blood-brain barrier (BBB), interact with histamine receptors in the brain, and alter the balance of neurotransmitters, such as serotonin and norepinephrine. These changes can lead to anxiety symptoms.[84] Similarly, CRH stimulates mast cells to release neurotoxic and neuroinflammatory mediators, disrupting the BBB. This disruption activates glial cells, triggering the release of additional inflammatory mediators and driving chronic neuroinflammation in the brain.[85]

On top of these physiological effects, it's important to remember that living with MCAS can feel like the whole world around you has turned into a swirling vortex of potential triggers that can seriously harm you and even pose life-threatening risks. It's no surprise, then, that anxiety is a common experience for those affected.

With this in mind, it helps to know how you can cope with anxiety. There are many techniques you can use to calm down before or even during an anxiety attack. Some of the following are widely known methods, and some are from my own repertoire.

UNDERSTANDING THE ONSET

Recognize the early signs

The actual chain of events leading up to a bout of anxiety may be complex to identify at first, but it's a good idea to consider them. It helps to identify what triggers anxiety in you and what you can do to stem it. Anxiety is taxing for anyone, but I think it's even worse for those with MCAS because the stress it creates in the body significantly exacerbates mast cell activation.

Mast cell stabilizers, certain medications, and natural herbs can help alleviate anxiety, but I find taking it into your own hands is even more effective. You can sometimes overcome anxiety by intentionally using the power of your mind—a tool that's always available, has no undesirable side effects, and costs you nothing.

Anxiety doesn't just set in without warning. The signal might come on suddenly or slowly, but there is often some clue. It's probably very individual, but in my experience, there's a general feeling of unease, claustrophobia, or a creeping sense of fear that precedes a full-blown anxiety attack. Acting on these signals when you first become aware will likely give you enough time to prevent the anxiety from taking over completely.

CALMING TECHNIQUES

Limit stimuli

Find the quietest place available, whether at home, in the office, or in a public space. Sit where you feel safe and try to connect to the stillness within. If relocating to a quieter spot isn't possible, earplugs can help. I also use wired noise-canceling headphones in busy environments, which are fantastic at blocking overwhelming sounds.

Additionally, a cap and sunglasses can dim harsh lighting, and wearing a hoodie can provide a sense of protection. These minor adjustments make a big difference in creating a calmer environment, even when surrounded by activity.

Focus on your breath

Deep breathing is one of the most powerful tools you can use—and it's always available and completely free. It effectively brings your focus right back to the body. During an anxiety attack, we tend to go into fast and shallow breathing, which will only make things worse. Breathing slowly and fully has a calming effect on the nervous system.

A simple technique is to silently count to four while breathing out through the nose and then to four again while breathing in. Go as slow as you can and repeat until you feel calm. Breathing out first is additionally calming because when you inhale, your heart rate speeds up, and when you exhale, it slows down. Try to remember to focus on your breathing when you feel good, too; if you're already practiced, it will be much easier when you are agitated.

Connect to your senses

When you feel anxiety rising, pause and name four things that you can see, three things you can touch, two things you can smell, and one thing you can taste. This engages your senses and shifts your focus to the present moment.

Connect to the Earth

Taking your shoes off and walking barefoot on a patch of grass, soil, or sand has an immediate soothing effect. This simple practice is often referred to as "earthing" or "grounding" and helps calm the system.

Change of scenery

Getting out of the house or away from the location where the anxiety began to creep up has helped me before. Simply breathing in fresh air, feeling the warm sunlight on my skin, or sitting under a tree and taking in the scents of nature has done wonders for me.

Light exercise

Gentle movement can bring your attention back to your body and away from the mind.

Muscle relaxation

Tensing your muscles and then consciously releasing them has a very relaxing effect. You can progressively move up through the body, starting at your feet and ending at your head.

Mindfulness

Focus your attention on something other than the anxiety. Deliberately direct your thoughts away from the panicky feeling. By focusing intently on something else, you're not fueling the anxiety. This will help your mind calm down because you give it something to do; thus, it cannot intensify the panic.

Pick one object and try to see it as clearly as you can. Think about it—what it means to you, where it came from, how it was made, what it is made of, and so on. Continue thinking about it to keep your mind focused for a while. In effect, you are training yourself to be present.

Observe the anxiety

Once you've identified the signals at the onset of a panic attack, you can acknowledge them and then determine to go back to what you were doing. This takes a strong will, but I find it an exquisite technique to prevent the anxiety from manifesting. As you immerse yourself in whatever activity you have chosen, the feelings of unease will soon dissolve because you're simply not adding any fuel to them.

STRENGTHENING INNER SUPPORT

Acknowledge yourself

It can help to hug yourself and simply feel the love you have for yourself.

Know this will pass

Remind yourself that such moments of anxiety never last forever; knowing this can make coping a little easier.

Use your imagination

Picture yourself as both your loving, caring parent and the younger you. Do what an ideal parent would do for you. A parent would likely try to soothe the child's spirit while also staying objective and looking for solutions. Be both—the child and the parent—because you'll need to be able to listen to that wiser voice and follow its advice. In tricky situations, for example when a part of you wants to give up, this is a potent technique that can help you act prudently.

REACHING OUT

Ask for help

The support of a psychologist or psychiatrist can be invaluable, offering personalized strategies to help you navigate and overcome anxiety.

AVOIDING OVERWHELM IN THE FIRST PLACE

Set your boundaries

For the longest time, I felt so utterly responsible that if someone asked for help, I would always do it. If I had just a drop of energy, I felt obligated to be there for others, even when I was utterly exhausted or in considerable pain. I often pushed far beyond my limits and frequently ended up sick or in a state of oppressive anxiety. Learning to recognize and respect my boundaries and then clearly and confidently state them to others has helped me tremendously in maintaining my equilibrium and protecting myself against overextension.

Learn to say no

Oh my, saying no felt so wrong at first! It made me feel utterly guilty. The first time I tried to tell someone I wouldn't be able to help them, it almost felt like I was speaking a foreign language. I felt so uncomfortable squeezing that *no* across my lips that it was accompanied by a slight adrenaline rush and a vigorously pounding heart. I'm sure I was flushed, too.

Much to my surprise, it was perfectly okay with the person who had asked me for the favor. They just took my no as an answer and weren't upset about it at all. They simply understood that I had said no. It wasn't a *forever and ever no;* it was just a question that happened to be answered with a no. So, they would go and come back again, and we were still friends with no hard feelings thereafter.

In the long run, it's actually the nicest thing you can do to state your truth the way you really mean it. A half-assed yes is unfriendlier than a well-meant no. Being able to say no when you mean it helps tremendously in keeping overwhelm at bay.

Create space for your mind

Making lists of things that are continually floating around in your mind can enable you to feel calmer. It allows for structure, and you can get these things off your mind. Lists can be made of anything you keep thinking about repeatedly, such as questions for the doctors, what you need to accomplish for the week, things you want to learn, or even your long-time aspirations.

Recently, I made a list of everything that stressed me out. Then I took care of each item as I had the energy to do so. Of course, I had to go step by step, and it took quite some time to get all of it done, but in the process, I also learned to balance what had to be accomplished and the energy I could devote to it each day. Crossing off each completed item made me feel much calmer. Finally being done—and then tossing the list—is a glorious feeling! Finished, achieved, clear. And you'll see that you still make progress, even when this illness slows you down at times.

KEY TAKEAWAY

Anxiety and MCAS are linked. Mast cell mediators can cause neuroinflammation, and constant vigilance over potential triggers takes a psychological toll. Mindfulness, breathwork, meditation, and other anxiety-management tools are vital. Don't hesitate to seek professional mental health support—MCAS is heavy, and having someone to talk to can help lighten the load.

CHAPTER 24

Mindset

I had already been homebound for days in the aftermath of a reaction. When I tried to do anything around the house, things kept slipping out of my shaky hands. Even just standing on my feet hurt so much that it was pure torment. My vision was blurry, my head was pounding, and I was so incredibly exhausted that absolutely everything I tried to do took an incredible amount of effort and willpower. It's an unspeakable drag to be so utterly clumsy and lethargic when you could otherwise do pretty much everything swiftly and effortlessly.

Trying to navigate myself through this thick, seemingly impenetrable brain fog and debilitating pain, the only thing I could think was, *I'm so sick. I'm so tired. How the fuck am I supposed to do anything? Ouch, this hurts. My legs feel so heavy. I can't stand on my feet. I can't see. This sucks! My eyes hurt. Oh, gosh, I'm so sick! I'm so sick! Ugh. I'm so sick!*

Then, in one blessed moment, I realized what I was doing: I was telling my body how it felt—and it was listening! How on earth should my cells understand that I want to change this situation if I just keep contemplating how bad everything is?

SHIFTING THE NARRATIVE

The power of positive thought

In dealing with MCAS, we need to heal on a cellular level. Our bodies are miracles. They are incredibly intricate, interconnected systems. There are trillions of cells functioning within us, and they have their ways of understanding what's going on.

No matter how clever we are, humans still cannot heal an infection or mend a cut solely with intellect. We depend on the wisdom of our cells. What became clear to me then was that I couldn't possibly think these words and phrases and expect things to get better anytime soon.

With this realization, I decided that no matter how bad I felt, I would tell myself an entirely different story. Admittedly, this did feel rather odd at first—as though I were choosing to ignore reality. It felt a bit like I was trying to cheat. Nevertheless, I decided to give it a try. And so, whenever I noticed that I was mentally commenting on how bad I felt, I changed my thoughts to something positive. From then on, if I felt any pain, I'd tell myself, *I am getting better. It's getting better day by day. I am grateful. I am healthy.*

POSITIVE THINKING, REAL PAIN

Battling inner resistance

At first, part of me went up the walls! *No, you're not, you fool! Don't you feel it?! It hurts all over!* Then, *yeah, I know—but I will not stick to it.* And I kept repeating positive thoughts to myself: *This is getting better. I am thankful. I feel better and better. I am thankful the cramp is over. The inflammation will wane. I am going to be healthy. Healthy, healthy, healthy. I am happy, happy, happy....*

Even though I wasn't happy at all, I'd repeat the word like a mantra: *Happy, happy, happy, happy....* My mind changed it to: *Crappy!* And I'd snap right back: *No. Happy!*

Part of me was clearly rebelling against these statements, but after some time, I felt a bit lighter. It's wild how much these reactions hurt, and telling yourself the opposite may sound ridiculous, but finally, who cares if it makes you feel better?

Caution: toxic positivity?

All that said, while this new perspective has helped me adopt a lighter outlook, it may not be the ideal path. As Dr. Rejmer pointed out, this mindset might lead to what could be termed *factual delusions* or *toxic positivity,* which can be dangerous when taken too far.

Truthfully, on the first day after embracing this new mindset, I left the house determined to think nothing but, *I am healthy, healthy, healthy...* but I collapsed before I'd even walked three minutes, and it took me an entire day to recover from that setback. So, remain hopeful and focus on the positive as much as you can, but be realistic enough to respect your limits.

HELPFUL HABITS

Focusing on the good

I believe it's vital to focus on all the good that happens. No matter how small, every uplifting detail deserves to be celebrated. Fixating solely on our discomfort only intensifies the pain and prolongs our suffering, while focusing on how we want to feel can help us get there more quickly.

Our cells might be more attuned to our thoughts than we realize. Positivity is contagious. So, I decided to do everything in my power to make myself feel better. Training myself in this positive mindset has significantly helped me feel better sooner and cope with this disease—and with life in general—in a much more pleasant way.

Daily gratitude practice

To further ground myself in positivity, I've started a gratitude journal. Every day, I find things I'm grateful for and write them down in a designated notebook. Writing them down feels good in the moment, and it's also uplifting to read through it when I feel down. Sometimes it takes a bit of brainstorming, but ultimately, it's always sweet to see on paper how much good stuff happens, even if you're homebound.

For example, the comfort of having a bed and a roof over our heads, the sunshine outside, the beautiful clouds drifting by, the enchanting sound of the rain, the clean water we have at home, that we have at least one friend who loves us, or even the simple fact that we're able to breathe… There is always something beautiful to be grateful for.

Even just deliberately deciding to focus on things you're grateful for helps you notice them more readily. Moreover, a regular gratitude practice naturally lifts your mood. Feeling calm and happy has a soothing effect on the nervous system and will also help calm the mast cells. Simply put, the better you feel, the better you'll feel.

Finding gratitude amidst the struggle

If you're reading this while still in the early stages of your diagnosis, then I understand that you might feel like you want to kick my ass. Talking about gratitude while you're suffering intense pain can feel infuriating. Yet, please bear with me, because I've been there too, and I'm telling you it helped me, so I think it is worth trying.

We can nearly always find things to be grateful for. If there's not one big and obvious thing, we can start with the *little* things. Maybe you felt frustrated reading the "little things" I mentioned above. *Like, yeah, beautiful sunshine, but I react to it! Sure, it's nice that I have running water, but I can't take a shower without passing out each time! Yeah, I have one friend who bears with me, but everyone else turned their backs on me!* Believe me, I do understand that this all sucks! But if you can find the courage to do so, try to stop paying attention to the negative. It's like a fire that you don't keep feeding with new wood. You starve it out so it can cease to be.

Being thankful resonates throughout our whole being and all of our cells, including the mast cells. The more you can make yourself feel good, the calmer these little guys become, and the better you will feel. There are no adverse side effects to this practice. With this, you really can't lose.

> **KEY TAKEAWAY**
>
> Your thoughts can influence your body. Cultivating a healing mindset helps redirect focus toward recovery. Emphasize what's going well and keep a gratitude journal. Expect inner resistance—and gently push through it.

CHAPTER 25

Days of Exhaustion

Yes, there are these days of exhaustion—unconquerable, debilitating exhaustion! Days on which you feel like you weigh tons and gravity seems somehow amplified. Being so incredibly exhausted is unquestionably challenging, and I have yet to find a solid remedy. Ultimately, this gets better once we can avoid reactions in the first place, but until we're there, we might have to accept that we feel completely drained on some days.

WHAT CAN HELP

Boosting energy levels

In the meantime, it helps to learn what we can do to boost our energy levels. Sufficient water and nutrient intake, movement, fresh air, and adequate sleep are all crucial. As strange as this might sound, these things can easily be overlooked when you're so very sick. Additionally, it helps to keep vitamin C and electrolyte levels up.

Supplements

If you're low on vitamin D, B12, or iron, supplementing with these nutrients could help boost your energy levels. As discussed in Chapter 39, "Iron Infusions," my energy levels increased significantly once I learned how to tolerate the infusions.

During my research, I encountered a woman who combats lethargy with daily high doses of vitamin B12. I agree that vitamin B12 is crucial for energy; I noticed a significant improvement after receiving a series of VitaRubin injections to address my deficiency. Later, I discovered a supplement called Hydroxo B12 from Seeking Health, which I tolerated well. I now prefer it over the shot because it's completely painless, and I don't have to go to the clinic to get it, unlike the injection. Additionally, it's more affordable, and I can take it weekly.

A word of caution: Excessive vitamin B12 supplementation, especially when combined with high doses of vitamin B6, may have negative health impacts if intakes exceed daily recommendations.[86,87] I've found that taking the supplement once a week improves my energy without putting me at risk for toxicity.

REST IS KEY

Some days, you simply must rest

There are still days when I feel completely exhausted. In a way, I've come to terms with it and learned to just rest on these days. I might do some super light activities, like listening to podcasts, because even watching a movie would be too much. I now know that if I don't give my body the rest it needs, I'll just drag it out, and the lethargy will win itself another day. Unless I try to push myself beyond my limits, I usually feel better after a day or two.

It certainly is frustrating to watch friends frolic outside while you're stuck in the same old bed you've been stuck in for way too long already, but you've got to take things as they are. Fighting this fatigue will only make you more tired on top of being tired already. In my opinion, it's best to rest on such days: sleep as much as you need, try to maintain a positive outlook, and remind yourself that better days lie ahead.

> **KEY TAKEAWAY**
>
> To fight fatigue, prioritize hydration, nutrient-dense food, gentle movement, fresh air, and restful sleep. Maintain your intake of vitamin C and electrolytes, and consider supplements to address deficiencies. Respect your limits and rest when needed.

CHAPTER 26

Tracking Reactions

Tracking and understanding all of your triggers takes time and perseverance. It can also be challenging to distinguish the initial cause from the symptoms that may follow because each reaction has an aftermath.

Triggers vary from person to person—and they can even change for an individual from time to time. There's no official guideline you could adhere to, and you'll likely have to engage in some trial and error until you know all your triggers and how to handle them. Some reactions are so "loud" that, for a while at least, you might think it's the only thing that sets you off. And then—just when you think you've got it all figured out—the next alarm bell might go off.

WHERE TO BEGIN

Start with what hurts the most

Initially, I thought all my symptoms were connected to reactions to food, but the better I understood what, when, and how to eat, the calmer my digestive system became. As a result, I began to notice other triggers like noise, perfume, different odors, dust, and more. It took me about two years to finally understand most of my triggers. Actually, it's pretty simple: you'll notice the most intense reactions first, so start by addressing those. Once they're under control, subtler culprits become more apparent.

Remain vigilant and patient

All these reactions can feel overwhelming, but identifying triggers is a gradual process, so you'll need to take it step by step. Understanding how they affect you takes time, so patience is key.

TRACK & DETECT

Journaling

It can be helpful to track your reactions in a journal. I did this in the beginning, but once I'd learned what set me off, I decided to stop journaling about my ailments and focus instead on the things that helped me feel better. However, in the early stages, a journal can be crucial for making sense of your reactions. Note down the time, symptom severity, and possible triggers. Over time, you'll notice patterns that will help you identify your key triggers.

Look for patterns

For example, if I've been triggered by food, the first sign is a distinct reddening of my facial skin within minutes of ingestion. Then bloating sets in, followed by severe cramps. Within twenty minutes, my typically flat belly swells to the size of a basketball. These symptoms can last anywhere from seven hours to two days and are often accompanied by hot flashes, cold sweats, a feverish feeling, irregular heart rate, shaky hands, severe headaches, blurry vision, eye pain, pain in my kidneys, legs, and arms, and irritating skin reactions. And just when I think I've made it through the worst, the inflammation phase begins!

Recognizing such patterns makes coping with reactions more bearable. Over time, they become less intimidating because you learn to anticipate how they typically unfold.

Track the aftermath

At first, this was quite confusing, but I soon realized there is often a delayed response, especially after an intense flare. Mast cells are present in nearly every type of vascularized tissue, and stress can trigger them. Once activated, they release an array of mediators into these tissues. Ironically, this response could help protect us from pathogens—if only the trigger had been a real threat! But with nothing to fight, the body gets flooded with these mediators, causing pain and inflammation throughout.

So, while I writhe in pain from food my body couldn't tolerate, the mast cells detect this stress and keep releasing their "ammunition," which, unfortunately, only amplifies the pain. Depending on the severity of the reaction, inflammation can last anywhere from a week to a month. Understanding that each response has its life cycle helps one cope during recovery.

RECOVERY & RESILIENCE

Simplify and avoid

During the heightened sensitivity phase, it's essential to keep things as simple and gentle as possible. After a strong flare, I'm much more easily triggered by other things. My sensitivity to all kinds of stimuli increases quite drastically. Noise, harsh lights, dust, smells, and perfumes can become unbearably overwhelming, and I also react to more foods than usual. To prevent triggering another wave of reactions, it's crucial to avoid further triggers and maintain a gentle, low-stimulus environment until the body has calmed down.

Keep perspective

One thing that has made it easier to cope is understanding that every reaction will eventually end. Nowadays, when I go into a flare, my first thought is still, *shit*, of course, but it only takes me a few seconds to remind myself: *This will pass. I'll be fine.* I then focus on the horizon and do my best to calm the reaction. The worst reaction I've experienced to this day lasted about 48 hours, and the subsequent inflammation subsided within a month.

If I get triggered by perfumes, I might feel off for a few hours or up to three days. Thus far, by day four I've always been okay again. If I get triggered by dust, my skin will be irritated for a few days, but once I have a clean space to calm the reaction and take care of my skin, I usually start feeling better soon. Every anaphylactic shock takes some time to recover from, but the body always returns to balance eventually.

In the beginning, I felt much more anxious because I didn't know if all of this would last forever. Now I know that even the most painful reactions decline in time. Just knowing that makes it substantially easier to cope.

> **KEY TAKEAWAY**
>
> There are no universal MCAS triggers; everyone reacts differently, and individual sensitivities can shift over time. Keep a reaction journal to track symptoms, severity, timing, and suspected triggers. Start by addressing the most obvious ones. Once those settle, subtler triggers become easier to detect. After a strong flare, you often enter a phase of heightened sensitivity, so it's important to minimize stressors during this time.

SECTION IV

Daily Survival Tactics

CHAPTER 27

Working Around Triggers

To work around your triggers, you must learn to listen attentively to your body and remain cautious. I've found that I can often avoid a full-blown reaction by keeping a safe distance from my triggers. Over time, I've learned how to quickly assess whether something is harmful and how to lessen its impact.

THE FIRST SIGNS OF A REACTION

- Burning in my eyes or on my facial skin
- Reddened skin
- Burning or tightness in my throat
- Shortness of breath
- Rapid heartbeat
- Blurry vision
- Itchy skin
- Nausea or stomach discomfort
- A tingling sensation in my stomach—like gentle fireworks or a mild adrenaline rush
- A rush of pain throughout my nervous system
- Sudden exhaustion
- Brain fog
- Tinnitus

MY IMMEDIATE RESPONSE

- I move away from the trigger as quickly as possible.
- I cover my mouth using a mask, scarf, jacket collar, sleeve, or hand.
- I breathe shallowly and slowly until I can get fresh air.
- Once in a safe spot, I sit down and relax until I feel calm again.

- Most importantly, I stay as calm as possible the moment I notice a reaction coming on.

OUTDOOR SCENT STRATEGY

If someone's perfume triggers me outdoors, I immediately check which direction the wind is coming from and swiftly adjust my position to ensure I'm breathing fresh air and not the perfume. It often suffices to take a step to either side to ensure I'm upwind from the trigger. It can also help to turn my back to them and take a quick breath while my body blocks the perfume.

PROTECTION

Masks

Wearing a mask is undoubtedly one of the safest and easiest ways to reduce the impact of airborne triggers. Masks are explicitly built for this purpose, and some come with good filters—but who wants to walk around with a mask all the time? I've worn them before, but after a few unpleasant encounters with strangers, I began exploring alternatives.

That said, public attitudes toward masks have certainly shifted due to the COVID-19 pandemic. Nowadays, unpleasant encounters should be relatively rare, and masks built for this purpose will surely work better than clothing or your hands.

Alternatives

Clothing can act as a barrier, and even using your hand as a shield against triggers can provide a sense of safety. And although these measures don't work as well as masks, they can block out smells and provide a sense of safety—which is helpful because staying calm often prevents reactions from worsening.

I know the idea of breathing through your hand sounds strange; I honestly didn't believe it would help when another patient first suggested it. But after trying many times, I must say it does help quite a bit, likely because the smell of my hand covers the triggers and is recognized as safe and familiar.

KEY TAKEAWAY

To recognize triggers, stay alert for early warning signs such as burning eyes, throat, or skin, nausea, exhaustion, or brain fog. At the first signal, remain calm, cover your mouth and move away while breathing shallowly until you reach fresh air. Outdoors, position yourself upwind so that perfumes and scents drift away rather than toward you.

CHAPTER 28

Reducing Physical Stress

Stress is a very potent trigger. Learning how to reduce it—and even better, avoid it in the first place—can make a big difference in managing MCAS and life in general. Here are some strategies that might help.

HELPFUL HABITS

Set limits

If you're genuinely exhausted, postpone anything you don't have the energy for. Don't stress about being unable to accomplish everything you want. Go as far as you can, but respect your limits. Trying to be faster will slow you down more often than not. Whenever you overdo something, the mast cells freak out and knock you out for the count, likely setting you back for another few days. So, be gentle with yourself—it will help you maintain equilibrium.

Avoid known triggers

Knowing your triggers and thus being able to avoid them will greatly help reduce stress. While this may seem nearly impossible at first, it will get easier as time goes on.

Ask for help

If you don't have enough energy to get everything done, don't be afraid to ask for help. Friends, family, or even neighbors might be happy to lend you a hand. Your doctors may also be able to arrange for home care to assist you with your daily needs. It can't hurt to ask.

Plan ahead

Schedule your tasks in a way that doesn't leave you overwhelmed. See which activities you can combine and prioritize what's most important. Tackle these things first so that it won't be such a big deal if you run out of energy.

Shop less frequently

Shopping can be very stressful for people with MCAS due to all the potential triggers in a store. To reduce exposure, you can order your supplies online or purchase larger quantities to store or freeze what you can. Consider which foods stay fresh the longest and eat the ones that spoil more quickly first.

Eat a wholesome diet

Make sure to supply your body with the nutrients it needs to function. If you're still reacting to too many foods, try finding supplements you can tolerate. They can provide the essential nutrients your body needs until you can reintroduce more foods into your diet. Try to be mindful when you eat and avoid eating when you're agitated.

Sleep hygiene

Try to establish healthy sleep patterns. Go to bed and get up around the same time each day. Reduce—or better yet, avoid—screen time in the evenings, and try to get some natural light early in the morning. This will help set your circadian rhythm so you'll sleep better at night.

Additionally, set up your bedroom so it's solely used for sleeping (and your love life), but keep all work-related items out. Your bedroom should be a relaxing, soothing environment where you feel completely at ease. For more information on optimizing sleep, refer to Chapter 31, "Improving Sleep."

GROUNDING PRACTICES

Center yourself

If you notice you're starting to feel off balance, take action as soon as you sense the scales beginning to tip. Sit down and take a breather. If possible, wash your face with cool water. Use earplugs to block out the surrounding noise in busy environments. And if necessary, signal to others that you need a moment of silence or whatever helps you regain your balance. Try not to be ashamed of having to take these moments—they're essential for your well-being, especially when living with MCAS.

Breathing and humming

Breathing practices and humming are simple yet effective techniques for managing stress and anxiety. Slow and deep breathing activates the parasympathetic nervous system, helping the body transition from "fight-or-flight" mode to a more relaxed and calm state.

Humming, similarly, activates the vagus nerve, a key component of the parasympathetic nervous system and the brain-gut axis. Activating the vagus nerve lowers heart rate and blood pressure, enhances cognition, and improves bowel function. Additionally, humming increases nitric oxide levels in the nasal cavity, increasing airflow and supporting relaxation.[88]

MOVEMENT & BODY AWARENESS

Posture

Maintaining good posture not only reduces strain on the body but also improves mood and confidence. To support your body's alignment, try to be mindful of how you sit, stand, and move. Invest in a good mattress and a pillow that supports your neck. All this can help your body feel more at ease.

Exercise

I genuinely miss it tremendously. Before I got so sick, I was super active. Still, I believe it's essential to keep moving anyway, even—and especially—if you're low on energy. Exercise releases endorphins that boost mood, improve sleep, and reduce stress. Just go as gently as you need to. Life is movement, and movement creates energy. If we don't move enough, our muscles begin to atrophy, and every bit of muscle we can retain is an asset. While bed-bound, I did my best to stretch and flex to at least get some movement in.

Exercises that may work well for people with MCAS include walking, gentle yoga, Pilates, tai chi, or qigong. If you feel strong enough to get into resistance training, this is a good option, too. Swimming is another excellent choice, provided you have access to an unchlorinated pool or clean natural waters. Just make sure someone is with you, since people with MCAS can potentially become lightheaded or even faint in the water. Stay in the shallow area so you can stand and take breaks as needed. In their book *Die Systemische Mastzellerkrankung*, Molderings and Mücke recommend avoiding any sport that causes strong jolting or shaking of the intestines. Examples include running, horseback riding, tennis, and golf.[4]

Massages

Therapeutic bodywork can help relax our muscles and bring blood flow to areas that need it. This can be a good alternative to exercise when physical activity isn't possible. I usually bring my own oil to ensure I won't get triggered by the oil the therapist usually uses.

Craniosacral, osteopathy, and Zen-shiatsu are all gentle bodywork techniques that are done with clothing on. They require neither oil nor rubbing, so they may be a good choice because friction on the skin and oil can potentially trigger mast cell reactions.

> **KEY TAKEAWAY**
>
> Stress is a major trigger, so respecting your limits is key. Ask for help when needed, consolidate tasks to avoid overextension, emphasize nutrient-dense whole foods, and make sure you get enough rest. Gentle exercise, good posture, therapeutic bodywork, and grounding practices like breathing or humming can help ease tension.

CHAPTER 29

Reducing Mental Stress

First of all, know that things can get better. Hold onto that hope and keep it steady. Once I learned how to navigate life with MCAS, things got a lot better for me.

Also, look at what can happen to cancer patients: in some cases, cancer goes into remission and essentially disappears. I once read an article that stated only patients who believed in healing and had the will to live were able to beat the cancer—but, hey, that should be telling us something: healing is sometimes possible even if it doesn't look like it, and our mindset plays an important role!

Some people walk again after being told they never would. Others with severe vision problems have restored their eyesight to 20/20. Some people with supposedly terminal illnesses have fully healed. So, why shouldn't we also be able to feel better and recover from our ills?

To heal—or at least feel better—I believe it's essential to make an effort to feel as good as you can on as many levels as possible. Eliminating stress is crucial because any kind of stress can trigger mast cells, but also because a calm mind will allow you to focus on what you truly need, and you'll make better decisions. Below are some examples of what I've done to reduce stress in this situation.

MINDSET MATTERS

Accept the diagnosis

Once you know it's MCAS, try coming to terms with the fact that you have it. Instead of getting stuck on being upset about how hard it is to be affected, learn more about the condition and how you can help yourself feel better.

Embrace the present

Stop worrying about what other people say, think, or do. Stop comparing yourself to others. Stop worrying about what happened in the past. Stop blaming others for your circumstances. Blaming others or yourself will make you feel worse every time you do it. It never gets you out of misery and will even work against your ability to resolve the issue. Blaming is like putting wood into a fire that doesn't need to be. Focus on the present instead. Surrendering attachment and blame for the past can significantly reduce stress.

Experience the journey

You will find much helpful information on this journey. You'll inevitably learn a lot about your body—but also about people, communication, relationships, the medical system, nutrition, and everything that triggers you. You are experiencing a learning curve, and there are good things to come, no matter how it may seem. While missing out on many things, you also have the chance to delve into your own life much deeper than many other people likely ever will. You might discover a lot of valuable insights. Try to see this condition as an opportunity to grow and improve your life and health.

Cultivate compassion

Everyone is going through their own struggles, and if you could see in depth what others are dealing with, you might not want to change roles. There are millions above you and millions below you; accept where you are right now and keep moving forward.

CLEAR YOUR HEADSPACE

Limit information input

Designate specific times to check your emails, social media, and the news. Some things don't need to be done multiple times a day, and I'm telling you that every bit of energy you can save will make a difference. Instead, spend that time engaging in nourishing activities. Unsubscribe from newsletters you no longer need and cancel any outdated subscriptions, both email and physical mail.

Turn off notifications

Constant alerts on our phones clutter our headspace, even if we don't check them right away. Disabling notifications, banners, and quick alerts helps create a calmer mindset. It also lets us check messages on our own terms, when we actually have the time for it.

Build in downtime

Learn to appreciate and cherish the quiet moments. For example, leisurely savoring your favorite hot beverage while cradling the warm cup in your hands, watching a sunset, or deliberately pausing to admire a beautiful view can do a lot for your well-being.

Practice reacting less

There are many occasions in life that we have little to no control over. I'm not saying we should be completely indifferent, but rather that it's helpful to learn not to worry about things we cannot change or influence in any way, as this will free up room for us to change the things we can.

Stay centered

Whatever happens around you, do your best to stay as centered as possible. Reaching for the stillness inside you may take some practice, but it's an extremely helpful trait to foster. Being able to remain calm during emotionally stressful situations is like pure gold for those affected by MCAS.

Use weekly to-do lists

Writing things down can be an excellent tool for reducing stress because it helps free up your mind, and once you cross off what you've accomplished, you'll see that you still get stuff done. Acknowledging such little victories is vital because being so incredibly sick can make you feel utterly useless.

Because of this, I prefer weekly lists over daily ones, as I can never know how I'll feel on any given day and whether I even have the energy to accomplish anything at all. Weekly lists allow me to simply move unfinished items to another day, helping me feel less like a failure if I am too weak to complete what I had planned. Of course, you can also list all your long-term goals. Crossing off what you've accomplished is always a celebration of goals met.

FIND INNER CALM

Breathing

Paying close attention to your breath inevitably brings your focus back to the body—a powerful way to quiet the mind. When you're feeling agitated, sit and breathe for a few minutes. Breathing in and breathing out—that's all. There is tremendous power hidden in this simple exercise.

Meditation

Meditation doesn't have to mean sitting cross-legged with a straight spine and eyes closed in complete silence. And, by all means, incense is not required to reach a blissful state! Instead, meditation is about cultivating mindfulness to provide your mind and body with moments of calm. Thoughts are very powerful, and they keep our entire system busy. The object of meditation is simply stillness and connecting to the present. There are likely as many ways to reach that state as people on this planet. Maybe a gentle walk in nature, listening to beautiful music, or enjoying a hot cup of tea will do it for you.

You can try this simple exercise to experience how thoughts connect to the body: Close your eyes and feel your body—your arms, hands, belly, and chest. Now, say the word *up* and notice what happens. Return to neutral, and this time, instead, say the word *down* and notice what happens.

You most likely felt a subtle upward motion throughout your body when you said *up* and a downward motion when you said *down* to yourself. This happens because your entire system is interconnected and functions as an integrated whole. Your body anticipates the movement when you say the word—a small but noticeable physical response. That's why meditation can feel so refreshing: our constant stream of thoughts is mirrored in the body, and when we quiet the mind, even briefly, the body can begin to relax.

Look for the good

While intentionally focusing on the positive may take some willpower at first, this exercise is uplifting in every way, and before long, it feels like second nature. Keep an open mind, and you'll always learn something new.

Of course, some things are just downright bad. But once you've seen them clearly for what they are, you can make a good choice and walk away—whether it's a person, a situation, a habit, or a food you don't tolerate. In that choice, you'll have found something good: your decision to be kind to yourself.

Gratitude

Gratitude is such a powerful feeling that when you're fully immersed in it, stress has no place to stay.

KEY TAKEAWAY

A hopeful mindset can make a big difference. Viewing your diagnosis as an opportunity for growth may lighten the emotional burden. Build in downtime, limit overwhelming information, and remain flexible with tasks in case you need to rest. Meditation, mindfulness, and gratitude nurture inner stillness, while compassion toward yourself and others supports resilience.

CHAPTER 30

Optimizing Your Living Environment

Your home is your primary place to recuperate, so it's crucial to keep it trigger-free. First, identify your triggers, and then clear your home of them to ensure your safety within your dwelling. Some adjustments might be necessary, but I promise you it's worth the effort. It's so important to have a safe space where you can sleep well and recover in case you've just gone through a flare. Given the abundance of triggers in the outside world, your home is most likely the only place you can guarantee to be a trigger-free zone.

Make your home a safe refuge

You can't control the world outside, so at times your home might be the only safe place for you to be. It's essential that it feels comfortable to you, because after a bad episode, it's best to stay home and not risk any further triggers until the reactions wane.

ELIMINATE IMMEDIATELY

Scented products

Soaps, candles, laundry detergents, and cleaning products are often scented, and fragrances can trigger mast cell responses. I wholeheartedly recommend skipping incense, air fresheners, and dryer sheets altogether. Scented personal hygiene or household products, like sanitary pads, toilet paper, and garbage bags, should also be avoided.

If you don't want to toss everything, maybe donate such items to a thrift store, put them in a free box on the sidewalk, or host a giveaway party for your friends. You'll make others happy and do yourself a huge favor, too. Just one caveat: if you give these things to your friends, you'll probably still have to deal with them whenever you visit.

CHOOSE SAFE PRODUCTS

Body care

Pay attention to whether you get any reaction on your skin, eyes, or respiratory tract, or if you feel nauseous or dizzy when smelling it. I recommend scent-free, hypoallergenic products with as few ingredients as necessary.

Cleaning agents

You'll likely feel better once you switch to scent-free products. Even simply reducing your use of detergents may make a difference. I use cleaning agents only where they're truly needed: one product for lime in the bathroom, one for grease in the kitchen, plus an all-purpose cleaner and a disinfectant. I wash my laundry with a scent-free detergent and use white vinegar as a fabric softener and odor remover. I also use scent-free tabs for the dishwasher and scent-free dishwashing liquid.

INFRASTRUCTURE & MATERIALS

Mold

Mold is a potent mast cell trigger, so we need to make sure we're not exposed to it, especially in our homes. To test for mold, you can purchase a DIY mold test kit online or at a hardware store or, even better, hire a specialist to test it for you. When hiring a specialist, choose someone who doesn't also offer renovation services to ensure their assessment is unbiased and accurate.

Textiles

Many textiles, such as blankets, bedding, mattresses, carpets, couches, and so on, can have toxic components that may trigger reactions in you. It might be a good idea to replace those with natural options.

Building materials

Remember that new floors, paint, and furniture made with toxic materials, glues, or finishes may also cause reactions. Examples include vinyl flooring that emits phthalates, PVC products, and formaldehyde-containing materials such as plywood, MDF, and particleboard. Furniture and upholstery can be problematic if treated with flame retardants, water repellents, or other chemical components.

Heating systems

Some heaters can trigger mast cell reactions by emitting smells or harmful particles. The most problematic types include gas heaters, quartz tube infrared, fan heaters, oil-filled radiators, and electric convection heaters, which can also stir up dust, mold spores, and allergens.

Safer alternatives include infrared panel heaters, radiant tile heaters, hydronic radiators, central heating systems, and geothermal (earth-warmed) solutions.

Electrical appliances

Avoid electrical appliances in your bedroom. If that's not possible, at least unplug them at night. It's better than only turning them off, because they still emit electromagnetic frequencies (EMFs) even in standby mode.

Lighting

Harsh lighting can trigger mast cells. Choose comfortable lighting and avoid fluorescent lamps if you can.

CLEANING STRATEGIES

Simplify cleaning

Set your home up so it's easy to clean. Keep your surfaces clear of clutter so you can quickly dust them, and keep the floors free so you can easily mop them.

Cabinets with doors or drawers

Declutter your house because every little thing accumulates dust, and a chaotic environment is never supportive of healing. Cabinets with doors and drawers make it much easier to keep things clean, dust-free, and tidy—and they also save you a lot of time and energy when cleaning. Keeping stuff stashed away means you won't always need to clean everything.

Microfiber cleaning rags

Microfiber is highly effective at trapping dust and minimizing allergic reactions while cleaning. Regular dusting will also reduce your need for cleaning agents. I always use two rags: a wet one for the first wipe and a dry one to dry off and remove the rest of the dust. I dust all surfaces, preferably multiple times a week if I have the energy. If I don't, I try to do it at least once a week. Dust might seem insignificant, but I feel significantly better when it's clean.

Vacuum cleaner with HEPA filter

I prefer mopping over vacuuming because mopping effectively binds dust. In contrast, some vacuum cleaners blow out heaps of tiny dust particles and disperse them into the air—a recipe for disaster if you're sensitive to airborne triggers. HEPA stands for high-efficiency particulate air, and these filters are specifically designed to trap microscopically small particles.

Steam vacuums

Steam cleaners with a vacuum function are a great way to freshen upholstery and remove odors, especially from fabrics. They also cut down on the need for detergents, since the steam loosens dirt on its own.

Carpets

Carpets accumulate dust, attract dust mites, and hold onto scents. If you prefer to keep rugs, consider having them cleaned periodically. Replacing wall-to-wall carpets with alternative flooring may be worth the effort. If removal isn't an option, regular steam cleaning can help maintain cleanliness.

Curtains

Curtains accumulate dust, which can be an irritant. Wash them regularly, or use outside shutters instead.

HELPFUL HABITS

Change your bedding often

Tiny dust particles, dead skin cells, pollen, and bacteria are invisible, but they can easily aggravate the mast cells—better to keep those little guys happy, or they won't let you sleep.

Change your clothing daily

Fabrics accumulate dust, pollen, scents, and sweat. Get out of contaminated garments as soon as possible. For example, if someone who wore perfume hugged you (which unfortunately does happen), you'll feel better in a fresh set of clothes. Since scents cling to fabrics, I always change upon coming home, especially after being out in public.

Air out your place often

Airing out your home regularly reduces air pollution, enhances oxygen, gets rid of smells, and prevents condensation, which can cause mold inside houses. Just make sure to do it when the air outside is clean and fresh.

UPGRADE WHEN POSSIBLE

Water filters

Good water filters remove harmful contaminants such as lead, pesticides, and chlorine from the water, which are all potential mast cell triggers. I've heard of mast cell patients who lived in an area with bad water quality and used to get reactions simply from the water in the shower. Once they installed a good filter, their symptoms improved.

Air filters

Air filters are designed to help remove harmful indoor air contaminants such as fungi, mold, viruses, dust, and allergens, all of which may potentially trigger mast cells.

Dishwasher

A dishwasher will be a great aid if you're dealing with inflammation, fatigue, or time pressure. If there is a machine designed to do a job that you would have to do daily anyway, why not use it? Our energy is often so limited that every bit of relief is helpful. Additionally, it's common that we react to smells, so leaving your dirty dishes out can potentially trigger the mast cells again.

Food processor

Most of us deal with inflammation repeatedly. This can make cooking difficult because some days, our hands might hurt so much that even holding an object is nearly impossible—let alone cutting, grating, or mashing! A good food processor that does the grating, chopping, and blending for you saves time, energy, and strength.

For a quick reference, you'll find a *Safe Home Checklist* in the backmatter of this book.

KEY TAKEAWAY

Your home should be your trigger-free sanctuary. Eliminate scented products, test for mold, and check textiles, building materials, and heating systems. Use non-harsh lighting and avoid electrical appliances in the bedroom. Keep your home decluttered and dust-free with a HEPA-filter vacuum and regular washing of fabrics. Air out your place frequently, but only when outdoor air is clean, and consider buying air and water filters, along with supportive appliances to conserve energy.

CHAPTER 31

Improving Sleep

Sleep is tremendously important to our overall well-being. It is a vital part of the recovery process, protects our mental and physical health, and dramatically affects how we feel while we're awake. What we do during our waking hours in turn affects how we sleep, and if we don't manage to get a handle on our sleep patterns, it can quickly turn into a vicious cycle. Sleep deprivation can even be linked to an increase in inflammation.[89]

When your body is in agony, it can be very difficult to get good rest. For example, if your skin is itchy and burning to the point where you might wish you could just take it off, it's of course challenging to wind down. The same goes for any pain. Other times, it's hard to fall asleep because maybe you felt so weak during the day that you finally didn't move around very much, so your body simply isn't tired enough to sleep. Sleep and wakefulness are intrinsically interconnected. Insomnia is awful for anyone, even for otherwise healthy individuals, but it's even worse for those affected with a disease like this because it very likely intensifies all our other symptoms.

The two years before my diagnosis were grueling, as I could rarely sleep more than three hours per night. My sleep improved after I split from my ex-husband and moved into my own apartment, but mast cell reactions still prevented restful sleep until I identified my triggers and learned how to manage them. I also researched how to improve sleep quality. Nowadays, I usually sleep well by using my gathered clues and sticking to effective strategies. The following solutions have helped me improve my sleep.

CORE SLEEP HABITS

Create a bedroom sanctuary

Your bedroom should feel peaceful, relaxing, safe, and comfortable. Keep work-related items like your cell phone and computer in another room to support that. As for televisions, they emit everything but calm. I wholeheartedly recommend keeping them out of the bedroom.

Consider using mellow lighting and maybe even painting the walls in a color that feels soothing to you. For example, blue is said to be calming, while green is said to be rejuvenating. White or purple could work well, too. It's probably best to avoid bright and invigorating colors such as red and yellow because they stimulate our nervous system to be more alert, creative, and productive.[90] And as a note of caution: If you decide to paint your bedroom, make sure to use certified non-toxic paint.

If you tolerate them, you could make use of essential oils. Melissa (lemon balm) and lavender can be calming by placing a few drops into a small bowl of water near your bed.[91,92] However, I'd like to note that with MCAS, I often start reacting to scents after longer exposure, even to the ones I initially tolerated.

Mind your triggers

You could react to the fabric of the sheets, the material of the mattress, your blankets and pillows, or even your pajamas. Natural materials are less likely to cause reactions. I use a non-toxic mattress made from natural materials, pure cotton sheets, a down comforter, and down pillows with a dust mite-proof casing.

Remember that even building materials and furniture can cause reactions. Vinyl flooring, carpets, off-gassing glues or finishes, formaldehyde-containing furniture, or water damage inside walls might trigger your mast cells. Airborne pollutants coming through your window could be another cause. Keeping your bedroom clean and scent-free is a must, and avoiding any lights while trying to sleep also helps greatly.

Change your bedding frequently

Sheets accumulate dust, oil, sweat, dead skin cells, and pollen. If I have enough energy, I change my bedding twice a week because I sleep so much better in fresh bedding.

Reduce screen time before bed

Before bedtime, it's crucial to log off and avoid screens for at least one to two hours. The short-wavelength blue light of monitors and tech screens interferes with our circadian rhythm. Blue light is stimulating, and the movements on the screen make us more alert by signaling the body for readiness. However, exposure to these wavelengths in the evening makes it much harder to fall asleep and can significantly reduce overall sleep quality. If you cannot avoid screens in the evenings, use programs that filter these lights (blue light blocker/nighttime settings) or wear blue light-blocking amber-lensed glasses.[93]

Turn off electrical devices

Electromagnetic frequencies can affect sleep negatively. Electric home appliances emit electromagnetic radiation in low and high frequencies (ELF/EMF). Wi-Fi and other wireless devices, microwave ovens, cordless telephones, refrigerators, and air conditioning compressors all emit these frequencies. Your bed shouldn't be placed near such devices—not even on the other side of a wall from an ELF/EMF source. It might also be a good idea to turn off the Wi-Fi inside your apartment during sleep time.[94,95]

Air out the room before you sleep

Fresh air promotes better sleep, so air out the room before you go to sleep—or keep the windows cracked during the night if it's safe and there aren't high levels of noise, light, or pollution in your area.[96]

Keep your feet warm

If you notice your feet are cold, putting on warm socks can help you fall asleep faster. When your feet are cold, your body automatically increases blood flow to warm them up. However, during the transition to sleep, our bodies typically slow down. So, if your body suddenly starts pumping more blood again, you'll likely feel restless simply because of this additional energy expenditure.[97]

Mind the room temperature

Maintaining a comfortable temperature in your bedroom is crucial for quality sleep. Studies suggest that the optimal room temperature for sleep falls between 60°F and 72°F (15.6°C and 22°C), with many experts agreeing that temperatures around 60.8°F to 64.4°F (16°C to 18°C) are ideal. You could also try silk sheets, as they help regulate body temperature.

Catnaps improve energy and alertness

While sleeping for several hours during the day can make it challenging to get good rest at night, a nap of as little as twenty minutes early in the day can help you be more alert without adversely impacting your sleep.[98]

Get early sunlight exposure

Getting natural light in the mornings helps regulate your circadian rhythm. For best results, expose your skin and eyes to the light without wearing sunglasses. Even just a few minutes of natural light can make a difference.[99]

HELPFUL TOOLS

Grounding sheets

The science of grounding/earthing products is still preliminary, but many users report remarkable improvements in sleep quality and, in some cases, significant reductions in pain and inflammation.

Weighted blankets

Although research on weighted blankets is still in its early stages, existing studies and user reports suggest they may help with falling asleep faster, improving sleep quality, reducing stress and anxiety, and potentially even boosting our mood by promoting relaxation through deep-pressure stimulation.

SUPPLEMENTS

Melatonin: the darkness hormone

Close the shutters and use good lightproof curtains in your bedroom to ensure it's pitch dark when you sleep, especially in areas with bright streetlights. If you must use an alarm clock, try to find one without a light.

Melatonin, often called the *"sleep hormone"* or sometimes the *"hormone of darkness,"* is created in the pineal gland. As these names suggest, melatonin plays a crucial role in regulating sleep by acting as a biological clock, signaling the body when it's time to sleep in response to darkness. Bright lights at night can interfere with melatonin secretion.

Melatonin also exhibits protective effects in treating some neurodegenerative disorders and is known to have antioxidant, anti-inflammatory, anticoagulation, and endothelial-protective effects. Additionally, it aids with pro-inflammatory cytokine inhibition.[100]

A melatonin supplement can improve sleep onset and quality and is generally considered safe. A theory goes that long-term supplementation can lead to even worse insomnia because the body stops reacting to not only the supplement itself but also to the melatonin produced naturally, but I couldn't find any scientific evidence supporting that claim. However, you shouldn't take melatonin supplements during the day, as they can result in fatigue, drowsiness, and diminished performance a few hours later.[101]

Further below, I mention certain foods that contain relatively high melatonin and/or tryptophan levels. Consuming these regularly may help you sleep better, but their sleep-enhancing effect could also be due to their relatively high content of vitamins and minerals.

Magnesium supplements

Magnesium can help improve sleep by optimizing blood pressure and circulation, balancing blood sugar levels, reducing pain, promoting muscle relaxation, and calming the nervous system.[102,103]

FOOD & SLEEP

Tea before bedtime

A cup of herbal tea before bed, such as chamomile, hops, valerian, or passion-flower, can have beneficial effects on sleep.

Chamomile

Chamomile is calming and helps diminish muscle spasms and rheumatic pain. It can also aid with anxiety, sleeplessness, and gastrointestinal conditions. Members of the self-help groups reported that a cup of chamomile tea before bed eased their skin reactions, resulting in less redness and itching. Some studies have also proposed that it prevents histamine release from mast cells.[104,105]

Since chamomile can be contaminated with pollen from other plants, people who react to pollen or members of the daisy family might experience adverse reactions to chamomile.[106]

Hops

Hops tea benefits sleep and helps diminish nocturnal activity.[107] Beer also contains hops, but it's high in histamine and contains alcohol, so it's best avoided—especially before bedtime.

Valerian root

Valerian is typically consumed as tea, extract, or as a supplement and is generally considered safe for improving sleep onset and quality.[108] However, it can enhance the effect of sedatives and anesthesia, and it may interact with certain drugs that are broken down by the same liver enzymes as valerian, including antihistamines, antifungal medications, and statins.[109] I've found that valerian helps exceptionally well when combined in a supplement with hops.

Passionflower

In traditional herbal medicine, passionflower is sometimes used to treat anxiety and insomnia. Clinical studies of passionflower showed weaknesses, and it has been suggested that new clinical trials should be conducted. Nevertheless, the plant is believed to have a reasonably good safety profile, and its sleep-enhancing qualities have been confirmed in animal studies.[110,111]

As stated in Beaufort Memorial Health Library, no studies have examined the effects of passionflower on children, so do not give passionflower to a child without a doctor's supervision, and don't use it if you are pregnant or breastfeeding. Furthermore, passionflower can enhance the effects of certain blood-thinning medications and may boost the impact and the side effects of monoamine oxidase inhibitors (MAOIs).[112]

FOODS TO AVOID

What you eat also matters greatly when it comes to improving your sleep quality! Eating the wrong foods in the evening can quickly interfere with your sleep, and your overall daily diet plays an important role, too. Caffeine, deep-fried foods, alcohol, cheese, and spicy foods should all be limited—and ideally completely avoided before bedtime.

High sugar and saturated fat intake have been associated with lighter, and consequently generally less restorative, sleep. Carbohydrate and/or protein deficiencies are also linked to shorter sleep durations. Furthermore, diets that are low in fat and high in carbohydrates are also associated with reduced sleep quality compared to diets high in fat and low in carbohydrates.[113]

FOODS TO EMPHASIZE

Foods rich in tryptophan and melatonin

Certain foods, such as barley, rice, walnuts, olives, and tomatoes, contain melatonin and its precursor, tryptophan. Research shows that consuming these foods can increase melatonin levels in the bloodstream, although this may be due to their high mineral and vitamin content rather than the melatonin itself.

Animal studies show that magnesium, zinc, polyunsaturated fatty acids, and

B vitamins are important for melatonin production. Deficiencies in these nutrients cause melatonin levels to drop. Additionally, deficiencies in DHA have been shown to reduce nocturnal melatonin secretion, while supplementation restores the levels to normal.

While this connection is less studied in humans, there are some findings: one study in children (aged eighteen months to eight years) found that intravenous vitamin B6 (pyridoxine) doubled melatonin levels. However, a small study in adults showed that taking B6 orally had no effect.[114]

Sleep-enhancing foods

Cherries, especially cherry juice, are known to help increase melatonin and reduce inflammation. Regularly eating kiwifruit promotes better sleep.[115] Maca, a root vegetable from the Andes, is high in potassium, calcium, and fatty acids and can also promote better sleep. Barley grass powder may have similar effects, likely due to its magnesium, calcium, GABA, and B-vitamin content. Walnuts may also help improve sleep due to their notable amounts of serotonin, melatonin, and total polyphenols.[116]

Another option is "night milk," a special type of milk obtained from cows milked in the dark. It contains more melatonin than regular milk. Dietary tryptophan also supports better sleep. While it's often associated with turkey, tryptophan is also found in chicken, eggs, grass-fed beef, rolled oats, beans, and lentils.[117,118]

MY FAVORITE REMEDY

When I am tired AND wide awake

My favorite go-to remedy when I am ready to sleep but just can't fall asleep is to get up again, head to the kitchen, and cook a bowl of white rice. I eat it steaming hot, drizzled with a bit of canola oil. While I have no scientific evidence to back this method, it has unfailingly worked to knock me out within minutes.

It's important to go back to bed immediately after eating this meal because waiting more than twenty minutes would likely result in a surge of energy that could keep you awake for several more hours. Although this approach is based purely on personal experience, research does suggest that consuming a high glycemic index carbohydrate meal around four hours before bedtime may help you fall asleep faster.[113]

KEY TAKEAWAY

Sleep is often disrupted by mast cell reactions. Improve sleep quality by creating a soothing, trigger-free bedroom. Wash bedding frequently, air out the room before sleep, and keep it around 61–65°F. Avoid screens before bed and get early morning sunlight to support your circadian rhythm, and skip caffeine, alcohol, sugar, and spicy foods in the evening. Nutrient-dense foods, calming teas, supplements, grounding sheets, or weighted blankets may further enhance sleep.

CHAPTER 32

Taking Showers and Baths

It's mind-boggling that something as ordinary as taking a shower can suddenly require adjustments. Yet, with this disease, even the most common day-to-day tasks can become challenging, and we've got to find new ways to deal with life on so many levels.

Shortly after receiving my diagnosis, I moved to a new apartment that had a shower but no bathtub. One day, one of my vertebrae dislocated, and I had to resort to an emergency visit with my doctor. He worked on my back for an hour, trying to adjust it, but the muscles had become so tense that he couldn't get the vertebra back in. Finally, he did some dry needling so the muscles would eventually relax. After this session, I decided to walk home because walking can help loosen things up.

It was early winter, with temperatures around freezing. When I arrived home, I decided to take a hot shower. However, as if my day hadn't been challenging enough already, the boiler wasn't working that day, and there was no hot water in my house!

At this point, I figured it would probably be even better to take a hot bath instead, so I went to a friend's house to use his tub. I took a long, hot bath, letting my back unwind in this soothing heat. It felt wonderful—until I came out of the bathroom and unexpectedly almost fainted!

Within seconds, everything started to spin. I was drenched in sweat, my heart pounding wildly, and I got so incredibly dizzy that I could only flop onto a chair in front of the open window and breathe the cold winter air. That poor friend of mine must have felt so helpless, because I was completely unable to explain to him what was happening to me or tell him how he could have assisted. Besides, I didn't even understand what was happening to me. All I could see were smears of colors floating around the room, and all I could do was wait until this roller coaster stopped. It took about an hour until I was steady enough to walk home.

Arriving at my house, utterly exhausted, I went to bed immediately. I was lying there, ready to drift off to sleep, when suddenly this incredible pain started surging through my muscles, just like how muscles ache sometimes when you have the flu. This phenomenon lasted for the rest of the night and a few days afterward.

When I finally asked in the self-help group what might have happened, I got at least twenty answers, all saying that my bath was *too hot* and caused a reaction. Following are a few helpful insights I've learned since then.

HELPFUL HABITS

Find the right water temperature

Both too hot and too cold can potentially cause reactions. It seems to be more common that people react to heat rather than cold, but everyone is different, so you'll have to see what works best for you.

Take shorter showers

Experts recommend keeping showers brief; they should last only a few minutes to prevent your skin from losing too much moisture. Dry skin can intensify skin-related symptoms. Baths shouldn't last much longer than it takes for your fingers and toes to wrinkle.

Choose body care products carefully

To determine whether a product has a negative effect on you, pay attention to how it feels on your skin and whether its scent gives you a headache, irritates your eyes or airways, or makes you feel nauseous or dizzy.

Be deliberate about soap

Limit the use of soap to the areas that need it: your private parts, armpits, feet, hands, and face. Our arms and legs don't produce as much oil, so warm water is usually sufficient to clean them.

Use a clean towel

Towels can be germ magnets; let your towel dry thoroughly after each use, and change it often. Also, be sure to wash your towels with a laundry detergent you don't react to, and don't use dryer sheets.

Pat yourself dry

Patting yourself dry is gentler on the skin than rubbing. Friction can trigger the mast cells, and rubbing can dry out your skin and potentially even damage it.

Apply moisturizer, ointment, or cream

Moisturizing your skin after a shower will help lessen reactions by keeping it soft and well-nourished. Dry, crackly skin is more prone to irritation.

MOLD & MAINTENANCE

Mold in the bathroom

Mold spores proliferate in moist environments and are a major trigger for mast cells. Bathrooms are particularly vulnerable, so airing out the bathroom after each shower can help reduce moisture buildup and prevent mold growth.

If mold does appear on non-porous surfaces, bleach can kill it. However, bleach is toxic when combined with specific other cleaning agents, and its fumes can cause significant irritation to the eyes, mouth, and throat. Never mix bleach with ammonia or other cleaners. If you need to bleach out your bathroom, it's best to have someone else do it for you. Leave the house until the job is done and only return once it's been aired out properly.

If you have to do it yourself, take precautions: wear a mask, gloves, and preferably safety goggles to protect your skin and eyes. Open the windows first. Instead of using a spray bottle, carefully put the bleach directly onto a rag and apply it to the moldy areas. Leave the bathroom promptly to avoid inhaling the fumes. Let the bleach soak in for a few minutes before rinsing it off. Lastly, dry everything thoroughly.

Wash the rags right away so the smell won't irritate you later. Wash them separately to avoid staining your other laundry, or use old rags you can throw out. If you toss them, take the trash out immediately to avoid getting triggered by the smell whenever you open it.

Showerheads

Make sure your showerhead is clean. Since showerheads are constantly damp, they are a perfect breeding ground for mold and harmful bacteria. Replacing it with a new one may be worthwhile if yours is old.

KEY TAKEAWAY

Even showering can be challenging with MCAS. Use scent-free products, keep water at a comfortable temperature, and keep showers brief. Always use a clean towel, pat skin dry instead of rubbing, and moisturize afterward to prevent irritation. A mold-free bathroom is essential!

CHAPTER 33

Body Care Products

Finding the right body care is essential to feeling better. Sometimes we don't even realize a product affects us negatively until we stop using it for a while. Taking a break can bring clarity—once you reintroduce the product, it's often easier to tell if it has an adverse effect. This can be true even for people without MCAS.

Now, body care products—if you start looking into the ingredients some companies put in their stuff, you might be surprised. All those complicated words on the ingredient lists can be looked up in a Cosmetic Ingredient Dictionary. The first time I did this, long before I knew of mast cell issues, I tossed almost everything I had at my house. Some of the ingredients were outrageously toxic. After that, I mostly used all-natural personal care products for years—but nowadays, even these can be a trigger!

CORE GUIDELINES

Scent-free and safe ingredients

Finding scent-free products is undoubtedly a good first step. Additionally, some mast cell patients may be triggered by salicylates, which are often found in personal hygiene and cleaning products.

Hypoallergenic options

Ask your pharmacist for hypoallergenic products with minimal ingredients. Less, indeed, can be more. Many pharmacies offer samples, allowing you to test a product before purchasing a whole bottle so you don't end up spending money on something you can't use.

Adverse reactions

Signs of an adverse reaction could include rashes, flushing, itching, nausea from the smell, dizziness after use, a burning sensation in the eyes, and irritation in the throat.

Shared environment

Remember that everyone in your household should follow the same guidelines. Even if you carefully choose safe products, exposure to your partner's or family member's products can still trigger reactions. A shared commitment to scent-free body care helps create a truly safe environment.

I'm not sponsored, but I'll share the products I've used for several years without any adverse reactions. While they might work well for you, it's important to remember that everybody reacts differently. However, I hope this can provide a helpful starting point for your product research.

WHAT WORKS FOR ME

Splat toothpaste

Splat is simply the best toothpaste I've ever used, and I highly recommend it. Its ingredients include plant enzymes, bioactive calcium, and charcoal. Their toothpaste gets your teeth super clean while protecting and restoring the enamel, unlike many other all-natural oral care products that clean your teeth but also erode the enamel. I also tolerate Parodontax, a sentiment echoed by others in the self-help community.

Avène skin care products

Great company for soap, shower oil and gel, facial cleanser, face cream, body milk, sunscreen, and thermal water spray. Avène is a village in southern France, with a thermal water spring called Sainte-Odile dating back to the 1700s.

I am so grateful to have found their hypoallergenic line, because not only do I not react to these products, but they also help make my skin feel better. The thermal water spray helps soothe my skin more quickly than any other product or medicinal ointment I've used—it reduces redness and stops itching within minutes! That said, I only tolerate their hypoallergenic products (not others), but I swear by them.

Weleda

I'm okay with some Weleda products, like the Arnica Shower Gel, but I react to others.

Free & Clear hair care

It took me a long time to find shampoo and conditioner that are free and clear of perfumes, fragrances, and substances that can cause reactions, and I'm happy with them. In her book *My Crazy Life: A Humorous Guide to Understanding Mast Cell Disorders,* Pam Hodge shares that she's also using the company's shower gels and soaps.

Innersense hair care

I also tolerate the hypoallergenic line from Innersense. Their products are on the pricier side, but for lovely curls, they're worth it.

Moisturizers

Some members of the self-help groups use jojoba and vitamin E oil for moisturizing. I recently found a cream called Rovectin Skin Essentials Barrier Repair Cream, a scent-free moisturizer that feels amazing on my skin.

Deodorants

Here's a tip from my friend Ellie, who also suffers from mast cell issues: she makes her own deodorant by diluting food-grade hydrogen peroxide (3%) in a spray bottle. It helps kill the bacteria that cause body odor without relying on fragrances or irritating ingredients. After spraying it on, she applies a small amount of moisturizer to soothe and moisturize the skin. Even diluted 3% hydrogen peroxide can irritate sensitive skin, so always patch-test first.

UNDERSTANDING INGREDIENTS

Cosmetic ingredient dictionary

Being vigilant about the ingredients in body care products is crucial, especially for highly sensitive individuals. If you come across terms you don't understand, you can look them up in the *Cosmetic Ingredient Dictionary,* an online resource that explains the function and safety of cosmetic ingredients (https://cosmeticsinfo.org/Ingredient-dictionary).

Salicylates

Dr. Tania Dempsey's website offers an overview of salicylate sensitivity, including where they are found and what to avoid (https://drtaniadempsey.com/salicylate-sensitivity/).

KEY TAKEAWAY

Body care should be hypoallergenic and scent-free, since both synthetic and natural products can cause reactions. Request samples before buying, and watch for warning signs such as nausea, flushing, or throat and eye irritation. Use a Cosmetic Ingredient Dictionary to check unfamiliar terms, and be mindful of salicylates, which are common in hygiene products. For safety, all household members should follow the same guidelines.

CHAPTER 34

Clothing and Fabrics

It took me quite some time to realize that using and wearing the right fabrics greatly affects how I feel. Some days, I felt awfully fatigued, but when I came home and changed my clothes, I felt better: I could suddenly breathe more easily and feel my energy return.

Finally, I recognized that I felt decidedly better when wearing clothing made of 100 percent cotton or pure linen. Other natural fabrics include bamboo, hemp, flax, and silk. Calico is an unbleached, undyed fabric made from 100 percent cotton, which makes it less likely to cause allergic reactions in highly sensitive individuals. Semi-synthetic fabrics such as modal and lyocell could also be good options.

After coming to this realization, I sorted out my wardrobe, eliminated any synthetic blends, and replaced them with clothing made of natural materials. This simple change alone resulted in significant overall improvement!

HIDDEN TRIGGERS IN CLOTHING

Synthetic fabrics

Any kind of fabric can be an irritant due to friction on the skin, but clothes made with synthetics such as spandex, polyester, rayon, nylon, and rubber are more likely to cause reactions. These textiles prevent the skin from breathing and increase sweating, which can also be a trigger. Friction can aggravate skin problems, so one thing you can do is to wear loosely fitting clothing that lets your skin breathe and doesn't constrict you in any way. Even just removing tags can help a lot.

Dyes and chemicals

It's also possible that dyes, glues, and chemicals such as p-phenylenediamine (PPD) and formaldehyde resins, which are sometimes used to make fabrics waterproof, wrinkle-free, or resistant to shrinkage, could be the culprits that cause reactions.[119]

Some mast cell patients reported using only non-dyed clothing because they react so much to dyes. I learned that the brighter the colors are, the more likely they've used harsher chemicals in the dyes. It is recommended to wash new clothing four to five times before wearing it.

WHAT YOU CAN DO

Test different fabrics

Just try it out for yourself! Put on a loosely fitted cotton shirt and keep it on for some time. Later the same day, switch to something made of synthetic fabrics or something tight and compare how you feel in each one. For me, the difference is enormous—I feel my energy crash pretty much instantly. I know they say we all react differently, but many other MCAS patients have also stated that pure cotton is their preference.

Check labels

When buying clothes, look for allergen signals. If any of the following are mentioned on the tag, consider skipping the purchase: wrinkle-resistant, permanent press, colorfast, stain-resistant, flame retardant, or wash separately. If these fabrics aren't touching your skin directly, it might not be a problem. However, if you have ongoing skin reactions and you're still wearing such fabrics, it might be worth putting them aside to see if you notice any improvement.

Seamless underwear

Switching to seamless underwear has helped me tremendously! The friction from that little seam on the bra and undies always caused rashes, which would intensify many other symptoms like heart palpitations, flushing, and exhaustion. Oh, it made me feel almost crazy for a while!

To get some relief, I initially just turned my underwear inside out to avoid this stupid friction. But who on earth wants to wear their underwear inside out? Not me—and probably not you. Naturally, I sought a better solution and eventually found perfectly comfortable seamless panties from Sloggi's Zero Feel line. Since getting these, the rash around my hips has disappeared, and with it, many of my other symptoms calmed down a notch.

Every little bit of improvement makes a difference, but wearing the right kind of clothing was a game-changer for me! Keep in mind that your bedding material is just as important as your clothing.

> **KEY TAKEAWAY**
>
> Natural fabrics like cotton, linen, bamboo, and silk are usually safest—synthetics may trap heat and moisture that may trigger reactions. Dyes, glues, and chemical treatments like flame-retardants may also cause problems. Wash new clothing several times before wearing, and choose loose, breathable, and seamless options to reduce friction. Bedding and sofas should also be made from natural, non-irritating materials.

CHAPTER 35

Laundry

Washing laundry is usually a no-brainer, but if your mast cells have gone mad, you must be extra careful. There are a few things I have learned about doing the laundry, which greatly helped me lessen my reactions. Since I began applying these methods, my skin is less itchy and less prone to rashes, my eyes don't sting and burn so much, my stomach feels better, and my throat is less inflamed. Additionally, both the feeling of dizziness and my overall energy have improved.

DETERGENTS & ALTERNATIVES

Detergents

Use a dye-free, fragrance-free, hypoallergenic laundry detergent. You can get such products in pharmacies, health food stores, or buy them online. Some stores have them in the baby section. If you desperately want fragrance in your laundry, you can find an essential oil you tolerate and add a few drops to your detergent.

Fabric softeners

Avoid fabric softeners and dryer sheets. These products often contain a mix of synthetic fragrances, preservatives, and chemicals like silicones, which can transfer onto your skin and be absorbed into your body simply by wearing treated clothing. Even "natural" or "eco-friendly" options may still contain irritants.

Alternatives: baking soda or white vinegar

If you live in an area with hard water, try adding baking soda or white vinegar during the washing cycle. These work like fabric softeners, without the chemicals and fragrances. Both baking soda and vinegar also neutralize odors, and vinegar additionally prevents colors from fading. However, be careful not to inhale the vinegar fumes, as they can cause irritation.

HELPFUL HABITS

Hygiene program

Many modern washing machines have a hygiene or drum-cleaning program. Running this cycle from time to time helps remove detergent buildup, mold, and odors inside the washer. I now always run it before washing my clothes, especially when using a shared machine.

Make sure the washing machine is clean

If the machine you use isn't clean, or even moldy, the substances will wash right into your clothes and can be very difficult to get rid of. You may have to stick your head into the machine to inspect the inside thoroughly. Mold can also cling to the door seal, which is a concern for dishwashers as well, and detergent residue can accumulate in the soap compartment and drum—both of which can cause reactions.

Cleaning the washing machine

While wearing a mask and, ideally, eye protection to minimize contact with the fumes, use a cleaning agent specifically designed for washing machines to soak and rinse the soap compartment and wipe down the laundry drum, door, and door seal. Next, put the remaining detergent into the soap compartment and do one empty run at a high temperature.

These washing machine cleansers are designed to remove detergent residues, odors, and microorganisms that are usually not eliminated at lower temperatures. Although this is quite a bit of extra work, it's ultimately easier and saves a lot of time, money, and frustration, because having reactions to your own clothing is like wearing a trigger suit!

Use an extra rinse

Many washers have an "extra rinse" setting, which helps remove detergent residues and smells from your clothes after the wash.

Remove scents and mold from clothing

If your clothes have been exposed to mold or scented detergents, you could soak them in a vinegar solution for a few hours and then wash them out. Be sure to wear a mask when doing this, not only because of the mold but also because the fumes of the vinegar can potentially trigger a reaction.

One time, I washed my clothes in a machine that had just been used with a scented detergent. As a result, I had severe reactions to my clothing and finally had to wash my stuff eight times to get these smells out. Since then, I always clean the machine before using it.

Hang-dry your clothes to prevent static

Maybe this is minor, but I've noticed that less static charge in my clothing also means less irritation on the skin. Hanging clothes to dry should only be done in well-ventilated areas to avoid condensation and, thus, also mold. The best option is to dry your clothing outside in the fresh air.

> **KEY TAKEAWAY**
>
> For laundry, use fragrance-free, hypoallergenic detergents, and replace fabric softeners and dryer sheets with baking soda or diluted white vinegar. Keep your washing machine clean to prevent mold and detergent residue, and run an extra rinse to remove irritants. When possible, hang clothes to dry in fresh air to reduce static that may trigger reactions.

CHAPTER 36

Getting the Itching Under Control

The first and most helpful step for me in controlling this unbearably intense itching was to take quite heavy doses of antihistamines. After several months of testing, I received my diagnosis and was finally allowed to take antihistamines. I couldn't take them during the testing phase, as they could have skewed the results. Initially, I was advised to take two pills per day, which I then had to increase to four pills per day to alleviate the itching. While it didn't completely resolve the issue, it helped improve my symptoms to the point where I could finally sleep again.

The downside to taking so many pills is that pretty much all medications come with side effects, and as helpful as they are, they usually tax our bodies in other ways. I inevitably noticed the pharmacists' astonishment when they saw how many of those pills I was instructed to take. They always asked how on earth I could stand the drowsiness, to which I would reply that I was just glad I could finally sleep again! I mean, I had barely slept more than two hours a night in the two years before my diagnosis, and I was desperate to catch up on rest. Fexofenadine is a third-generation antihistamine known for its minimal impact on drowsiness, but taking four pills per day definitely made me sleepier.

So, antihistamines are an integral part of MCAS treatment and help reduce itching, but proactive measures can address the issue at earlier stages and potentially even prevent the reactions in the first place.

THE BASICS

Keep your environment trigger-free

- Change your clothing daily
- Change your bedding at least once a week
- Keep your apartment clean and dust-free
- Use an unscented, allergy-friendly laundry detergent
- Wear clothing (fabrics) that won't trigger you
- Eat a histamine-free diet
- Use good-quality cookware, pans, and utensils
- Use a good mattress made from natural materials
- Get mite-free pillowcases, blankets, and mattress covers

Take care of your skin

- Moisturize your skin often, or at least after you get out of the shower
- Use unscented, hypoallergenic body care products
- Avoid hot showers and baths. Warm is okay, but too warm can be a trigger

Breathe deeply, and don't scratch!

I've woken up with bloody sheets and scratches all over my skin, too. I know all too well how it feels. Just remember that the scratching itself will trigger the mast cells even more. It takes willpower and determination—but try to breathe through it. It's worth the effort!

SOOTHING SKIN REACTIONS

Antihistamines

Zyrtec (cetirizine), Benadryl (diphenhydramine), Claritin (loratadine), Allegra (fexofenadine), and Clarinex (desloratadine) help reduce itchy skin.[47]

Mast cell stabilizers

Mast cell inhibitors like cromolyn sodium or quercetin can help prophylactically control mast cell activity, resulting in less itching due to reduced mast cell reactivity.

Other medications

Some medications, like prednisone, have also reportedly helped reduce itching.

Skin ointments

Topical medications like Benadryl, corticosteroid creams, and cromolyn sodium lotions can relieve symptoms. I store them in the refrigerator so that, in addition to the soothing active ingredients, the coolness of the lotion upon application offers immediate relief.[47]

Fresh aloe masks

I have found that aloe masks can help soothe itching. Aloe is high in salicylates and some people react to it, so it's advisable to test it on a small patch of skin first. Finding what works for you often involves trial and error. I apply this remedy when the hives have already broken out. I use fresh aloe leaves, cut out the flesh, blend it in a blender, and rub the gel over the affected area twenty to thirty minutes before showering.

Cabbage leaves

Cool cabbage leaves can serve as soothing compresses for irritated skin. Store them in the fridge and rotate them when a leaf gets warm.

Witch hazel

Some members of the MCAS self-help groups have reported that witch hazel has helped them calm their skin reactions.

Thermal water sprays

This is my personal favorite remedy for itching, as it has worked wonders for me! When someone first told me about this, I thought it sounded like complete nonsense. However, since I couldn't possibly focus on anything else due to that burning pain, which drove me absolutely nuts, I finally gave it a try and quickly realized that it really does work.

I use "Eau Thermale" from Avène, which you can buy in a big, medium, or small travel-sized bottle. I keep a big bottle at home and always carry a small one with me whenever I get a reaction while I'm out. It usually takes the itching down within minutes.

Other things that might help

- Avoid dietary triggers and foods you're allergic to
- Avoid histamine-rich and histamine-liberating foods
- Include foods with mast cell–stabilizing properties
- Drink lots of water
- Drink chamomile tea (if tolerated)
- Baths with chamomile extract
- Baths with baking soda (short term)
- Baths with lactic acid
- Alkalizing baths
- Cool compresses
- Cold packs (too cold can be a trigger)
- Compresses with yogurt
- Stay calm

KEY TAKEAWAY

For itching, antihistamines can help, but often come with side effects, so preventive measures are key. Keep your environment clean, change clothing and bedding regularly, and use hypoallergenic detergents and products. Nourish your skin, follow a low-histamine diet, and consider mast cell stabilizers. Avoid scratching, breathe through the discomfort, and try supportive options like topical creams, thermal water sprays, soothing masks, cool compresses, or tolerated baths. Staying well hydrated and calm can further ease symptoms.

CHAPTER 37

Calming Reactions in the GI Tract

The most vital step in managing your GI symptoms is to determine which foods you don't tolerate so that you can avoid them.

Identifying trigger foods

In the beginning, it's helpful to keep a food diary to determine which foods you react to. Write down everything you eat, with the time and date—then follow up with how you feel.

Remember that some allergic reactions to foods can be delayed by hours or even days after ingestion, making it challenging to pinpoint the specific trigger. Keeping a food journal can help you identify patterns and determine your triggers.

For myself, a water fast has been the most effective way to reset and identify what I can tolerate. I feel it helped clear my body of any lingering irritants in the digestive tract that might have contributed to reactions, allowing me to start from a clean slate. This approach has been invaluable in helping me identify my trigger foods. Once you've been symptom-free for a while, you can start reintroducing foods one by one. This way, you'll quickly notice if a food triggers a reaction in you. If you attempt a prolonged fast, it is best to do it under medical supervision.

IMMEDIATE RELIEF FOR GI REACTIONS

Calming down an immediate reaction can be done by medications like Benadryl or prednisone, but I've personally never tolerated any of these pills, so I had to find alternatives. My personal emergency protocol includes:

- *Boswellia serrata* extract
- Stomach acid–resistant peppermint oil capsules
- Antihistamines
- Chamomile tea
- Water

When I notice a reaction to food coming on, I immediately take two or three pills of *Boswellia serrata* extract. *Boswellia serrata* is a potent anti-inflammatory believed to possess mast cell–stabilizing properties. Additionally, I take two capsules of stomach acid–resistant peppermint oil, which effectively alleviates bloating. Peppermint is high in salicylates, and although I do react to salicylates, the positive effect clearly outweighs the negative in this case.

I take additional antihistamines, drink plenty of water to help move things along, and drink lots of tea. Ginger tea for its anti-inflammatory and pain-relieving benefits, and chamomile tea for its anti-inflammatory, antispasmodic, and carminative properties. Chamomile is a digestive relaxant and aids in the treatment of stomach cramps, indigestion, diarrhea, flatulence, vomiting, and nausea. Chamomile's bioactive ingredients include flavonoids such as terpenoids, coumarins, and quercetin, giving it some mast cell–stabilizing action as well.[105]

I usually repeat this protocol three or four times a day and continue it during the following days. Besides a possible reaction to the salicylate from the peppermint, I don't experience any undesirable side effects. The salicylates may prompt some inflammation and pain during the following days, but these reactions taper off in time and are nothing compared to the pain of a severe GI reaction.

Apart from that, I do my best to maintain steady and deep breathing. If I can pull myself together, I go for a walk, because it helps move things along and takes my attention away from the pain. I walk slowly with steady, deep breathing and focus on all the beautiful things I see.

COPING WITH A REACTION

The emotional aspect of GI reactions

Whenever the pain roars at me, I keep reminding myself that no reaction lasts forever. These GI cramps usually go on for about seven hours, but once they lasted forty-eight hours straight—and even then, they eventually stopped.

Of course, there's an aftermath to each episode. You might feel extra tired and experience inflammation, brain fog, and increased sensitivities for a while, but it greatly helps to know that this pain will pass in time.

I've learned to just take it for what it is, neither beating myself up about it nor pitying myself for having to go through this because of a simple mistake in eating the wrong food. I try to view it as a matter-of-fact thing that I have to deal with right then. It's just the next hurdle to overcome.

Healing and recovery

During the next several days, it's crucial to eat simply to avoid adding anything that could aggravate the symptoms. I usually consume just small portions of steak until my system has calmed down. I know this doesn't sound very appetizing, but since I'm certain that beefsteak doesn't cause any symptoms for me, this is my best option. It's just super important to give the digestive system enough time to recuperate and not add anything that could worsen it. Some people don't tolerate meat, but from what I understand, it's mostly folks who have been affected by Lyme disease. In this case, I would go for a diet as bland as possible for a few days and strictly avoid foods that might cause bloating and irritation.

REMEDIES

Natural remedies

Apart from the remedies mentioned in my emergency protocol, ginger may also help calm gastrointestinal distress. It acts as a pain reliever with anti-inflammatory properties and has been seen to improve gastrointestinal health. Cannabis could also be beneficial, thanks to its potent anti-inflammatory action and its ability to reduce nausea.

Long term

Managing your GI symptoms over the long term requires a personalized approach—there's no one-size-fits-all protocol, as numerous factors play a role in how your body responds to food. While there's no guaranteed solution to fully resolve these symptoms, a few general tips may help: Variety is key to a healthy microbiome, so once you're stable, carefully start reintroducing new foods. Prioritize hydration and incorporate anti-inflammatory and mast cell–stabilizing foods. DAO supplements help break down histamine from food, and adding probiotics, prebiotics, and resistant starches may further support gut health.

Probiotics

Probiotics are living microorganisms (bacteria and yeasts) that can help restore balance in the gut flora. They are naturally present in fermented foods like yogurt, kefir, sauerkraut, tempeh, natto, kimchi, and kombucha. Unfortunately, these foods are high in histamine and may need to be avoided.

Probiotics can also be taken as supplements, but it's important to know that some strains can increase histamine levels, while others may help reduce them. My experience with probiotics has been mixed—at times, they've been beneficial, but other times, they've caused tremendous discomfort. This sentiment is frequently echoed in self-help groups, highlighting the importance of choosing the strains carefully.

Products and strains mentioned in the self-help groups as tolerable include:

- Probiota Histamine X (Seeking Health)
- Low Histamine Probiotics (VitaMonk)
- MegaSporeBiotic (Microbiome Labs)
- Flora Symmetry (Vitanica)
- Florastor (Biocodex)
- Culturelle (iHealth)
- L. *rhamnosus*

POTENTIAL ROOT CAUSE

SIBO stands for small intestinal bacterial overgrowth, a condition in which bacteria normally found in the large intestine migrate to the small intestine, where they don't belong. SIBO can cause various complications and is frequently discussed in self-help groups. If you're experiencing persistent GI symptoms, testing for SIBO may be worthwhile. Diagnosis typically involves breath tests, clinical assessments, or small intestine fluid collection.

During my research, I came across Dr. William Davis, a cardiologist and author of the book *Wheat Belly*. He developed a yogurt recipe using L. *reuteri* strains, which has reportedly helped some individuals overcome SIBO. I have personally used this yogurt for about eight weeks. While I cannot be entirely sure that my symptoms improved solely because of it, it has definitely helped my gastrointestinal symptoms, as I could tolerate a broader range of foods after using it.

KEY TAKEAWAY

GI reactions in MCAS can be brutal. Management starts with avoiding trigger foods, but once stable, foods should be carefully reintroduced to support the microbiome and prevent malnutrition. For acute relief, medications like Benadryl, prednisone, and antihistamines can help, though individual responses vary. Alternatives include *Boswellia serrata* extract, peppermint oil capsules, chamomile, ginger, cannabis, and water, alongside steady breathing and gentle movement. Support recovery with bland, well-tolerated foods. Long-term management is highly individual; probiotics can be helpful, though tolerability varies by strain, and testing for SIBO may be worthwhile.

CHAPTER 38

Managing Joint Pain

Even though joint pain is not a common symptom of MCAS, it's widespread in general. I've been dealing with it since I was fourteen, and along the way I've picked up a few useful tips. Traditional medical treatments never gave me lasting relief, despite trying everything doctors recommended. Cortisone, creams, and casts sometimes eased the pain temporarily, but nothing managed the symptoms long-term. So, I kept searching and gradually found a few things that really made a difference.

MOVEMENT & MECHANICS

Training

Building muscle is one of the best ways to improve your joint health. Strong muscles give crucial support and stability to your joints, better than anything else. Start slowly and carefully, and always prioritize proper form and ergonomics.

Ergonomics

Be mindful of how you use your joints when moving, lifting, or pushing. Keeping your joints in alignment helps prevent injury and inflammation. Learning about body mechanics and proprioception goes a long way toward protecting your joints and improving everyday function.

Keep moving

Staying still for too long can increase stiffness and pain. Gentle movements like stretching, walking, or even just shifting positions can make a big difference.

TRIGGERS & INFLAMMATION

Avoid triggers

Any mast cell trigger can intensify joint pain. For example, I did a little experiment with red food dye. I tried a beverage containing it three times, spaced well apart to be sure. But each time, my joints hurt so much the next day that it became crystal clear the food dye was, in fact, the cause. It's a good reminder that even seemingly unrelated triggers can significantly impact symptoms.

Mind your diet

What you eat can have a major impact on joint health. Diets high in refined carbs tend to intensify inflammation, so it helps to keep sugar and processed foods to a minimum. On the other hand, eating healthy fats and sufficient protein supports tissue repair and helps regulate inflammation, which is essential for joint health. Including a variety of colorful foods in your diet also makes a difference, as they provide beneficial plant compounds that support the body's natural defenses.

RELIEF STRATEGIES

Quick relief

As odd as it may sound, wraps with quark or cabbage can help soothe joint inflammation. I swear by them. For a quark wrap, place about a cup of quark in a double-folded kitchen towel, wrap it around the painful area, and wait for it to dry. After about thirty minutes, open it over a sink or tub—and the dry quark crumbles off. Repeat once or twice a day for a few consecutive days. It's amazing how quickly this draws out inflammation. If you prefer cabbage, roll the leaves with a bottle or warm them slightly to soften them, then wrap them around the inflamed area for about thirty minutes. It's a simple and incredibly soothing remedy.

Supplements

Although research on glucosamine is mixed, it's my go-to whenever my joints hurt. Glucosamine is often combined with MSM, chondroitin, and hyaluronic acid—all of which are popular in joint support formulas. While the evidence may vary, I find this combo incredibly helpful.

KEY TAKEAWAY

Although not a hallmark symptom of MCAS, many people experience joint pain. Beyond traditional treatments like cortisone, creams, and casts, self-management strategies can make a big difference: strengthen muscles to stabilize joints, practice body awareness, and avoid triggers in food and the environment. Limit sugar and processed foods, emphasize anti-inflammatory foods, and consider supplements like glucosamine, MSM, and chondroitin.

CHAPTER 39

Iron Infusions

I received my first iron infusion around age twenty-seven, shortly after moving back to Switzerland. When my doctor suggested it, I didn't hesitate, because a friend had recently marveled at how amazing she'd felt after hers, calling it one of the best days she'd ever had. So, I booked the appointment for my lunch break without much thought. The treatment would take only twenty minutes, giving me enough time to grab something to eat and bike back to work.

Yet, shortly after leaving the doctor's office, I was hit by a crushing lethargy. My legs felt so heavy it hurt to pedal uphill, and by the time I arrived at work, my knees were so weak I could barely stand. Drenched in sweat, with my entire body in pain and my vision blurred, I was alarmed! I called the doctor's office right away, but they said it was unlikely to be related to the infusion and suggested I might have caught the flu.

Whatever it was, I felt so miserable that my boss sent me home for the rest of the day. For the next ten days, I truly felt as if I had the flu, just as they'd suggested. My body ached, I was exhausted, and psychologically, I felt like absolute crap. I felt depressed, angry, useless, and completely hopeless.

MY EXPERIENCE WITH IRON INFUSIONS

"It's just the flu."

At my follow-up visit, I asked again if the iron could have caused my symptoms. My doctor shook her head, insisting it was the flu. Still, I couldn't shake the feeling the infusion was to blame, so I pressed further. Clearly annoyed, she grabbed a medical reference book and began reading. Then, suddenly, her tone shifted. She found that 0.01–1 percent of patients experience the exact reactions I had described. Taken aback, she paused, then turned the question over to me: Did I want to proceed with the second dose or hold off? Having just recovered from the first one, I decided against it.

Returning to iron infusions

Ten years later, my iron count was still ridiculously low, so Dr. John suggested trying it again—this time starting carefully with the amount typically administered to infants. Yet my body still couldn't handle it! After that, I swore off iron infusions because they obviously had the opposite effect on me from what they were meant to do.

However, a few years down the line, Dr. John nudged me into trying it again, insisting it would really help with my energy. Despite years of oral supplements, my levels had never exceeded 30, while the healthy range is 50–170. By then, I had better control over my mast cell reactions and a more stable baseline, so I mustered the courage to go for it. Unfortunately, it backfired again, leaving me wrecked for another two weeks.

Preparing for success

After that, I gave it some thought. By that point, I understood that iron infusions can trigger severe mast cell reactions and need to be administered with caution—but how could we achieve that?

By then, I had learned a lot about vitamins and minerals and knew that some foods inhibit iron absorption while others enhance it. So I decided to give it another try—but this time, prepared. For the two weeks before the treatment, I avoided foods that hinder iron absorption and focused on those that support it. Additionally, we diluted the iron in twice the usual amount of sodium chloride solution (NaCl) and let it drip in slowly over 1.5 hours instead of the usual twenty minutes. Lastly, my partner came with me for support in case I reacted again.

With these adjustments, I finally tolerated the infusion. After that, we went on to complete six sessions, gradually increasing the dose from 50 to 100, then 200, and within a few months, my iron levels had climbed above 120.

One time, I skipped the protocol and reacted again, but the next time, following it properly, I was fine. I later found that I could prep for just three days instead of two weeks and still tolerate the infusion, though I'm not sure if that would've worked in the beginning, when I wasn't as stable yet.

The benefits of adequate iron levels

Reaching adequate iron levels has made a staggering difference for me. I have more energy, fewer reactions to triggers, and I can tolerate a wider range of foods. I feel stronger, which allows me to exercise regularly—and that, in turn, gives me even more energy. It's been an absolute game-changer for me.

NAVIGATING IRON INFUSIONS WITH MCAS

In the ten days leading up to the infusion, aim to:

- Get plenty of vitamin C throughout the day
- Include freshly made juices daily
- Focus on iron-rich foods
- Take oral iron supplements (if tolerated)

Avoid or cut back on:

- Coffee
- Grains
- Dairy
- Alcohol
- Oxalates

Additionally, it's essential to:

- Slow the infusion down significantly. Diluted in twice the amount of NaCl, mine typically takes 1 to 1.5 hours. This gradual approach helps minimize the risk of reacting to the sudden iron influx.
- Avoid coffee right beforehand. It significantly hinders iron absorption, and as tempting as it is to perk up before the procedure, skipping that cup can make a real difference.
- Have someone with you, or at least on standby. Knowing someone's there to help if needed provides peace of mind and support in case you react.

> **KEY TAKEAWAY**
>
> Iron infusions can trigger intense reactions in MCAS. Improve tolerance by boosting intake of vitamin C and iron-rich foods, avoiding foods and drinks that block iron absorption, and diluting the infusion so it drips slowly over 1–1.5 hours instead of the standard twenty minutes. For safety, have someone pick you up in case you still react despite the preparation.

CHAPTER 40

Temperature

Temperature changes can affect the mast cells. Sudden extreme changes can cause anaphylaxis, while being too cold for too long can sometimes leave you feeling icy cold for hours following. Some people react to heat, while others respond to cold.

Based on my experiences and reading in the self-help groups, impaired temperature sensation is also a common symptom. Sometimes, we feel like we have a fever with no actual fever present, and other times, we feel well, even though we do have a fever. Sometimes, we might feel shiveringly cold when it's hot out, and other times we might feel hot when the temperature is mild.

Histamine influences body core temperature, primarily through its action on H1 and H3 receptors.[120] So maybe it's the excessive histamine release from mast cells or the antihistamines we must take to manage symptoms that cause our temperature perception to be off—but this is just a guess. What's clear, though, is that questions regarding temperature regulation frequently come up in the self-help groups, and it has been a burdensome issue for me until I discovered effective coping methods. Below are a few simple ideas that may help. While many of these tips may seem like common sense, I've included them because people with MCAS need to make so many adjustments that it's easy to overlook certain things—and because every one of these insights has genuinely helped me feel better.

DRESSING SMART FOR TEMPERATURE CONTROL

Wear ski pants or rainproof pants

Whenever I go out in the cold, I wear ski or rain pants over my regular pants. That way, I'm protected from rain, wind, and cold while outside, and I can quickly just shed that one layer when I go back indoors.

Wear leggings or long underwear

While they may seem more fashion-conscious, tight clothing can sometimes trigger reactions. It restricts the skin's ability to breathe and may lead to friction and heat buildup. Additionally, leggings worn under regular pants can be inconvenient to take off in case you start feeling too hot.

Wear a hat

This helps keep you warm, and you can easily take it off when you get too hot.

Wear comfortable socks

If you're cold, putting on a pair of comfy, non-irritating wool socks can quickly warm you up. Socks with effective thermoregulation properties are also a good choice, as they keep your feet dry and prevent heat buildup.

Bring backup clothes

I always bring an extra shirt and socks so I can quickly change if necessary.

Dress in layers

Adjust swiftly as the weather changes: the sooner you adapt, the better you'll feel.

Wear shoes that breathe

Having heat accumulate in your shoes may leave you drained to the max. Wearing breathable shoes or walking barefoot can make a big difference.

Wear light-colored clothing

It helps you stay cool by reflecting more of the sun's rays than darker clothing.

TOOLS & TRICKS

Sip warm beverages

A wonderful way to warm up is to have a cup of tea or a bowl of hot soup. If you're out all day, you could carry a thermos and enjoy some whenever you like.

Use a pocket warmer

If your hands are often cold, pocket warmers can provide quick relief and are easy to carry.

Protect yourself from the sun

An umbrella, a parasol, and a hand fan can be great tools to help you stay cool.

Eat cooling foods

Salads, dark leafy greens, watermelon, peppermint, cherries, cucumber, bananas, berries, and coconut are all said to have cooling qualities. However, some of these foods are high in histamine and may need to be avoided.

Cool your wrists, face, and neck

If you get too hot, you can cool your wrists under cold, running water for a few minutes and splash some on your face and neck. Alternatively, bring a light scarf with you, soak it in water, and then wear it wet around your neck.

Take cool showers

Gradually adjust the water to cooler temperatures rather than coming in from the heat and jumping right into an ice-cold shower. To avoid shock, it's also a good idea to start at the extremities—first feet, hands, legs, and arms—moving slowly toward your torso and then finally the trunk and head.

Whenever I do this, I breathe deeply, keep my mind calm and positive, and reaffirm to my cells that this is all good and helpful. Call me crazy if you want to, but I find it helps.

> **KEY TAKEAWAY**
>
> Shifts in temperature can trigger mast cell flares, even anaphylaxis. Support your body by dressing in layers to adjust quickly and using tools like fans, parasols, or pocket warmers. Warm foods can help in the cold, while cooling foods can help ease heat. To cool quickly, try short, cool showers, splash your wrists, hands, and face with cold water, or wear a damp scarf around your neck.

CHAPTER 41

Breathing Tips to Reduce Reactions

Reactions to smells are a common symptom in MCAS. Smells that may trigger us come from perfumes, laundry detergents, body care products, car exhaust, printer ink, paint, cleaning products, and various toxic fumes that could be lurking around every corner. Even natural substances, such as the smell of certain foods, can cause reactions!

Finding ways to work around such triggers is extremely challenging because there is simply no way for us to control what floats around in the air—and smells aren't visible.

However, we can diminish the severity of reactions to smells by practicing intentional control over our breathing. We can exercise at least some personal discretion in deciding exactly when to take a deep breath. When triggers are present, we can often avoid inhaling these substances, at least to some extent. These breathing techniques help me reduce the intensity of airborne reactions and limit their impact on the system. While they have helped me personally, they may not be appropriate for everyone.

I developed them out of necessity after fainting multiple times simply from exposure to smells my body couldn't tolerate. This happened while I was grocery shopping, near people wearing perfume, or inside facilities with off-gassing materials, machines, or products that triggered me. More than once, I had to return home without any groceries, only to try again the next day.

Once I adopted these skills, being in public became much less taxing. It isn't easy to explain, but I'll do my best to convey these techniques step by step.

A note of caution: If you have a heart or lung condition, or if you feel dizzy or faint, please do not try the following exercises, or talk to your doctor first.

BREATH & TRIGGER AWARENESS

How long can you hold your breath?

First, it helps to know how long you can comfortably hold your breath. It's probably longer than you think. I can easily hold my breath for one minute and fifteen seconds. I find it helps to know this, because sometimes I happen to walk into a situation where there are so many triggers around that I risk passing out if I inhaled them. In such settings, I've learned to just hold my breath and quickly get myself to a safer spot.

I've found that the best way to determine this is to get perfectly calm, close your eyes, and even think as little as possible. Slow down everything inside you. Breathe in and out a couple of times deeply and comfortably. When you feel ready, set a timer, breathe in, and hold your breath until you feel the need to breathe again. The calmer you feel, the longer you can hold it. It's good to have an idea of how long you can safely do this so that when you have to use this technique in the turmoil of everyday life, you won't panic.

What is the direction of the airflow?

You will need to learn to feel the wind or airflow to determine which direction it is coming from. Once you've locked this in, you can quickly position yourself upwind whenever triggers are present.

There's always some movement in the air, and you can make this an ally. To me, it has become like second nature to feel the air on my face. In doing so, I can quickly assess the direction of the airflow. Most people affected by MCAS seem to be quite sensitive, so we have an advantage in learning this quickly. With a bit of practice, you'll likely start to notice even the slightest changes in airflow without much effort.

In addition to feeling it, you can also see the wind direction by watching how things move: leaves on trees, dust on streets, and hair all move with the breeze and can often be seen all around you. The lighter the wind, the subtler these movements become, but once you are attuned to them, you'll pick up even the gentlest signs.

How does your facial skin feel?

We can use our faces as a kind of monitoring device because our facial skin is quite sensitive and almost always exposed. For example, when a perfume triggers you, you'll likely feel it first on your face. You may also experience a burning sensation in your eyes, lips, and nose. In such moments, it's best to avoid taking full breaths. Instead, keep moving until you feel the air becoming clearer.

Are your taste buds impacted?

Can you taste airborne smells on your lips, tongue, or in your mouth?

Are you experiencing watery eyes?

If your eyes suddenly get watery or sting, it's usually best to walk a few steps further before you take a full breath.

REDUCE REACTIONS

Expelling a trigger

I've found four ways to breathe out effectively before an airborne trigger gets too deep into my system. As soon as I notice I've inhaled a trigger, I breathe out forcefully, because I feel it helps reduce its impact. At first, this probably won't look very smooth, but over time you'll be able to do this so subtly that people around you won't even notice. Applying all these techniques together is an art, but with a little practice, it becomes as natural as riding a bike. The four options are:

- Breathing out quickly and forcefully through your nose, pushing air out from the lower part of your belly, can sometimes reduce the intensity of a trigger before it affects you more strongly.
- Breathing out slowly and deeply through your nose can help if a trigger has already reached deeper into your lungs. It can feel like clearing your airways from the inside out.
  This works well by applying gentle pressure to your throat, almost closing it, so that swallowing becomes difficult. Then apply some pressure from the diaphragm and slowly and steadily push the air out of your nose.

- If you catch a trigger through your mouth, it seems best to expel it back out through your mouth as well. Give it a quick push from your lower belly and diaphragm while puckering your lips with slight tension in your cheeks.
- Voluntary coughing can help quickly push out the air that contained the trigger. Additionally, rinsing your mouth with water can help wash away anything that may still be lingering in your mouth.

Dodging perfumes

Once you can tell the airflow, you can position yourself upwind from others so their perfume blows away from you while you are passing or conversing. If the wind shifts, simply stepping to either side is often enough to avoid the current.

When walking among people, you'll quickly notice that their scent carries on behind them in their wake, similar to the wind tunnel created by a passing truck. It begins to disperse only about ten meters behind the car itself. It's the same with perfumes, although some linger longer than others.

Try to avoid walking directly behind perfumed people. Instead, step to either side to ensure you're out of the danger zone, meaning the smelly trail where the perfume lingers.

Passing toxic storefronts

When you are about to pass by stores that sell perfume, shoes, clothing, paint, or other strongly scented or chemical products, keep as much distance as possible. Sometimes it helps to simply cross to the other side of the street.

What I personally do is take one deep breath before coming close to the doorway. I hold my breath while I swiftly move past the entrance, and then I use the sensations on my face to determine when it's safe to breathe again.

A short-term trick to manage reactions

I can sometimes avoid a reaction by "tricking" the mast cells: I cover my mouth with the palm of my hand and then breathe carefully through my mouth. This helps mask other smells with the scent of my hand. As strange as this may sound, I've found this method effective in the short term.

It won't help over a long period—you'll still need to relocate to a trigger-free place—but I believe it helps because my body feels safe with my own scent, and it masks other odors. As soon as you reach a place with clean air, take a moment to rest there, breathing deeply and slowly to take in fresh oxygen and recenter yourself.

Masks

There are situations when even all these methods combined won't suffice to keep you safe. For example, it's not possible to hold your breath long enough without passing out in crowds of people or inside stores, hospitals, or places that are basically saturated with triggers. In these environments, you'll have to wear a mask.

Stay calm

To get the best results from these techniques, it's essential to remain calm. In my experience, it becomes almost effortless after a while, but it takes some practice. And while I know that we're normally supposed to breathe continuously—and shallow breathing isn't ideal—I personally feel much better using these methods rather than being slammed by triggers again and again.

> **KEY TAKEAWAY**
>
> Scents are a tricky trigger in MCAS because they're invisible, but intentional breathing can lessen their impact. Learn early warning signs, know how long you can hold your breath, and attune to the airflow so you can position yourself upwind from scents. Avoid walking behind perfumed people, and hold your breath when passing toxic places. When surrounded by triggering smells, wear a mask or cover your face with your hand, scarf, or jacket collar until you reach fresh air.

CHAPTER 42

Shopping

Unless we have a big garden where we can cultivate everything we need or someone else to shop for us, grocery shopping is something we can't avoid. Everyone needs food and supplies, but, gosh, stores can be a terrifying place if you're living with MCAS! Grocery stores are so full of potential triggers that, as ridiculous as this might sound, the simple act of shopping can become a daunting experience.

I hate going into stores nowadays—there's just too much of everything in there! In addition to what they sell, there are overpowering smells from customers' perfumes, laundry detergents, fabric softeners, body care products, shampoos, conditioners, hair sprays, and aftershaves. Then come the cleaning agents used in stores, while harsh lighting and noise make it even worse. Stores are simply not a good place to keep overactive mast cells calm. That said, there are a few strategies that can make the experience more manageable.

SAFER ALTERNATIVES

Online shopping

One alternative to exposing yourself to the threat is simply ordering your supplies online and having them delivered to your home. Many companies offer this service at no extra cost if you buy a certain amount per delivery. Others charge a small additional fee, which might be worth the expense.

To avoid reactions to the delivery person's laundry detergent, perfume, or fabric softener—over which you obviously have little control—you can often request to have your order left at the door.

Farmers' markets and direct farm visits

Excellent alternatives for shopping are farmers' markets or buying directly from a farm. Not everyone can do this, but it's likely a less triggering experience than going into a conventional supermarket. Growing your own food sounds like heaven to me, but not everyone has a garden or a balcony, and not every climate allows for growing food year-round.

TRIGGER MANAGEMENT STRATEGIES

Avoiding triggers in stores

If you must go into a store, avoid the aisle with the cleaning agents! In time, you'll know exactly where things are in the shops you visit, and you can steer clear of the "stinky" sections. Whenever I pass by an aisle I know could trigger me, I hold my breath and sometimes even close my eyes for the few steps I must take to pass by. Wearing sunglasses can also help to protect your eyes from airborne triggers and reduce the strain caused by harsh store lighting.

In his book *Never Bet Against Occam*, Dr. Afrin states that our eye tissue has approximately 5,000 mast cells per cubic millimeter. That's a good explanation for why our eyes water, itch, or turn red almost instantly when triggers are present.

Minimizing time in stores

Given that most of us react to many foods and products, your shopping list will likely become very short, making it a bit easier to get the shopping done quickly. Most likely, you won't feel like spending lots of time browsing through shops anyway because it could be frustrating to see all the things you'd actually like but have to abstain from. I say make it quick and painless by getting in and out as fast as possible.

Priming before you go in

Before entering a store, I do my best to get centered and calm. I take a deep breath, envision the process going smoothly, and then walk swiftly to the sections with the required products. I pick up the few things I need and proceed to the checkout as swiftly as possible. Once back outside, I always take a moment to sit down and rest for a bit, catching my breath for a few minutes before I make my way home.

Handling smells on packaging

Smells from other items in the store can sometimes transfer onto packaging, and—believe it or not—even these can trigger reactions. Upon coming home, I usually wipe off the packaging, or transfer the contents to my storage containers or mason jars. I then toss the packaging immediately and may even go so far as to take out the trash. Otherwise, I risk triggering a reaction whenever I open the garbage. You might even want to wear a mask while doing this to minimize reactions, or you can just hold your breath.

Shopping less frequently

Shopping less frequently has helped me feel better. I limit my exposure to triggers as much as I can because I am painfully aware that just walking into the wrong kind of setting can set me back for days. To reduce the frequency of your shopping trips, plan ahead and store food optimally so it stays fresh longer, as discussed in Chapter 56, "Storing Food."

> **KEY TAKEAWAY**
>
> Stores are full of triggers—perfumes, cleaning products, packaging, harsh lighting, and noise. Limit time inside, avoid risky aisles, hold your breath when needed, and wear sunglasses for eye protection. Once home, wipe packaging or transfer items into your own containers. Safer options include farmers' markets, direct farm purchases, or online shopping.

CHAPTER 43

Travel

Traveling with all these restrictions is another major challenge. Nearly every time I tried to go somewhere in the past few years, I ran into problems! I reacted to dust, perfumes, and other scented products, or the carpets and new furniture in a hotel caused issues. In some places mold made me seriously sick; other times the heat got me. My attempts to eat out in a restaurant regularly resulted in anaphylaxis, or I'd end up convulsing with horrible cramps and debilitating digestive issues afterward. Trying to sleep at someone else's house, I'd often wake up with a sore throat and fever, hives, and nausea, and occasionally I couldn't even sleep at all. Sometimes, I could immediately pinpoint the culprit—such as off-gassing carpets, scented laundry, dust, mold, or incense stashed in a cabinet somewhere in the room—but other times I had no clue what made me sick.

The easiest solution to stay on the safe side when traveling with MCAS would probably be to have your own mobile home, fully equipped with a kitchen, a bed, and all the necessities for the journey. But if that isn't possible, you'll have to figure out how to go places without getting sick every single time. The following are a few ideas that I came up with for safer traveling experiences.

WHAT TO BRING

Travel cooking kit

The first step was to put together an easy-to-carry, lightweight travel kitchen. It took some tinkering, but the whole thing now fits neatly into two toiletry bags. One bag holds the cooking equipment and the cleanup kit, and the other bag contains various food items and cutlery.

(a) The kitchen bag holds a small fold-up camping gas stove, a small gas can, a small fold-up pan, a plate, a thin cutting board, a cleaning rag, a scrubby sponge, and a travel-sized bottle with dish soap. I stack them on top of each other, which saves a lot of room.

(b) The second bag holds a cutlery kit, seasonings, oil, rice, and some tea. I use travel bottles like those typically used for shampoo and soap to keep my favorite condiments: paprika, chives, sugar, and salt, with which I find I can make pretty much any food tasty. I transfer some oil into a small bottle and pack rice in a Ziploc bag to keep things light. The cutlery kit includes a kitchen knife, a fork, two non-toxic plastic spoons, and chopsticks.

Food

I usually buy veggies and fruits once I've arrived at my destination, as they are available almost everywhere. I bring just as much rice as I will use. While you can't make super elaborate meals with such a setup, you can still make tasty dishes. It's far better to eat simply rather than nothing at all, and it's for sure better than taking a chance on eating out and ending up suffering for the rest of the trip. It also feels great to know you're set and that you can care for yourself.

Body care products

I keep personal care products in travel-sized bottles. This helps reduce the weight and size of my overall luggage, and even a small bottle lasts me a week or two.

Bedding

I always bring my own bedding, because the reactions I experience to certain laundry detergents can be so intense that there's just no way I could sleep in such bedding and stay well. I bring my pillow, a mattress sheet, and a blanket cover.

Silk may be the ideal bedding material for travel because it's very light and packs down to an unbelievably small size, but if your budget is tight, cotton works well, too. You could also just bring your own sleeping bag, but depending on the length and location of your stay, a set of real bedding is likely more comfortable.

Medication

Of course, we also have to bring the medications we need. To reduce the volume of this package, I pack whatever I need in small Ziploc bags labeled with a ballpoint pen (permanent marker fumes can trigger reactions). That way, I carry only the amount required for the trip. I then keep all these little bags in a small waterproof toiletry bag to ensure everything stays dry.

Remember that some prescription drugs must be brought in their original package, and some might even require you to bring the actual prescription with you.

In addition to bringing the medications I need daily, I carry an emergency set that includes an EpiPen, painkillers, stomach acid–resistant peppermint oil capsules, *Boswellia serrata*, and chamomile tea. Whenever I travel with others, I inform them where these things are.

SETTING UP A SAFE STAY

Hotel stays

When considering a hotel stay, it's crucial to call beforehand to ask whether they use room fresheners or scented products and to inquire about non-carpeted rooms. Carpets can accumulate a lot of gunk that may trigger us, and depending on the material, even the carpet itself can cause reactions.

If these requests cannot be met, I'll choose another hotel. When I book a stay, I always inform the staff about my condition, and I'll also ask whether it's okay to bring some of my food and stash it in their fridge, which has never been a problem.

> **KEY TAKEAWAY**
>
> Traveling with MCAS requires careful preparation. Bring safe food, body care, bedding, and medications, and consider a compact travel cooking kit. Pack medications in labeled bags (or in the original packaging if required), carry your emergency kit, and tell companions where it is. When booking hotel stays, call ahead to request fragrance-free, non-carpeted rooms and permission to store your food.

CHAPTER 44

Eating Out

Eating out in restaurants? Honestly, I think it's risky. I tried for a while, but over the last few years I ended up in so much pain every single time, no matter how carefully I communicated my situation to the waiters and the chefs. If I react strongly to something I eat, it can take me weeks to get back on track, so I've finally come to accept that it's just not worth the trouble.

PREPARATION

Creating a list of tolerated foods

If you really don't want to miss out on restaurant experiences, I recommend writing a list of the foods you tolerate and those you must avoid. Keep it in your wallet or save it to your phone so you can easily share it. Including the things you tolerate can be helpful, as a list that only shows what you need to avoid might overwhelm others and leave them unsure of what they can prepare for you.

Calling ahead for safety

As with hotel stays, it's best to call a restaurant beforehand to ask if they use room fresheners or scented products, such as scented candles. If they do, it may be wise to choose another spot.

I would also always ask if you could speak directly with the chef to explain what might happen if the food becomes contaminated with something you react to. A responsible person will be careful, or they'll hopefully deny cooking for you—which I find considerate if they can't guarantee your safety.

Bringing your own salt

Always bring some salt you tolerate. Restaurants often use iodized table salt, which must be strictly avoided. Food without salt tastes awfully bland, so bringing your own will make it more tasty.

SAFETY PRECAUTIONS

Emergency medications

Always bring your emergency medications and have them handy in case you go into anaphylaxis. It's also a good idea to communicate this possibility to the people you're with and tell them where you keep your EpiPen.

Hand hygiene considerations

Lastly, bring your own hand soap in case you have to use the bathroom, and be cautious with hand towels. If they've been washed with a scented detergent, touching them may cause reactions. Paper towels are usually a safer option, or you can bring a small quick-dry microfiber travel towel, which comes in various sizes and packs easily.

AN ALTERNATIVE APPROACH

Cooking at home for social gatherings

To lighten the load on my family and friends, we've finally decided that I'll do the cooking whenever we visit. They'll pay for the groceries or organize what I need, and I take care of the meals. That way, nobody has to worry about making a mistake or dealing with the consequences. As a result, we can all relax and enjoy the simple pleasure of sharing meals again.

> **KEY TAKEAWAY**
>
> Dining out is risky, but preparation can help. Keep a list of tolerated foods, call ahead to ask about scented products, and speak directly with the chef about your requirements and what could happen if you react. Always bring your own salt, carry emergency meds, and let companions know where they are. Bring tolerated hand soap, and use paper towels instead of cloth towels that may carry detergent scents.

CHAPTER 45

Hair Loss

Hair loss is a common MCAS symptom. I have noticed that I frequently lose a lot of hair in times of ongoing reactions, but whenever I'm more balanced, things seem to go back to normal. It's important to remember that there is always a cause for any symptom, and it's best to tackle the problem at its root.

UNDERSTANDING HAIR LOSS

Addressing the cause first

I can absolutely relate to anyone who's suddenly losing a lot of hair and is desperate to make it stop. There are thousands of miracle hair growth treatments out there, and trying some of them can be tempting, but it's probably best to talk to a specialist about it first.

You could spend a fortune on such products, but it's entirely possible that they wouldn't help because the underlying cause of your hair loss persists. Also, many of these products contain substances and fragrances that might make your mast cells mad, which in turn might cause you to lose even more hair than before.

Additionally, supplementation can even be harmful if there is no actual deficiency. Over-supplementation of certain nutrients, including selenium, vitamin A, and vitamin E, has, in fact, been linked to hair loss.[121]

Common causes of hair loss

Deficiencies in iron, zinc, protein, or fatty acids, poor nutrition, malabsorption of nutrients, hormonal changes, hair treatments, heredity, and stress can cause hair loss.[121,122]

Hair loss in MCAS

Since I frequently experience significant hair loss during acute reactions—and it stops once I regain control—I believe that hair loss in MCAS patients may be linked to mast cells surrounding the hair follicles. Maybe the mediator release in the scalp causes hair loss, but, like I said, it's just a guess. It could also be linked to stress or nutrient deficiencies. However, the mast cell mediator prostaglandin D2 (PGD2) has been linked to hair loss.[123]

GETTING TO THE ROOT

Risk-free tips to reduce hair loss

While consulting a specialist is undoubtedly the most sensible approach to determining the best steps for preventing hair loss in your specific case, there are a few simple, inexpensive, and risk-free things you can do on your own that may help diminish hair loss.

- Use a leave-in conditioner or detangler and avoid tugging when combing to reduce breakage.
- Apply a moisturizing conditioner after each shampoo to keep your hair hydrated.
- Avoid harsh treatments such as chemical straightening, excessive heat styling, or bleaching.
- Avoid overwashing, as it can strip your hair of natural oils.
- Use a good, wide-toothed comb, preferably made from natural materials such as wood, to minimize breakage.
- Let your hair dry naturally or use the lowest setting if you use a blow dryer to reduce damage.
- Use a silk or sateen pillowcase, as soft fabrics will cause less breakage to your hair.
- Stay hydrated: drinking enough water helps maintain scalp health and keeps your hair hydrated.
- Eat a balanced diet: ensure your diet includes sufficient vitamins and minerals, particularly biotin, zinc, iron, and omega-3 fatty acids, which are essential for healthy hair.

KEY TAKEAWAY

Hair loss may be linked to stress, nutrient deficiencies, or mast cell activity. Quick fixes often contain triggers, and over-supplementation of certain nutrients can even worsen symptoms. Risk-free strategies include consulting a specialist, gentle hair care, avoiding harsh treatments, using wide-toothed combs and soft pillowcases, staying hydrated, and eating a nutrient-rich diet.

CHAPTER 46

Dark Circles Under the Eyes

Dark circles under the eyes are a consistent and stubborn symptom of MCAS for several reasons: most of us experience chronic pain, have very restricted diets, and struggle with poor sleep. Additionally, side effects from medications could be a culprit, and the strain of constant reactions takes a toll on the body. This disease is simply stressful!

Doctors sometimes refer to these circles as "allergic shiners," and self-help group members often ask what they can do about them. Typical advice includes drinking more water and getting more sleep, but for me it seemed like no amount of water or sleep would ever make them go away. I often looked like a tired ghost, even when I felt reasonably good. So, what can you do about them?

Covering them with cosmetics?

You could try covering the dark circles with cosmetics, but that doesn't get rid of them, and you might even get a reaction from the makeup, which would likely make things even worse.

SUPPORTIVE STRATEGIES

What helps with dark circles

- Drinking enough water is certainly a good idea.
- Getting sufficient nutrients is crucial.
- Maintaining good sleep hygiene is tremendously important.
- Keeping your electrolytes balanced is definitely beneficial.
- Avoiding triggers of all kinds will surely help.

A surprisingly simple solution

I found this tip on YouTube: treat the dark circles with ice cubes! The idea sounded a bit strange to me, but since I really longed to see my face without these ugly dark circles under my eyes, I decided to try—and it worked! After about three weeks, the dark circles started to fade away, and, as a nice side effect, my face felt very refreshed.

Gently rub an ice cube over your face, especially the area under your eyes, until it melts away. Do this a few times per day for a week or two and see whether you notice any improvement. This method stimulates blood circulation and leaves your skin feeling refreshed and invigorated.

> **KEY TAKEAWAY**
>
> Dark circles, sometimes called "allergic shiners," may come from poor sleep, stress, or ongoing reactions. Instead of covering them with cosmetics that may trigger reactions, emphasize hydration, electrolytes, nutrients, trigger-avoidance, and good sleep. A simple method that helped me was gently rubbing an ice cube under the eyes several times a day to improve circulation.

SECTION V

Diet & Nutrition

CHAPTER 47

Fundamentals

I've certainly been there—when eating became a downright frightening burden, a necessity I would've much rather dodged altogether. Before each meal, I'd sit in front of my plate, pondering whether I should be brave enough to try and risk another avalanche of pain, or whether I should just starve myself to death. Either way, it would probably hurt, and for a while it felt like I'd die soon, regardless.

I know many mast cell sufferers who, at one point or another, wished they didn't have to eat anymore. This makes sense once you understand that food reactions in MCAS can bring on excruciating pain, not just for hours, but sometimes for days or even weeks. If you've gone through that more than once, it's only natural to want to avoid the pain altogether. But quitting food isn't an option, so we must eventually figure out which foods we can tolerate. From my experience, things get much easier once you've solved this riddle. I'm not saying it'll be easy, but it will calm your system and help you tackle the next steps more comfortably.

How, then, do we approach this issue? How can you find out which foods you can tolerate?

While diet is highly individual, I believe some basic principles can help almost anyone with this condition. For me, it caused years of pain, suffering, and confusion. I searched and researched, trying advice from countless doctors, healers, and nutritionists—and while some approaches made me feel better, none fully fixed my GI problems. I kept reacting to the simplest, healthiest foods and could never find the culprits. On the bright side, none of it was wasted. At least I learned a lot, and my cooking skills improved!

The following steps helped me navigate this maze and ease my symptoms to the point where I can finally enjoy food again without always dreading the consequences.

- Test for long-term allergies
- Go gluten-free
- Eliminate dairy
- Make water your main beverage
- Prepare every meal yourself
- Cook fresh with wholesome ingredients
- Eliminate processed foods
- Use the right salts
- Read labels carefully
- Stay unyieldingly strict about diet
- Keep it simple

NAVIGATING DIET WITH MCAS

Allergy tests

I underwent prick tests, patch tests, and blood tests over about sixteen years, but they consistently came back negative. Only when I tested specifically for long-term allergies were my allergies finally revealed. IgE responses happen immediately, but IgA and IgG responses can occur hours or even days after eating, making them nearly impossible to identify through food diaries, elimination diets, and self-observation.

Gluten and milk

I've personally seen many people experience significant health improvements after cutting out these two foods. Some people find that avoiding milk and gluten helps them feel less inflamed or experience less GI distress, and some also notice weight loss. If you're dealing with ongoing digestive discomfort, a common approach is to avoid these foods for about six weeks to see whether you notice any changes. Additionally, research suggests that some individuals with MCAS tolerated new medications better when they avoided gluten, milk, and yeast for the first few weeks of treatment.[29]

Pure water

Water may be your best choice of beverage, since it's highly unlikely to cause allergic reactions. That said, I've read in the self-help groups that some people experience reactions to water. I'm unsure why this happens; it could be due to water treatments, contamination in the plumbing system, bottling materials, or certain minerals. However, it's likely the safest option if you have access to pure, clean water.

It might take some time to adjust if you're used to flavored drinks, but your palate will adapt. Much to my surprise, I even started noticing subtle differences in the taste between different waters. Another benefit of primarily drinking water is that you won't have to deliberate about what you want. I guess that's a bit of a silver lining: fewer choices can at least simplify life in some ways!

Preparing food yourself

This isn't just wise for your own well-being but also makes things easier for those around you. It's a lot to ask someone else to follow all the rules we've had to adopt. Leaving that responsibility to others can be inconsiderate, because if they're cooking for you, they likely care deeply and would feel awful if you got sick from something they made.

I stopped letting others cook for me after getting seriously sick multiple times and feeling their regret and concern afterward. Nowadays, if I want to have a meal with friends, I cook. If I'm invited, either they reimburse me for the groceries I bring, or I let them know what I need so they can shop ahead of time. Since handling it this way, I haven't gotten sick, and I can finally enjoy meals with friends again.

Preparing each meal freshly

It's crucial to eat fresh, because even low-histamine foods can accumulate histamine over time, so eating leftovers is just not safe. To avoid wasting food, learn how to prepare the right amounts.

Ready-made meals

Processed foods, frozen dinners, and take-away options should be avoided altogether. If you're used to eating this way, this might seem like an overwhelming lifestyle change at first. However, preparing your own food isn't as hard as it might seem. Cooking isn't rocket science, and the taste and nutritional value of a wholesome, freshly made meal is just so much better than anything you can buy.

Packaged foods usually contain many stabilizers and additives and are often made with cheap table salt. To make matters worse, they were prepared *who knows how long ago*, so they're unlikely to be low in histamine. I'd say processed foods should be avoided by anyone, but especially by those whose mast cells have gone mad!

Using the right salts

Your choice of salt is crucial. Table salt is often fortified with iodine and fluoride, both of which can trigger mast cell reactions. It may also contain anti-caking agents that can exacerbate symptoms. However, salt is essential: it supports the nervous system, maintains fluid balance, helps muscles contract and relax, and helps prevent low blood pressure. While too much salt can raise blood pressure, too little can cause it to drop.

I like to use Himalayan crystal salt, rock salt, desert salt, fleur de sel, and untreated sea salt. Each has its own distinct taste, and pure, untreated salts contain a wide range of trace minerals. As with most things in MCAS, you'll need to experiment to find what works for you. Sea salts can contain traces of heavy metals and iodine, so if you have an underlying issue with heavy metals, you may react to them. Similarly, Himalayan salt can contain minerals like zinc that might cause reactions.

Reading labels

You need to know what's in your food. If you haven't started reading labels, you might be surprised by how many extra ingredients are hidden in some products. It's essential to be aware of these ingredients and stay selective about what you buy. At first, you might need to do some research. Downloading an app that explains E-numbers and other additives can be helpful, or you can look up unfamiliar terms online.

It's startling how many products contain additives, even more so when you realize many are linked to potential health issues. If an ingredient is associated with any health concern, I wholeheartedly recommend avoiding it, at least until you can tell what does or doesn't affect you. Reading every label can be time-consuming, but being diligent will help you feel better faster.

Being strict about your diet

Sticking closely to your dietary plan will help you avoid unnecessary setbacks. I know it's frustrating when you can't join your friends for an occasional night out, and it really sucks to always be the person who has to say no to foods you'd actually love to eat. On top of that, you'll likely have to keep convincing those around you that these foods truly do hurt you, which is exhausting as well. Still, it's tremendously important that you take care of yourself, and being strict about your diet is a big part of that. It gives your body the space it needs to heal.

The easiest way to explain why you can't eat certain foods—and avoid endless questions—is to simply say you're allergic to them. No need to go into detail—just let them know these foods will make you sick. Period. End of story. No further discussion is necessary. I've found this works better than trying to explain MCAS to someone who's never heard of it, because allergies are more widely understood.

Keeping it simple

It's a good idea to keep things simple when you don't know all your triggers yet. I understand this might sound ridiculous when you must keep so many guidelines in mind, but it gets easier once you know precisely what to avoid. Having only a few foods to choose from makes deciding what to eat much more straightforward.

If your digestion is out of balance, it's best to stick to very basic meals until your system has had a chance to reset. Whenever I start reacting to food, I retreat to one to three foods I definitely tolerate and stay with those until my symptoms calm down.

Reintroducing foods when possible

To avoid malnutrition and support a balanced microbiome, your diet must have some diversity. Once you've figured out which foods are problematic and which you tolerate well, reintroducing foods—slowly and carefully—is an essential next step. For extra guidance, you can download the *Food Reintroduction Toolkit* by Bonnie Nasar at tmsforacure.org under Patient Resources.

KEY TAKEAWAY

Eating with MCAS becomes easier once you know your safe foods. Test for long-term allergies, avoid gluten and milk, and prepare your meals yourself with fresh ingredients. Processed, packaged, and leftover foods are best avoided. Avoid iodized salt, and read labels carefully. Stay strict with your diet, as it helps prevent painful setbacks. Once stable, carefully reintroduce foods to support nutrition and a balanced microbiome.

CHAPTER 48

Histamine-Free Cooking

Certain foods are naturally high in histamine and should be avoided altogether. The tricky part is that nearly any food can accumulate histamine over time, so it's essential to be mindful—not just of the products you use but also of how you prepare them. Even foods typically low in histamine can become "histamine bombs" if they have been cooked for too long, reheated, aged, or over-ripened. This might sound complicated at first, but it actually becomes quite simple: just stick to raw or freshly prepared foods with ingredients low in histamine.

General guidelines for a low-histamine kitchen

- Eat fresh. The fresher the food, the better.
- Become savvy about histamine content in foods.
- Choose low-histamine ingredients.
- Foods that are naturally high in histamine must be avoided altogether.
- You cannot decrease histamine in any way; cooking cannot remove it from food.
- Do not reheat food, as reheating increases histamine.
- The longer something sits, the more histamine it accumulates.
- Freezing fresh food halts the process of histamine accumulation. For example, you can freeze fresh meat to keep it longer, but you shouldn't freeze leftovers to reheat later, because reheating increases histamine content.
- Avoid all processed foods, as you have no control over their freshness.
- Avoid processed meats and meats cured for a long time.
- Avoid fermented products.
- Avoid all aged food products.
- Fish is only safe if absolutely fresh. Ideally, it should be eaten within an hour of being caught, or frozen immediately.

Meat preparation and safety

Meat is generally tolerable, but processed meats must be avoided. This includes ground beef, pre-cut chicken, lunch meats, or sausages.

Buy meat as fresh as possible, portion it into the needed amounts, and freeze it immediately. When buying meat or frozen foods, bring a cooler bag with ice packs to maintain the cold chain until you can put them in your freezer. Hermetically sealed meat is generally safer than meat from an open counter. The safest option is likely to buy directly from farmers, as some slaughter based on individual orders. That way, they can portion and freeze it right away. Lastly, purchase organic, grass-fed meats because they offer more nutritional value, and antibiotics used in commercial meat production can potentially cause gastrointestinal upset.

Ground meat

If you want to eat ground meat, it's best to get a meat grinder and make it yourself to ensure freshness and low histamine content.

> **KEY TAKEAWAY**
>
> Histamine-free cooking means choosing low-histamine ingredients, prioritizing freshness, and avoiding anything aged, processed, reheated, or fermented. Histamine builds up in foods over time and cannot be removed, so eat fresh and never reheat leftovers. Freezing is the only method that halts histamine accumulation. Buy meat sealed or directly from a farmer to ensure freshness. Fish must be fresh-caught or frozen immediately after catch.

CHAPTER 49

Histamine Liberators

Histamine liberators are foods that aren't necessarily high in histamine, but they can trigger its release in the body. To help minimize your total histamine load, it's essential to avoid them. Certain food additives, medications, and various external factors can also act as histamine liberators.

Based on Sigrid Nesterenko's *Histaminintoleranz – die unentdeckte Krankheit*[124] and the histamine food compatibility list from SIGHI (Swiss Interest Group on Histamine Intolerance),[125] the following pages list the most significant known histamine liberators.

HISTAMINE LIBERATORS IN FOODS

Fruits

- Avocado
- Banana
- Citrus fruits
- Grapefruit
- Mango
- Orange
- Papaya
- Pear
- Pineapple
- Plum
- Raspberry
- Strawberry
- Kiwi (possible)
- Chocolate

Vegetables

- Tomato
- Sauerkraut
- Pickled cabbage
- Button mushrooms
- Porcini

Legumes

- Soybeans

Dairy

- Aged cheese
- Mold cheeses
- Milk (possible)

Meat / Fish / Eggs

- Processed meat
- Seafood
- Egg whites

Grains / Seeds

- Wheat germ
- Sunflower seeds
- Nuts
- Cashew
- Walnut
- Condiments
- Mustard
- Vinegar
- Beverages
- Alcohol
- Red wine
- Black tea
- Green tea
- Yerba mate
- Cocoa
- Energy drinks

Other foods

- Licorice

OTHER LIBERATORS

- Medications
- Food additives
- Bacterial toxins
- Insect venoms
- Snake venoms
- Toxic processes
- Allergic processes
- Inflammation
- Heat
- Cold
- Stress
- Injuries

Vitamins, minerals, and stimulants

- Iodine
- Potassium iodate
- Potassium iodide
- Folic acid / folate / vitamin B9
- Theobromine (also known as xantheose)
- Caffeine

Color additives

E100	curcumin
E101a	riboflavin
E102	tartrazine
E104	quinoline yellow, food yellow 13, C.I. 47005
E110	sunset yellow FCF, orange yellow S
E120	carmine, cochineal, crimson lake
E122	acid red-14, azorubin, brilliant carmoisin 0, food red 3, carmoisine, C.I. 14720
E123	amaranth (azo dye amaranth artificial food coloring, not the grain)
E124	cochineal red, C.I. acid red 18, ponceau 4R, C.I. 16255
E127	erythrosine
E128	red 2G, acid red 1, azogeranine, azophloxine
E129	allura red, food red 17, C.I.16035, FD&C Red 40, naphthalene sulfonic acid
E131	patent blue V, sulphan blue
E132	indigotine, indigo carmine
E151	brilliant black BN, brilliant black PN, brilliant black A, black PN, food black 1, naphthol black, C.I. food black 1, C.I. 28440
E154	brown FK, kipper brown, chocolate brown FK, C.I. food brown 1
E155	brown HT, chocolate brown HT, food brown 3, C.I. 20285
E160b	annatto, bixin, norbixin
E180	lithol rubine BK, pigment rubine, carmine 6B, brilliant carmine 6B, permanent rubin L6B, lithol rubine, C.I. pigment red, C.I. pigment red 57:1, D&C Red No. 7, C.I. 15850:1

Preservatives

E200	sorbic acid
E202	potassium sorbate
E203	calcium sorbate
E210	benzoic acid
E211	sodium benzoate
E212	potassium benzoate

E213	calcium benzoate
E231	2-hydroxybiphenyl, ortho-phenylphenol
E232	sodium orthophenylphenol
E239	hexamethylenetetramine, hexamine, methenamine, urotropine, 1,3,5,7-tetraaza adamantane, formin, aminoform

Parabens (Preservatives)

E214	ethyl paraben
E215	ethyl p-hydroxybenzoate
E218	methyl parahydroxybenzoate
E219	sodium methylparaben

Sulfites (Preservatives)

E220–228	sulfites (sulphites)
E220	sulphur dioxide
E221	sodium sulfite
E222	sodium bisulfite, sodium hydrogen sulfite
E223	sodium metabisulfite, sodium pyrosulfite
E224	potassium pyrosulfite
E225	potassium sulfite
E226	calcium sulfite
E227	calcium bisulfite
E228	potassium hydrogen sulfite, potassium bisulfite

Antioxidants

E310	propyl gallate, propyl 3,4,5-trihydroxybenzoate, gallic acid propyl ester, n-propyl gallate
E311	octyl gallate
E312	dodecyl gallate, lauryl gallate
E320	butylated hydroxyanisole
E321	butylated hydroxytoluene (BHT)

Thickeners, stabilizers, and emulsifiers

E400	alginic acid, algin, alginate
E401	sodium alginate
E402	potassium alginate
E403	ammonium alginate

E404	calcium alginate
E405	propylene glycol alginate
E407 + 407a	carrageenan, processed seaweed
E410	carubin, carob gum, carob bean gum, locust bean gum, LBG
E413	tragacanth
E452	polyphosphates: sodium-, potassium-, calcium-, sodium-calcium polyphosphate

Flavor enhancers

E620–625	glutamates, glutamic acid, and its salts

Other problematic substances

- Quinine (bitter lemon or tonic water)
- Salicylic acid (forbidden as a food additive)

Medications that liberate histamine

- Pain medications / anti-inflammatories: diclofenac, flurbiprofen, ketoprofen, naproxen
- Antirheumatic agents: indometacin, mefenamic acid
- Other: acetylsalicylic acid (aspirin), codeine (cough/pain medicine), heparin (blood thinner), opiates

Medications that block diamine oxidase (DAO)

- Antidepressant: amitriptyline (ATC N06AA099)
- Anti-arrhythmic drug: propafenone
- Antibiotics: cefotiam, clavulanic acid, cycloserine, isoniazid
- Antirheumatic agents: chloroquine, indomethacin, mefenamic acid
- Antiseptic agent: acriflavine
- Asthma medications: aminophylline, theophylline
- Beta-blocker: alprenolol
- Calcium-channel blocker (cardiovascular agent): verapamil
- Expectorant drugs: acetylcysteine (ACC), ambroxol
- Gastrointestinal drug: metoclopramide (MCP)
- General anesthetic: propanidid, sodium thiopental
- Local anesthetic: prilocaine
- Tranquilizer: diazepam (Valium)

- Pain medications: metamizole, pethidine
- X-ray contrast medium

KEY TAKEAWAY

Histamine liberators are foods and substances that don't necessarily contain high levels of histamine but can trigger its release in the body. They occur in foods, medications, additives, preservatives, sulfites, colorings, thickeners, and flavor enhancers. Stress, heat, cold, injuries, infections, and inflammation can also provoke histamine release, and even certain vitamins and minerals may contribute. Avoid these triggers to help reduce your total histamine load.

CHAPTER 50

Biogenic Amines

Biogenic amines are naturally occurring nitrogen-containing compounds derived from amino acids. Foods high in biogenic amines (BAs) are normally listed in high histamine food charts, but understanding what they are and where they're found is helpful. BAs, such as histamine, serotonin, dopamine, octopamine, and phenethylamine, occur in foods like fish, cheese, beer, wine, meat, fermented vegetables, soy, fruits, chocolate, and nuts.[126,127]

The most relevant BAs are histamine, putrescine, tyramine, cadaverine, β-phenethylamine, and tryptamine.[126] They mostly form through microbial decarboxylation of amino acids.[128] While small amounts are necessary for specific physiological functions, high levels can be toxic,[126] causing symptoms like palpitations, hypertension, diarrhea, nausea, headache, inflammation, and flushing. Severe intoxication can be fatal,[126] depending on ingestion amount, type, and detox capacity.

BAs are usually broken down in the gut by enzymes like MAO, DAO, and PAO. If these are deficient or the system is compromised, BA levels can rise, especially in those who are taking MAO inhibitors or drinking alcohol.[126,128] Some BAs release histamine, while others block DAO, hindering breakdown. BAs are processed before histamine, potentially reducing histamine degradation. Those on low-histamine diets should avoid foods high in biogenic amines.[124]

The following are relevant biogenic amines and their typical food sources, adapted from *Histaminintoleranz – die unentdeckte Krankheit* by Sigrid Nesterenko (chapter: *Biogene Amine*, pp. 65-67)[124]:

BA:	Found in:
Agmatine	Cheese
Cadaverine	Spoiled meat
Diethylamine	Beer
Dopamine	Banana
Ethylamine	Beer
Histamine	Cheese, wine, vinegar, fish, yeast, tomato, banana, sauerkraut
Noradrenaline	Banana
Phenethylamine	Chocolate, cheese, cocoa
Putrescine	Banana, pineapple, papaya
Serotonin	Banana, pineapple, papaya, walnut, avocado, chocolate, tomato,plum, cashew
Spermidine	Pear, cashew, legumes, wheat germ
Spermine	Pear, cashew, legumes, wheat germ
Theobromine	Chocolate
Trimethylamine	Spoiled fish
Tryptamine	Cured fish, tomato, cheese
Tyramine	Cheese, wine, cocoa, chocolate, yeast, fish, sausage, tomato, avocado, citrus fruits, spinach, kohlrabi, sauerkraut, raspberry, banana

KEY TAKEAWAY

Biogenic amines (BAs) are naturally occurring compounds formed mainly by microbial breakdown of amino acids in food. Small amounts serve important physiological roles, but excessive intake can be toxic, causing various symptoms and even life-threatening reactions. BAs occur in many foods, especially fermented, aged, or spoiled products, and certain fruits and vegetables. When the enzymes that normally break down BAs are impaired, levels can rise. Some BAs directly release histamine, while others block its breakdown, compounding intolerance.

CHAPTER 51

Foods Low in Histamine

Since I find it much less discouraging to see your safe foods listed—rather than just all the good stuff you must avoid—I've included a chart of low-histamine foods you can potentially enjoy. This list might even inspire new recipe ideas! Please keep in mind that these foods may still trigger reactions due to individual allergies or sensitivities to substances like salicylates, oxalates, fructose, lectins, or FODMAPs.

The following information is sourced from SIGHI's regularly updated website www.histaminintoleranz.ch[125]:

Meat

- Beef
- Chicken (skinless)
- Duck
- Minced meat (fresh)
- Ostrich
- Quail
- Tongue (veal, beef)
- Turkey
- Fresh veal
- Lard

Fish

- Freshwater trout (fresh or frozen)

Eggs

- Egg yolk
- Quail eggs

Dairy

- Sweet cream butter
- Additive-free sweet cream
- Plain cream cheese
- Curd cheese
- Farmer's cheese
- Geheimrat's cheese

- Goat milk
- Young gouda cheese
- Milk (pasteurized or UHT)
- Mozzarella cheese
- Quark
- Raw milk
- Sheep milk
- Whey

Fruits

- Acerola
- Apple
- Apricot
- Blackberry
- Blackcurrants
- Blueberry
- Carambola / starfruit
- Cherry
- Cocoa butter
- Coconut
- Common sea-buckthorn
- Cowberry
- Cranberry
- Desiccated dates
- Goji berry
- Gooseberry
- Grapes
- Jostaberry
- Kaki / persimmon
- Lingonberry
- Lychee
- Melons (except watermelon)
- Morello cherries
- Nectarine
- Peach
- Pitaya / dragon fruit
- Pomegranate
- Quince
- Raisins (sulfite-free)
- Red currants
- Sour cherry

Vegetables

- Artichoke
- Asparagus
- Beetroot
- Sweet bell pepper
- Bok choy
- Broccoli
- Cabbage (green, red, white)
- Carrot
- Cauliflower
- Celery
- Corn salad
- Lamb's lettuce
- Courgette / zucchini
- Cucumber
- Endive
- Fennel
- Gourds
- Iceberg lettuce
- Marrow
- Napa cabbage
- Parsnip
- Pumpkin
- Radish (red, white)
- Romaine lettuce
- Squashes
- White onion

Nuts

- Brazil nuts
- Chufa / earth almond / tiger nut
- Macadamia
- Pistachio (additive-free, no iodized salt)
- Nutgrass
- Seeds
- Chia
- Hemp
- Psyllium husks

Starches

- Amaranth
- Chestnut
- Additive-free cornflakes
- Kamut / khorasan wheat
- Maltodextrin
- Millet
- Oats
- Pearl sago
- Potato
- Quinoa
- Rice
- Rice biscuits, cakes, and noodles
- Sago / spelt
- Sweet corn
- Sweet potato
- Wild rice
- Yam

Sweeteners

- Agave
- Birch sugar / xylitol (E967)
- Caramel
- Dextrose
- Sorbitol / glucitol (E420)
- Fructose
- Glucose
- Honey
- Inverted sugar syrup
- Lactose
- Maltose
- Maple syrup
- Stevia
- Sucrose
- Sugar
- Beet sugar
- Cane sugar

> **KEY TAKEAWAY**
>
> Low-histamine diets can still be varied and enjoyable. Chapter 51 includes a chart with tolerable options to inspire your recipes.

CHAPTER 52

Foods Rich in Quercetin

Quercetin is a flavonoid found in many plants. It helps stabilize mast cells when used prophylactically, has anti-inflammatory, anticarcinogenic, and antiviral properties, and influences platelet aggregation, capillary permeability, and lipid peroxidation—a process where free radicals damage cells.[51,129]

Quercetin should not be combined with digoxin (digitalis), an older cardiac medication. Caution is also advised when taking it with cyclosporine, diclofenac, phenytoin, tolbutamide, and vitamin K antagonists.

Clinical studies typically use 500–1000 mg daily, divided into smaller doses. Higher doses above 1000 mg daily may cause kidney toxicity.[130] Although foods contain far less quercetin than supplements, regularly consuming quercetin-rich foods may still offer benefits and gradually improve your overall well-being. The following information is sourced from quercetin.com[131] and superfoodly.com.[132]

Since many of these foods are known to be either high in histamine or act as histamine liberators, I've included a curated list in the *Resources and References* section, where safe items and problematic ones are visually separated. Printable PDFs are also available at www.mcas-book.com

> **KEY TAKEAWAY**
>
> Quercetin is a flavonoid with mast cell–stabilizing, anti-inflammatory, antiviral, and antioxidant properties. Clinical studies use 500–1000 mg daily; higher intakes can cause kidney toxicity. While foods provide much smaller amounts, regularly eating quercetin-rich foods may still support well-being.

Food	Quercetin mg per 100g/ml
Capers	233.84
Capers, canned	172.55
Lovage leaves	170
Elderberry juice concentrate*	108.16
Dock	86.2
Radish leaves	70.37
Wild rocket	66.19
Dill	55.15
Cilantro	52.9
Banana peppers	50.63
Fennel leaves	48.8
Juniper berries	46.61
Mexican oregano	42
Yellow onion, cooked (general)	41.9
Red onions	39.21
Carob flour	38.78
Radicchio	31.51
Red leaf lettuce	30.6
Spring onions (red bulb)	30.6
Watercress	29.99
Hartwort leaves	29.3
Ancho peppers	27.6
Elderberries	26.77
Hawthorn leaves**	24.1
Asparagus cooked	23.6
Kale	22.58
Okra	20.97
Bee pollen	20.95
Cocoa powder	20
Apples, skin only	19.36
Chia seeds	18.42
Moringa	16.65
Saskatoons	16.64
Annual sow thistle	16
Serrano peppers	15.98
Buckwheat	15.38

Food	Quercetin mg per 100g/ml
Hot green chili pepper	14.7
Cranberries	14
Goji berries dried	13.6
Red spring onion leaves	12.6
Black diamond plums	12.45
Romaine lettuce (source 1)	12
Yellow onion cooked (summer)	11
Scallions	10.68
Red leaf lettuce (winter)	10.3
Tarragon	10
Green chili pepper cooked	9.9
Sweet potato leaves cooked	9.84
Mustard greens	8.8
Arugula	7.92
Blueberries	7.67
Sea buckthorn	7.58
Red Swiss chard	7.5
Lingonberries	7.4
Oregano	7.3
Red kidney beans boiled	6.82
Chicory greens	6.49
Long yellow peppers	6.45
Figs	5.47
Yardlong bean, cooked	5.3
White sweet onion	5.19
Jalapeno peppers	5.07
Turmeric steamed	4.92
Chives	4.77
Acerola	4.74
Brussels sprouts cooked	4.33
Green leaf lettuce	4.16
Tomato products (no salt added)	4.12
Apples, all varieties, w/skin	4.01
Spinach	3.97
Tart or sour cherry juice	3.88
Blackberries	3.58

Food	Quercetin mg per 100g/ml
Celery	3.5
Cherry tomatoes	3.3
Broccoli	3.26
Bay leaves	3.19
Concord grapes	3.11
Bilberries	3.04
Snap green peas	2.73
Butterhead lettuce	2.73
Green tea brewed	2.69
Collard greens	2.57
Black grapes	2.54
Cayenne peppers	2.48
Broccoli rabe	2.25
Green bell peppers	2.21
White Swiss chard	2.2
Romaine lettuce (source 2)	2.2
Black tea brewed	2.19
Japanese green tea brewed	2.1
Applesauce, canned	2
Garlic	1.74
Apricots	1.63
Pistachio nuts	1.46
Red potatoes with skin, baked	1.43
Iceberg lettuce	1.42
Oolong tea brewed	1.3
Cherries	1.2
Strawberries	1.11
Apples, all, fruit without skin	1.05
Broccoli rabe cooked	1.05
Red raspberries	1.05
Red grapes	1.04
Red wine	1.04

* Elderberry juice may provoke flare-ups in autoimmune diseases.

** Hawthorn leaves are not recommended for low blood pressure.

CHAPTER 53

Anti-Inflammatory Foods

Certain foods are known to reduce inflammation. If they're low in histamine and you're not allergic to them, eating them regularly may help support your overall well-being.

Although nonsteroidal anti-inflammatory drugs (NSAIDs) are often used to manage inflammation, they are contraindicated for MCAS patients and have been associated with serious gastrointestinal, cardiovascular, and kidney-related side effects, especially with long-term use.[133-137] In contrast, anti-inflammatory foods are generally safe for long-term use and may provide a more sustainable approach.

Foods that fuel inflammation

Highly processed foods, refined carbohydrates, sugary and artificially sweetened foods, red and processed meats, fried foods, and trans fats are generally considered pro-inflammatory. Gluten and dairy may also be problematic for some, while others tolerate them well.

Foods that fight inflammation

Generally regarded as anti-inflammatory are green leafy vegetables, fresh fruits, vegetables, herbs, healthy oils, nuts, fatty fish, and poultry.

ANTI-INFLAMMATORY COMPOUNDS IN FOODS

Many plant-based foods contain natural compounds that support health and help protect the body from chronic inflammation. These compounds, known as phytonutrients or phytochemicals, have been shown to exert a wide range of beneficial effects, including antioxidant, anti-inflammatory, antimicrobial, antiallergic, anticancer, neuroprotective, cardioprotective, and immunomodulatory actions.

Some may also support liver health, blood sugar regulation, cholesterol balance, and protection against UV damage and age-related decline. Phytochemicals are also the foundation of functional foods and nutraceuticals, which are increasingly used to help prevent or manage chronic diseases.[138,139]

Phytonutrients are classified into broad categories such as polyphenols, carotenoids, terpenoids, resveratrol, limonoids, phytosterols, phytoestrogens, and glucosinolates. Each category includes subtypes that contribute to specific physiological functions.[139]

Polyphenols

Polyphenols are a large group of phytochemicals primarily known for their antioxidant activity, though many also provide anti-inflammatory, antiallergic, and protective cardiovascular effects. They include subgroups such as flavonoids, phenolic acids, stilbenes, and lignans. Polyphenols are especially abundant in fruits, vegetables, herbs, teas, legumes, and whole grains.[138,139]

Flavonoids (Polyphenols)

Examples:

- Flavones like ***apigenin*** or ***luteolin*** have cardioprotective, anticancer, and free radical-scavenging properties, and may help reduce age-related decline. Found in: oregano, parsley, rosemary, green olives, bell peppers, pumpkins, watermelons, honey, chickpeas, fava beans, and field peas.
- Flavanones offer protective effects against cardiovascular diseases and may help prevent inflammation and allergic responses. Found in: lemon, mandarin, pomelo, and grapefruit.
- Flavanols like ***quercetin*** and ***kaempferol*** help neutralize free radicals and may aid in preventing inflammation and allergic reactions. Both also help inhibit mast cell activity. Flavonols are generally found in chocolate, tea, and grapes. Quercetin is especially abundant in red onions, apple skin, red grapes, green tea, and buckwheat.
- ***Anthocyanins*** and ***anthocyanidins*** may help reduce inflammation and allergic reactions and offer protective effects against cardiovascular diseases. Found in: blueberries, raspberries, cranberries, red grapes, pomegranate, purple corn, red cabbage, and black soybeans.

Phenolic acids (Polyphenols)

Phenolic acids are known for their potent antioxidant and anti-inflammatory properties. They include caffeic, ferulic, p-coumaric, gallic, rosmarinic, vanillic, and carnosic acids, which have demonstrated protective effects against inflammation-related conditions, including cardiovascular and liver problems, cancer, neurodegeneration, and microbial and even coronavirus-based infections. They help neutralize reactive oxygen species (ROS) and modulate inflammatory pathways.[140]

Examples:

- ***Caffeic acid*** and its derivatives may help suppress pro-inflammatory markers and support vascular and neurological health. Found in: yerba mate, thyme, oregano, sage, rosemary, mint, moringa leaves, and some tea.
- ***Ferulic acid*** has shown beneficial effects in metabolic syndrome and lipid regulation. Found in: flaxseeds, black beans, oats, whole grains, and angelica root.
- ***Gallic acid*** and ***rosmarinic acid*** have been linked to reductions in oxidative stress and improved cognitive performance in animal studies. Found in: tea, blueberries, thyme, sage, rosemary, oregano, and certain medicinal plants like *Salvia* species.
- ***Vanillic acid*** and ***p-coumaric acid*** have shown antioxidant and cytoprotective effects, particularly in liver and brain tissue models. Found in: whole grains, garlic, basil, amaranth leaves, acai berries, and black sesame.

Stilbenes (Polyphenols)

A small but powerful class of polyphenols, best known for their anti-inflammatory, antioxidant, neuroprotective, cardioprotective, and anticarcinogenic effects. The most researched stilbene is *trans*-resveratrol, but others may have even more potent or specific effects.[141]

Examples:

- ***Resveratrol*** (trans-resveratrol) offers anti-inflammatory, cardioprotective, neuroprotective, antithrombotic, anti-aging, and anticancer effects. At dietary levels, it may support heart and brain health, while experimental research suggests it could help inhibit tumor growth and metastasis. Found in: red wine, grapes (especially skins), with smaller amounts in peanuts, pistachios, and berries.[142]

- ***Piceatannol*** offers stronger anti-inflammatory activity than resveratrol; modulates immune response, and inhibits T-cell activation and cytokines (TNFα, IL-1β). Found in: passion fruit, red grapes, blueberries, and rhubarb.
- ***Pterostilbene*** offers antioxidant, neuroprotective, and anti-inflammatory effects, supports brain and intestinal health, and has higher bioavailability than resveratrol. Found in: blueberries and Indian kino tree.
- ***ε-Viniferin*** offers anti-inflammatory, anticancer, and antioxidant effects and has stronger free-radical-scavenging activity than resveratrol. Found in: grapevine stems and roots.
- ***Mulberroside A*** offers protection against liver and intestinal inflammation; helps calm immune overactivation and maintain the intestinal barrier. Found in: mulberry.
- ***Rhapontigenin / Rhaponticin*** offers anti-inflammatory and antioxidant effects, inhibits histamine release from mast cells, and supports kidney and liver health. Found in: rhubarb.
- ***Polydatin*** offers antioxidant, anti-inflammatory, and mitochondrial-supportive effects; suppresses COX-2 and cPLA2 activity. Found in: grape skin, Japanese knotweed.
- ***Oligostilbenes*** (e.g., ampelopsin A/C) offer cytokine-inhibiting effects and may help modulate cartilage and joint inflammation via PGE2 inhibition in human chondrocytes. Found in: wild grapes.

Lignans (Polyphenols)

Lignans are a class of phytoestrogens found in flaxseed, sesame, whole grains, fruits, and vegetables. They may help reduce the risk of cardiovascular disease, osteoporosis, menopausal symptoms, depression, and certain cancers by influencing inflammatory and hormonal pathways.[143]

Examples:

- ***Secoisolariciresinol*** helps reduce inflammation and oxidative stress by increasing antioxidant enzymes and inhibiting NF-κB activation, a key signaling molecule in inflammation. Found in: flaxseeds.
- ***Pinoresinol*** exerts anti-inflammatory effects via inhibition of NF-κB signaling. Found in: sesame seeds, olives, and whole grains.

- ***Matairesinol*** may support cardiovascular health. Found in: flaxseeds and sesame seeds.
- ***Medioresinol*** supports antioxidant defenses and may help protect against cancer. Found in: whole grains and plant-based foods.
- ***Sesamin*** shows anti-inflammatory, antioxidant, and bone-protective properties. It may help reduce cardiovascular damage and depression. Found in: sesame seeds.
- ***Syringaresinol*** suppresses pro-inflammatory cytokines and shows promise in inhibiting prostate cancer progression. Found in: sesame seeds.
- ***Lariciresinol*** may protect against oxidative damage. Found in: flaxseeds, vegetables, fruits, and whole grains.
- Metabolites: ***Enterodiol*** (END) and ***Enterolactone*** (ENL) are gut-derived from dietary lignans and provide systemic anti-inflammatory and anticancer effects. Produced during the digestion of flaxseed, sesame, and other lignan-rich foods.

Other Polyphenols

- ***Polyphenol amides*** may help prevent inflammation and allergic reactions. Found in: chili, pepper, and oats.[139]
- ***Tannins*** offer antioxidant, antidiabetic, antimicrobial, and antiparasitic effects. Found in: tea, wine, grapes, coffee, cider, cereals, cacao, nuts, peas, legume seeds, and some leafy greens.[144]
- ***Oleocanthal*** has antioxidant, anti-inflammatory, antidiabetic, antimicrobial, and antiparasitic properties. It acts similarly to ibuprofen in its anti-inflammatory effect. Found in: olive oil.[145]
- ***Curcumin*** offers anti-inflammatory, antioxidant, and immune-modulating effects. Found in: turmeric.[146]
- ***Epigallocatechin gallate*** (EGCG) offers antioxidant and anti-inflammatory effects and anti-obesity, antidiabetic, antiatherosclerosis, and anti-cancer benefits. Found in: green tea.[147]

Carotenoids

Carotenoids are pigments that give many fruits and vegetables their yellow, orange, and red colors, and they also create the deep green shades in leafy greens. Found in foods like carrots, spinach, mangoes, sweet potatoes, and seaweed, they provide antioxidant support and may help protect the eyes, skin, lungs, and cardiovascular system.[148,149]

Examples:

- ***α-carotene*** supports gene regulation, may help protect against lung and prostate cancer, and promotes eye health. Found in: avocado, banana, butternut, chard, collard greens, green bean, mango, okra, peach, pear, pumpkin, squash, and tangerine.
- ***β-carotene*** enhances immunity and gap junction communication (direct signaling between neighboring cells). Found in: Brussels sprouts, carrot, grapefruit, mango, papaya, peaches, red pepper, romaine lettuce, sour cherries, and spinach.
- ***Lutein*** supports immunity and eye health. Found in: asparagus, broccoli, green beans, kale, lettuce, oranges, parsley, peppers, pistachio nuts, and spinach.
- ***Lycopene*** may improve eyesight, reduce pain, and support bone strength. Found in: tomato, apricot, papaya, pink grapefruit, pink guava, rosehip, sweet potato, and watermelon.
- ***Xanthophylls*** act as antioxidants, support eye health, and may help improve blood flow. Found in: mushroom, papaya, pepper, and pumpkin.
- ***Cryptoxanthin*** helps maintain lung health, supports immune function, and may help prevent arthritis and inflammation. Found in: apricot, papaya, peach, cashew apples, sea buckthorn, mandarin, tangerine, and lemon.
- ***Fucoxanthin*** may help reduce inflammation and offers antioxidant, antihypertensive, antidiabetic, anticancer, anti-obesity, and radioprotective effects. Found in: brown seaweeds, macroalgae, and microalgae.[139]

Terpenoids

Terpenoids, also called isoprenoids, are commonly found in herbs, citrus fruits, algae, and green foods. Their effects range from anti-inflammatory and antimicrobial to calming and neuroprotective actions.[150] Many terpenoids are also responsible for plants' distinctive scents and medicinal properties.

Examples:

- ***Limonene*** has anti-inflammatory, antioxidant, and anti-stress properties and may offer neuroprotective effects in Alzheimer's disease. Found in: lemon and lime.
- ***Myrcene*** has anti-anxiety, antioxidant, anti-aging, anti-inflammatory, and pain-relieving properties. Found in: mango, guava, thyme, parsley, bay leaves, lemongrass, cardamom, sweet basil, and juniper.
- ***Pinene*** offers antibacterial, antitumor, anti-inflammatory, and sedative effects. Found in: cannabis, turpentine tree, ironwort, and sage.

Glucosinolates

These are sulfur-containing compounds primarily found in cruciferous vegetables. When broken down during digestion, they form bioactive compounds such as ***sulforaphane*** and ***indole-3-carbinol***, which support detoxification and have been linked to anti-inflammatory and anticancer effects in experimental studies. Found in: brassica vegetables like broccoli, Brussels sprouts, cabbage, cauliflower, collards, kale, mustard, radish, rapeseed, and turnip.[151]

Other anti-inflammatory bioactives

- ***Gingerol*** is known for its anti-inflammatory, antioxidant, antimicrobial, antidiabetic, and anti-obesity properties. It also supports digestion by reducing nausea and diarrhea, promotes heart health by improving circulation, blood pressure, blood sugar control, and insulin sensitivity, and may also support brain health. Found in: ginger.[146]
- ***Capsaicin*** may reduce inflammation and pain perception by desensitizing sensory nerve pathways. Found in: chili.[152]

Omega-3 fatty acids

Although omega-3s do not belong to the class of phytonutrients, they exert powerful anti-inflammatory actions. Omega-3 fatty acids regulate immune signaling and may reduce inflammation in conditions like heart disease, arthritis, and MCAS-related inflammation. There are two types of omega-3s: EPA and DHA (from fish) and ALA (from plants). Found in: fatty fish (salmon, sardines), flaxseeds, walnuts, and chia seeds.

Since many of these foods are known to be either high in histamine or act as histamine liberators, I've included a curated list in the *Resources and References* section, where safe items and problematic ones are visually separated. Printable PDFs are also available at www.mcas-book.com

> **KEY TAKEAWAY**
>
> Anti-inflammatory foods can help reduce inflammation safely, unlike medications that often cause side effects. Avoid refined carbs, sugar, fried foods, trans fats, and highly processed products, and instead choose colorful, fresh whole foods, healthy oils, poultry, and fish. These provide phytonutrients with anti-inflammatory, antioxidant, antimicrobial, antiallergic, and protective effects.

CHAPTER 54

Creativity in the Kitchen

During my worst MCAS phases, I tolerated only three specific foods, and for over two years, I was restricted to eighteen options. Many fellow sufferers complain about this limitation and how boring it is to keep eating the same foods over and over again.

It definitely is boring to eat the same food every day, and it's also disheartening, as meals with loved ones are among life's greatest pleasures—a perfect chance to socialize. Constantly missing out on these gatherings is yet another reminder of how confining this condition can be.

Determined not to feel so limited, I took this as yet another challenge to overcome. With a bit of tinkering, I've developed so many recipes that delight both me and my friends. By simply preparing the same ingredients differently, I create varied and unique dishes. I thought about including recipes in this book, but instead chose to share ideas for making your own, as this is more of a manual for navigating life with MCAS rather than a cookbook.

Variations in preparation: The key to more options

To expand your meal options, *how* you prepare food is key. Suppose broccoli is the only food you can tolerate. Pretty boring, right? I agree! But it doesn't have to be, as it can be steamed, baked, fried, pureed, or even juiced. So, even though you're eating the same vegetable, the different textures will at least give you a bit of variety.

Combining methods, like baking it first and then briefly frying, can also help alter the taste and texture. Chopping vegetables differently also transforms the eating experience. I personally dislike zucchini in large chunks, but love it thinly sliced and fried until crispy. With this in mind, vegetables and fruits can be sliced, diced, grated, juiced, or blended, adding variety even with limited ingredients. So even if potatoes were your only safe food, you could still enjoy a different meal every day: baked whole, boiled, sliced into golden-brown wedges, mashed, crispy fried, as hash browns, in omelets, soups, salads, or as French fries.

I know someone who tolerated only three foods for over two years. Imagine how monotonous, and even repelling, that became after 700+ days! However, modifying texture and consistency can make repetitive meals more bearable.

Now, take just two ingredients, broccoli and potatoes, and suddenly, you have over ten menu options, such as:

- Mashed potatoes with roasted broccoli
- Boiled potato with roasted broccoli
- Baked potato with steamed broccoli
- Potato wedges with broccoli dip
- Potato soup with broccoli chunks
- Potato chips with creamy broccoli soup
- Potato cakes with steamed broccoli
- Potato slices with baked broccoli
- Potato omelet with crispy-fried broccoli
- Potato and broccoli salad
- Hash browns with steamed broccoli

Herbs and spices

Herbs and spices are an excellent way to add variety, as even small amounts can profoundly alter the flavor of a dish. Once you know which ones you tolerate, the range of tastes you can play with instantly expands. Adding spices to the water when cooking rice or potatoes profoundly changes their taste. For example, rice cooked with chives tastes different from rice with a pinch of paprika. Topped with a drizzle of oil and fresh herbs, it creates a satisfying, visually appealing meal—delicious, effortless, and ready in about twelve minutes.

Creative salad dressings

I don't tolerate vinegar, so I began making salad dressings with juiced fruits or vegetables. Instead of vinegar, I use freshly juiced apple, cucumber, or bell pepper and mix it with oil, salt, and chives. It's quick, easy, and delicious!

Creating substitutes for craving foods

If you miss a specific food, making something that at least looks similar can be surprisingly satisfying. It helps me feel less restricted, and every time I find a way to enjoy something MCAS has taken from my life, I feel a sense of victory.

If you're craving tomato sauce, try making something similar with bell peppers. It may not be the traditional spaghetti sauce you really want, but it looks the part and tastes great in its own right—plus, it's low in histamine. The result looks just like tomato sauce and, while not identical, is still tasty and satisfying.

Bell Pepper "Spaghetti" Sauce

A low-histamine alternative to traditional tomato sauce

Ingredients

- 2 bell peppers (1 for chopping, 1 for juicing)
- 1 white onion
- Olives
- Capers
- Oregano
- Thyme
- Rosemary
- A small amount of red wine
- Oil for frying

Instructions

1. Chop one bell pepper into chunks
2. Juice the second bell pepper and set aside
3. Fry the white onion until golden brown
4. Add the pepper chunks, olives, capers, oregano, thyme, and rosemary to the pan
5. Cook until the vegetables have absorbed the spices' flavors
6. Add a tiny sip of red wine
7. Pour in the juiced pepper
8. Let simmer until reduced to a pleasant, sauce-like texture

Craving pancakes? Try a rice-based alternative. It's not quite the real thing, but if rice is one of the few foods you tolerate, this can be a surprisingly comforting substitute. Add your favorite toppings and enjoy!

Rice-Based Pancakes

A satisfying option for those with dietary restrictions

Ingredients

- Cooked rice
- Pinch of salt
- Sugar
- 1 spoonful of potato starch
- A small amount of canola oil
- Neutral oil for frying

Toppings (optional)

- Butter
- Coconut butter
- Maple syrup
- Jam

Instructions

1. Cook rice as usual
2. Once cooked, puree half of the rice and mix it back with the remaining rice
3. Add a pinch of salt, sugar, potato starch, and a little canola oil
4. Let the mixture sit for thirty minutes to thicken
5. Form the mixture into small balls
6. Heat neutral oil in a pan
7. Fry the rice balls, using a spatula to flatten them in the pan
8. Fry well before flipping to prevent them from falling apart
9. Serve with your choice of topping

> **KEY TAKEAWAY**
>
> MCAS often limits food choices, which can feel monotonous and isolating. Creativity in preparation helps restore variety. Try different cooking methods, combine safe foods in new ways, and use herbs, spices, juices, and tolerated substitutes to expand flavors, boost nutrients, and satisfy cravings.

CHAPTER 55

Kitchen Tools

Kitchen tools can make life easier, especially when you have limited energy. If a machine can help with your daily tasks, why not use it? I'd say anything that simplifies life ultimately benefits the healing process. Additionally, if you are limited in the foods you tolerate, modifying their texture can make eating more enjoyable. Juicing fruits and vegetables, for example, is a great way to introduce more variety.

Tools I love using

- Juicer
- Blender
- Hand blender
- Bullet blender
- Food processor
- Steamer
- Rice cooker
- Dishwasher (countertop models connect to sink faucets—perfect for small spaces)

Allergen-free cookware

Good allergen-free cookware can help lessen reactions. I have a nickel allergy along with my mast cell issues, so I must be cautious with my cooking equipment. While this might not be an issue for you, allergy sufferers are often advised to avoid cookware containing nickel. I have fewer and less severe reactions since switching to allergen-free options, so it may be worth considering.

Stainless steel is an iron-based metal, often labeled 18/10, meaning it contains 18 percent chromium and 10 percent nickel. Chromium prevents rust, and nickel increases durability, prevents corrosion, and adds luster. Even if a nickel test shows negative results, stainless steel can still leach nickel into food when heated—especially when cooking with acidic or salty ingredients, since these ingredients can react with the metal surface.

Recommended allergen-free pans

- Glass pans
- Cast iron
- Ceramic-coated pans
- Titanium

Titanium is considered the safest non-stick option. However, some cookware marketed as "titanium" may actually use silicone, ceramic coating, titanium, or a combination of these materials. If you're allergic to silicone, use caution.

Non-stick frying pans

Non-stick frying pans, commonly called Teflon, have been free of PFOA since 2013. Polytetrafluoroethylene (PTFE), or Teflon, can degrade at high temperatures, releasing fine particles of perfluorooctanoic acid (PFOA), which can be toxic when inhaled. When using non-stick pans, ensure they don't contain PTFE or PFOA. PFOA has been included in the Stockholm Convention since 2019 and banned under the POPs regulation since July 2020. Importantly, discard any pans with damaged or matted surfaces.

Silverware

Like cooking equipment, silverware is often made from stainless steel, which typically contains nickel. If you react to nickel or other metals, or you suffer from contact dermatitis, allergen-free silverware may be worth considering. Alternatively, you could purchase allergen-free silverware made from titanium or high-grade plastics. I use chopsticks, wooden spoons, and allergen-free plastic spoons.

Smells in the kitchen

The AirHood is a portable device designed to reduce cooking odors, smoke, grease, and oil residue. It can be especially helpful for those who react to smells and smoke.

Storage solutions

Since some plastics can disrupt hormonal function, it may be wise to choose glass storage containers and drinking bottles instead.

KEY TAKEAWAY

Kitchen tools like food processors, juicers, and blenders save energy and add variety. Choose allergen-free cookware such as glass, cast iron, ceramic-coated, and titanium pans. If using non-stick, pick PTFE/PFOA-free options and replace damaged ones. Nickel-sensitive individuals may need to avoid stainless steel and use allergen-free silverware. For storage, glass containers are preferable to plastics, which may disrupt hormones.

CHAPTER 56

Storing Food

Knowing how to store food properly is especially useful when you're in a phase where you react to nearly everything, since stores can be full of triggers, and even stepping inside for a moment can set you back for days. To shop less often, I started buying in bulk. When I buy meat, I portion and freeze it immediately. I first eat salads, fruits, and vegetables that spoil quickly, and save the longer-lasting items for later in the week. Here are a few tips that can help keep food fresh a bit longer.

Bread

Best stored in a paper bag, cloth bag, wooden box, or pottery container. Avoid storing bread in plastic bags and in the fridge, as both trap moisture and accelerate mold growth. Moldy bread is highly toxic and should be discarded.

Cheese and dairy

Store in the middle of the refrigerator. Wax paper keeps the cheese from drying out and losing flavor. For hard cheeses, small mold spots can be cut off, and the rest is still safe to eat. For soft cheeses, the entire piece should be discarded.

Coffee

Store away from light, heat, and moisture in an airtight container in the pantry. Refrigerating causes it to lose flavor and absorb other odors from the fridge.

Cooking oils

Store away from heat and light, as both speed up spoilage.

Flours

Keep in an airtight container in a cool, dry place. Whole grain flours do better in breathable paper bags to prevent moisture buildup and pests.

Fruit

Most fruits keep best in the fridge, including figs and kiwi. Tropical fruits like bananas and mangoes are best stored at room temperature. Citrus fruits can be stored at room temperature or in the fridge.

Garlic

Best stored in a well-ventilated container, like a cardboard box or terracotta garlic keeper. Refrigerating it can cause it to mold more quickly.

Meat and fish

If not frozen, store in the coldest part of the fridge, which is usually the bottom shelf near the back, where cold air settles.

Mushrooms

Store in paper bags or wrapped in paper towels in the fridge. Avoid plastic as it traps moisture, causing them to mold quickly.

Onions

Keep in a cool, dark place, stored separately from potatoes. Refrigeration can cause them to mold more quickly.

Potatoes

Ideally stored at 45–50°F (7–10°C) in a dry and dark place to maintain freshness and prevent sprouting.

Rice and grains

Store them in airtight containers in a cool, dry place.

Salads

Keep best when wrapped in a slightly damp kitchen towel and stored in the fridge.

Tomatoes, eggplant, and pumpkin

Keep at room temperature for the best flavor and texture.

Vegetables

Most vegetables should be kept in the fridge's vegetable drawers, where the humidity is higher and the temperature is slightly warmer. Exceptions include onions, garlic, potatoes, squash, tomatoes, eggplant, and pumpkin.

Freezing

Meat, fish, and high-fat dairy products can be frozen for several months. Fresh herbs, chopped and frozen, keep for several months, though you could also grow plants on a windowsill and harvest them fresh.

Many fruits and vegetables can be frozen, but some need blanching first. These include asparagus, beans, broccoli, Brussels sprouts, cabbage, carrots, cauliflower, celery, corn, eggplant, kohlrabi, okra, peas, peppers, rutabagas, turnips, fennel wedges, kale, and Swiss chard. Blanching tutorials can be found on YouTube.

> **KEY TAKEAWAY**
>
> Proper food storage extends freshness and helps reduce trips to trigger-filled stores. Buy in bulk and freeze meat, fish, high-fat dairy products, suitable fruits, and vegetables. Store foods appropriately, and use perishable items first. Grow herbs on your windowsill for absolute freshness.

CHAPTER 57

Beneficial Diets

For most of my life, I was a vegetarian, but I also experimented with different diets—some out of curiosity and others to manage my GI issues and mast cell-related symptoms. Over the years, I tried raw food, vegan, keto, FODMAP, intermittent and extended fasting, food combining, and various detox approaches.

Honestly, I've found experimenting with different diets enjoyable and, at times, genuinely helpful, but in some cases, it made things worse. Some diets may lead to nutritional deficiencies, and rigorous approaches can negatively affect the microbiome, which is the community of bacteria living in our gut. These bacteria play a key role in digestion and help absorb and synthesize nutrients. A healthy gut flora is essential for overall well-being, so keep this in mind. That said, some diets have helped me feel better.

Gluten-free diet

According to Molderings et al. (2016),[29] avoiding gluten, cow's milk protein, and baker's yeast for three to four weeks at the beginning of a therapy is a precondition for the therapeutic effects of drug treatment in MCAS. Therefore, anyone with MCAS may benefit from exploring diets free of these ingredients.

I am allergic to gliadin, a protein in gluten, so eliminating gluten made a huge difference for me. When I switched to a gluten-free diet, I initially expected to feel deprived, because so many foods I was used to eating contain flour. However, I soon discovered so many great alternatives that my food options actually increased. Ultimately, I had more variety on my plate than ever before.

Importantly, I rarely tolerate commercially made gluten-free products, since they often contain stabilizers and additives my body can't handle. Yet, I do well with naturally gluten-free ingredients like potatoes, rice, or quinoa. When I crave bread, I make my own, but I've mostly stopped eating bread altogether.

Milk-free diet

Milk can be a good source of calcium, magnesium, and potassium. Still, as suggested by Molderings, dairy is best avoided for about a month when trying new mast cell medications. For me personally, cutting milk from my diet has dramatically helped reduce inflammation.

FODMAP diet

This diet is recommended for irritable bowel syndrome (IBS). FODMAP stands for fermentable oligosaccharides, disaccharides, monosaccharides, and polyols. These are sugar alcohols and short-chain carbohydrates that trigger symptoms like bloating, gas, stomach pain, reflux, and diarrhea. FODMAPs are found in many foods, and while there are plenty of resources available, it's easier to follow with the guidance of a dietitian or nutritionist.

Low histamine diet

Adhering to low-histamine foods is essential if you suffer from MCAS, especially in the beginning, until you've identified all your food triggers. A comprehensive low-histamine chart is available on the website of the Swiss Interest Group Histamine Intolerance (SIGHI) at histaminintoleranz.ch.[125] If you have additional allergies, you can print this list to add your triggers or use it as a template to create your own chart.

Low-salicylate diet

Many MCAS patients react to salicylates, a substance that occurs naturally in plants, where it helps protect the plant from stress and pathogens like insects, fungi, and bacteria. Salicylates are also synthetically produced and commonly used as preservatives in food, medications, body care products, and perfumes. While excessive salicylate causes adverse effects in anyone, those with intolerance react to even small amounts with symptoms like stomach pain, breathing difficulties, headaches, diarrhea, nausea, fatigue, swelling, sinusitis, and itchy skin, among others.

There are several books on the topic, including *The Salicylate Handbook* by Sharla Race and *Salicylate Intolerance* by Joan Tozzi Ablahani.

Low-carb diet

Eating fewer carbs has helped me reduce inflammation, shakiness, and heart palpitations. Remarkably, I feel more balanced and less anxious, allowing me to respond more calmly to mast cell symptoms. Staying composed during a reaction usually helps my symptoms subside more quickly.

Ketogenic diet

Originally designed as an alternative to fasting in the treatment of epilepsy, the ketogenic diet relies on fat as the primary fuel source, heavily restricting carbs and moderating protein intake. Typically, the body uses glucose for energy. However, by limiting carbohydrates for a few days until glycogen stores are emptied, the body begins using ketone bodies for energy, which the liver produces from stored fat.

I tried this approach after a few people, including one doctor, suggested it might help reduce my inflammation. Since many allowed foods are high in histamine, salicylate, or nickel, I had to follow a restricted version, but it proved beneficial in several ways: I experienced a significant reduction in inflammation, better focus, greater calmness, and my heart palpitations and dizziness improved. Because fat is so satiating, I ate fewer meals, which helped calm my GI symptoms. Reaching ketosis stopped my sugar crashes—a real eye-opener since I hadn't realized they had intensified my mast cell symptoms until then. I also lost a lot of weight, which wasn't my goal as I was already quite slim, but this could benefit others looking to lose weight.

The downside of the ketogenic diet is its restrictiveness, even if you can eat the full range of allowed foods. Prolonged restriction may lead to nutritional deficiencies, a compromised microbiome, and increased GI distress.

Mono meals

This means eating only one food at a time, which can help identify food reactions and calm the system. When I do this, I still eat a variety of foods, but space them apart—either between meals or from one day to the next.

Intermittent fasting

Intermittent fasting (IF) involves eating only within a designated timeframe each day, typically an eight-hour eating window followed by a sixteen-hour fast. It's simple to follow and effective.

IF allows the body to cleanse during fasting periods, offering benefits such as weight loss, improved blood sugar control, better cholesterol levels, enhanced brain health, reduced inflammation, and improved cellular repair. I believe IF is great for almost everyone, especially for those prone to inflammation or gastrointestinal issues, or those looking to lose weight.

For me, it feels great because it gives the body a break from processing food. When it's time to eat, you're genuinely hungry, and your body seems better prepared to absorb and process the food more efficiently.

A cautionary note: a 2024 study (not yet peer-reviewed) suggests that intermittent fasting might increase the risk of cardiovascular death. However, because the study relied on self-reported data and dietary tracking over only two days, more research is needed. These findings contradict earlier studies, but people with heart disease may need to be cautious with IF until more research is available.[153,154]

Fasting

Water fasting can be extremely helpful to calm the system, especially when you're reacting to nearly every bite of food. Giving the body a temporary pause from food may help it reset and begin healing. However, water fasting is intense and not appropriate for everyone. If you're considering a fast, it's important to do it under medical supervision.

> **KEY TAKEAWAY**
>
> Certain diets can help manage symptoms, though some may harm gut health or cause deficiencies. Helpful approaches include gluten-free, milk-free, FODMAP, low-histamine, and low-salicylate diets, while low-carb or ketogenic diets may reduce inflammation but can be overly restrictive. Simpler methods like mono meals, intermittent fasting, or water fasting can also calm the system, but fasting should always be medically supervised.

CHAPTER 58

Nutrients

Once you've identified your safe foods and your digestion has settled enough for you to think clearly again, it's time to start looking at nutrients and whether your diet provides enough. MCAS often leaves us with a minimal range of foods, increasing the risk of nutritional deficiencies. A prolonged lack of essential nutrients can cause entirely new health problems, adding to the already complex mast cell situation. Since it's easy to miss things when your whole system is under stress, it's wise to tackle this step with a dietitian or nutritionist.

Learning the basics of nutrition and what nutrients actually do for us helped me realize just how vital a balanced diet really is. Specific nutrients must come from food because the body cannot produce them, or at least not in sufficient amounts. These are called essential nutrients because they are crucial for good health, maintenance, growth, and disease prevention. Nutrients are broken down into two main categories: macronutrients and micronutrients.

- **Macronutrients**
  Proteins, carbohydrates, and fats are needed in large amounts, as they form the primary building blocks of the diet and supply the body with energy.
- **Micronutrients**
  Vitamins and minerals are required only in small amounts, but they're essential for overall health and support countless bodily functions.

Proteins

Protein is essential for good health. It's required for building muscle, bones, blood, cartilage, and skin, and is present in all cells and tissues, where it supports their growth and repair.

Proteins are composed of amino acids. Out of the approximately twenty amino acids, nine are considered essential because the body cannot produce them on its own and must obtain them through food. These include isoleucine, lysine, leucine, methionine, phenylalanine, tryptophan, threonine, histidine, and valine. Children may need additional amino acids, as their bodies may not yet produce enough of them.[155]

Carbohydrates

Carbohydrates are the body's primary fuel source. During digestion, they're broken down into simple sugars, which enter the bloodstream as glucose, also known as blood sugar. Glucose then moves into the cells, where it's converted into energy. When glucose intake exceeds the body's requirements, the surplus is stored in the liver, muscles, or other cells and may be converted into fat.[156]

Fats

Fat is a significant source of energy in our diets. It helps absorb specific nutrients, builds cell membranes and the sheaths surrounding nerves, and plays a role in inflammation. Body fat provides insulation against extreme temperatures and helps protect our organs from external stress. Some fats also support muscle function and blood clotting.

There are healthy fats and others that are best avoided. Good fats may help reduce inflammation, while bad fats may worsen it. Monounsaturated and polyunsaturated fats are considered healthy, while industrial trans fats are unequivocally harmful. Saturated fats should probably be eaten in moderation, as research offers conflicting findings: some studies link them to increased heart disease risk, while others find no clear evidence.

Vitamins

Vitamins are essential for a healthy immune system. They support growth and development, promote healthy skin and hair, and help ensure proper muscle, brain, and blood function. They also play a key role in converting food into energy.

Minerals

Minerals are essential for vital functions such as forming bones and teeth, transmitting nerve impulses, regulating metabolism, and supporting muscle contraction and relaxation. They also help maintain healthy blood pressure, regulate inflammation, balance hormones, and support wound healing.

Water

Water is crucial for every system in the body. It hydrates, carries nutrients to cells, and helps flush out toxins. It supports digestion, regulates temperature, boosts brain function, and even helps lift our mood.

> **KEY TAKEAWAY**
>
> Nutrients are life-giving substances in food. Essential nutrients must come from the diet and are divided into macronutrients such as protein, fat, and carbohydrates, and micronutrients such as vitamins and minerals.

CHAPTER 59

Vitamins

Vitamins are organic compounds essential for the body's proper functioning. Although needed only in small amounts, they are vital in maintaining health. Since our bodies cannot produce them, we must obtain them through the diet.

Water-soluble and fat-soluble vitamins

Vitamins are classified as either water-soluble or fat-soluble. Water-soluble vitamins must be consumed frequently, as excess amounts are quickly filtered out by the kidneys and excreted in the urine. Water-soluble vitamins are less likely to reach toxic levels than fat-soluble ones, but they still have upper intake limits. Over time, both deficiencies and chronic over-supplementation—especially with fat-soluble vitamins—can lead to significant health issues. Whenever possible, check your levels before supplementing, and always prioritize real food over supplements. Reaching toxic levels of nutrients through food is very unlikely, but it is easily possible with over-supplementation.

Water-soluble vitamins:	Vitamin C and all B vitamins
Fat-soluble vitamins:	Vitamins A, D, E, and K
Essential nutrient:	Choline

Caution: Beware of excipients in supplements

If you experience adverse reactions to vitamin or mineral supplements at reasonable doses, it's important to understand that the adverse reaction is almost certainly caused by an excipient, not the active ingredient itself. Since the body depends on these life-giving substances, the reaction is more likely triggered by fillers, binders, dyes, preservatives, contaminants, and other additives.

WATER-SOLUBLE VITAMINS

Vitamin C

Required for a healthy immune system, iron absorption, and protein metabolism. It also helps produce collagen, norepinephrine, and serotonin. As an antioxidant, it protects cells from damage, and long-term use may help lower cancer risk and protect against cataracts.[157,158,160]

A severe vitamin C deficiency causes scurvy. Due to its low toxicity, even high intakes are unlikely to cause serious adverse effects, with gastrointestinal disturbances being the most frequently reported symptom.[159]

Sources: fruits and fruit juices, especially guava, acerola cherries, papayas, kiwi, persimmons, lychee, strawberries, citrus, mangoes, and cantaloupe. Vegetables, especially peppers, cabbage, tomatoes, broccoli, snow peas, potatoes, cauliflower, and Brussels sprouts.[159,160]

Recommended Dietary Allowance (RDA) (ages 19+): men 90 mg,
women 75 mg (smokers should add 35 mg)
Tolerable Upper Intake Level (UL) (ages 19+): 2000 mg[159]

Vitamin B1 (Thiamine)

Essential for energy metabolism and cell function, growth, and development. It also supports nerve and brain function and healthy muscles, hair, and skin.[157,158,161]

Deficiency can lead to anorexia, weight loss, short-term memory loss, confusion, and other mental symptoms, as well as cardiovascular issues, muscle weakness, and other possible complications. Groups at greater risk include older adults, people with alcohol dependence, diabetes, HIV/AIDS, and those who've had bariatric surgery.

The Food and Nutrition Board (FNB) has not established tolerable upper intake levels (ULs) for thiamine, as high intakes have not been shown to cause adverse effects.[161]

Sources: nutritional yeast, macadamia nuts, sunflower seeds, meat, fish, fortified foods, flaxseed, navy beans, black beans, green peas, rice, oats, lentils, seaweed, asparagus, and Brussels sprouts.[160,161]

RDA (ages 19+): men 1.2 mg, women 1.1 mg
UL: not established[161]

Vitamin B2 (Riboflavin)

Essential for maintaining healthy blood, brain function, hair, and skin, as well as supporting vision and the function, growth, and development of cells. Vitamin B2 helps convert food into energy and plays a role in the metabolism of lipids, steroids, and certain drugs.[157,158,162]

Although rare, deficiency can result from inadequate intake or endocrine abnormalities such as thyroid hormone insufficiency and certain other diseases. Symptoms may include hair loss, skin disorders, cracked and swollen lips, angular stomatitis, sore throat, hyperemia, swelling of the mouth or throat, red and itchy eyes, reproductive issues, and, in severe cases, nervous system and liver degeneration.

ULs have not been established for riboflavin, as adverse effects from high intakes have not been reported. Still, the FNB cautions against excessive consumption.[162]

Sources: almonds, beef, organ meats (kidneys and liver), green leafy vegetables, whole grains and enriched grains, milk and dairy products, eggs, soybeans, avocados, and mushrooms.[160,162]

RDA (ages 19+): men 1.3 mg, women 1.1 mg
UL: not established[162]

Vitamin B3 (Niacin)

The term niacin encompasses nicotinic acid, nicotinamide, and related compounds like nicotinamide riboside. All body tissues convert absorbed niacin into the coenzyme nicotinamide adenine dinucleotide (NAD), which supports the activity of more than four hundred enzymes to catalyze reactions in the body. NAD also gets converted into nicotinamide adenine dinucleotide phosphate (NADP) in every tissue except skeletal muscle.[163]

Niacin helps convert food into energy and is essential for healthy blood cells, skin, brain function, and the nervous system. Its active form, NAD, plays a central role in breaking down fats, proteins, carbohydrates, and alcohol, transferring the potential energy from these sources to the cell's primary energy molecule, adenosine triphosphate (ATP). NAD also helps maintain genome integrity, control gene expression, and facilitate cellular communication.

NADP, in contrast, is primarily involved in anabolic reactions, including the synthesis of fatty acids, steroids, and essential building blocks for proteins,

DNA, and complex carbohydrates. NADP also plays a key role in maintaining antioxidant functions within cells.[157,158,163]

Severe niacin deficiency can lead to pellagra, a condition that causes a sun-sensitive rash, a bright red tongue, digestive issues, and neurological symptoms such as fatigue, depression, memory problems, and, in extreme cases, hallucinations or behavioral changes. While uncommon today, mild deficiency may still occur in people with poor diets, malabsorption, or certain medical conditions. Low intake of nutrients like vitamin B2, B6, or iron can also impair the body's ability to make niacin from tryptophan.

Consuming foods that naturally contain niacin doesn't cause adverse effects, but high doses from supplements can be seriously harmful.[163]

Sources: meat, poultry, fish, some nuts and seeds, avocado, potato, green peas, asparagus, mushrooms, whole grains, and tryptophan-rich foods.[160,163]

RDA (ages 19+): men 16 mg, women 14 mg
UL (ages 19+): 35 mg (from supplements)[163]

Vitamin B5 (Pantothenic Acid)

Vitamin B5 helps convert food into energy and supports the production of hemoglobin, neurotransmitters, steroid hormones, and fats. Its main role is synthesizing coenzyme A (CoA), a crucial compound for breaking down nutrients and building new molecules. CoA is also needed to transport small molecules like acetyl and acyl groups around the body.[157,158,164]

Deficiency is rare because pantothenic acid is present in nearly all foods. When it does occur—usually in cases of severe malnutrition—it often appears alongside other nutrient deficiencies. Symptoms may include burning or numbness in the feet and hands, fatigue, headache, restlessness, irritability, sleep disturbances, and digestive symptoms accompanied by anorexia.

ULs have not been established, as no toxic effects have been reported from high intakes. However, excessive supplementation may cause mild diarrhea or digestive discomfort.[164]

Sources: beef, organ meats, fish, egg yolks, shiitake mushrooms, whole grains, sunflower seeds, avocados, and tomatoes.[160,164]

RDA (ages 14+): men 5 mg, women 5 mg
UL: not established[164]

Vitamin B6 (Pyridoxine)

Pyridoxine refers to six related compounds (vitamers) that share vitamin B6 activity. It plays a key role in protein metabolism and supports the processing of amino acids, carbohydrates, and fats. Vitamin B6 helps maintain healthy brain function by regulating homocysteine levels and converting tryptophan into niacin and serotonin—a neurotransmitter involved in mood, sleep, and appetite. It also supports the production of hemoglobin, immune system function, and blood sugar balance.[157,158,165]

Deficiency is rare and usually occurs alongside other B vitamin deficiencies. Mild cases may go unnoticed for years. When symptoms do appear, they can include skin inflammation with cracked lips (cheilosis), a swollen tongue, weakened immunity, microcytic anemia, and neurological changes affecting mood, thinking, and brainwave activity.

While adverse effects from high intakes through food sources have not been reported, long-term use of oral vitamin B6 supplements (1–6 g/day over 12–40 months) may result in progressive and severe sensory neuropathy. Excessive intake may also cause photosensitivity, damaging and painful skin irritations, and gastrointestinal symptoms such as nausea and heartburn.[165]

Sources: fish, beef liver, organ meats, chickpeas, starchy vegetables, and fruits (except citrus).[160,165]

RDA (ages 19–50): men 1.3 mg, women 1.3 mg; (ages 50+) men 1.7 mg, women 1.5 mg
UL (ages 19+): 100 mg[165]

Vitamin B7 (Biotin)

Biotin is a cofactor for enzymes that help metabolize glucose, amino acids, and fatty acids. It plays a role in cell signaling, gene regulation, and modifying proteins (histones) that organize and protect DNA. Biotin also supports healthy hair, skin, and bones.[157,158,166]

There are no reports of severe deficiencies in healthy people who consume a regular, varied diet. Those at a greater risk for deficiency include pregnant or breastfeeding women, people with chronic alcohol exposure, and those who have biotinidase deficiency.

Symptoms of deficiency usually emerge slowly and can include thinning of hair that may progress to hair loss affecting the entire body, brittle nails, skin rashes and infections, acid buildup in the body, conjunctivitis, and neurological conditions such as tingling sensations, lethargy, depression, and hallucinations in adults. In infants, deficiency can cause lethargy, weak muscles, and delayed development.

ULs have not been established since there is no evidence that high biotin intake is toxic for humans. However, supplementation above the recommended levels can lead to false laboratory results, misdiagnoses, or improper patient management.[166]

Sources: whole grains, organ meats, egg yolks, soybeans, fish, sweet potatoes, seeds, and nuts. Biotin is also produced in the intestinal tract by bacteria.[160,166]

RDA (ages 19+): men 30 mcg, women 30 mcg
UL: not established[166]

Vitamin B9 (Folic acid, Folate)

Folate is the natural form of vitamin B9 found in foods, while folic acid is the synthetic version often used in supplements and fortified foods. It plays a key role in metabolism by helping break down amino acids, supporting the production of new cells, and assisting in the creation of RNA and DNA. It's especially important in early pregnancy to prevent brain and spine birth defects and is therefore recommended for all women of reproductive age, as pregnancy may not be immediately recognized.[157,158,167]

Poor diet, malabsorption issues, or chronic alcohol consumption may cause folate deficiency. Megaloblastic anemia, characterized by large, immature red blood cells, is an early indicator of deficiency. It can lead to fatigue, weakness, headache, difficulty concentrating, irritability, shortness of breath, and heart palpitations. In addition, folate deficiency may cause mouth sores, skin, hair, or nail pigmentation changes, and elevated homocysteine levels. Insufficient intakes during pregnancy may cause neural tube defects, low birth weight, preterm birth, and growth issues.[167]

There have been no reported adverse effects from high folate intake through foods, and as a result, no ULs have been set for food-derived folate. However, ULs are established for synthetic folate. Excessive folate supplementation can mask a vitamin B12 deficiency, which can be dangerous, as B12 deficiency-related neurological damage can become irreversible if untreated. Intakes of folic acid exceeding 1,000 mcg per day during the periconceptional period have been linked to lower cognitive scores in children aged 4–5. Excessive intake may also negatively impact immune function and contribute to cognitive decline in older adults.[167]

Sources: green leafy vegetables, legumes, liver, asparagus, Brussels sprouts, fruits, fruit juices, peas, seafood, eggs, dairy, meat, poultry, fortified grains, and cereals.[160,167]

RDA (ages 14+): men 400 mcg DFE, women 400 mcg dietary folate equivalents (DFE)
UL (ages 19+): 1000 mcg (for supplements) ULs differ for individuals taking high amounts of supplemental folate under the supervision of a physician.[167]

Vitamin B12 (Cobalamin)

Essential for the central nervous system, DNA synthesis, red blood cell formation, and lowering homocysteine levels.[157,158,168] Active forms include methylcobalamin and adenosylcobalamin.

Deficiency can result from poor diet, malabsorption, gastrointestinal surgery, or long-term use of medications like Metformin or acid-reducing drugs. It may lead to anemia, low blood cell and platelet counts, fatigue, palpitations, pale skin, infertility, neurological symptoms (tingling/numbness), dementia, and depression. During pregnancy or breastfeeding, a deficiency might cause developmental delays and anemia in infants.

Because Vitamin B12 has a low risk for toxicity, no UL has been set. Healthcare providers should monitor B12 levels in patients taking medications that interfere with B12 absorption (e.g., H2 blockers, proton pump inhibitors, Metformin).[168]

Sources: clams, beef liver, fish, meat, poultry, seafood, eggs, dairy, nutritional yeast, fortified cereals, and fortified soy milk. Vitamin B12 is not naturally present in plant foods.[160,168]

RDA (ages 14+): men 2.4 mcg, women 2.4 mcg
UL: not established[168]

FAT-SOLUBLE VITAMINS

Vitamin A (Retinol) and Carotenoids

Vitamin A supports immune function, reproduction, vision, and the normal development and maintenance of organs such as the eyes, lungs, and heart.[157,158,169] It is also essential for cell differentiation and communication.

There are two main forms of vitamin A in food: preformed vitamin A (retinol and retinyl esters from animal sources) and provitamin A carotenoids (alpha-carotene and beta-carotene from plants), which are converted into vitamin A primarily in the intestines. Carotenoids like lutein, zeaxanthin, and lycopene are classified as non-provitamin A carotenoids, as they cannot be converted into retinol. However, they have antioxidant properties and may support eye, heart, and cellular health.

In developed countries, deficiency is rare, but it is tragically common in low-income regions. Vitamin A deficiency is one of the leading preventable causes of childhood blindness. Chronic deficiency increases the severity of infections and has been linked to respiratory diseases, abnormal lung development, a higher risk of anemia, and even an increased risk of death.

Excess Vitamin A is stored in the liver and can accumulate, increasing the risk of toxicity. Very high doses (over 100 times RDA) may cause acute toxicity, with symptoms like muscle aches, blurred vision, nausea, dizziness, coordination issues, severe headaches, and potentially increased intracranial pressure or death. Chronic excess can cause dry skin, joint pain, fatigue, liver issues, and depression. Intake above the UL can also cause birth defects.

In contrast, beta-carotene is not toxic in large amounts, but may cause carotenodermia—a harmless orange skin discoloration that reverses when intake stops. However, long-term, high-dose supplementation has been linked to an increased risk of lung cancer and death in male smokers.[169]

Sources: retinol: liver, fish oils, fortified dairy, butter, eggs, beef, and shrimp.

Beta-carotene: carrots, winter squash, sweet potatoes, pumpkin, dark leafy greens, dark orange fruits like apricots, cantaloupes, and mangoes.[160,169]
RDA (ages 19+): men 900 mcg RAE, women 700 mcg RAE (RAE = retinol activity equivalents)
ULs (preformed vitamin A, ages 19+): 3000 mcg[169]

Vitamin D (Calciferol)

Essential for bone remodeling, growth, and calcium absorption, vitamin D maintains calcium and phosphate levels necessary for bone mineralization, and prevents involuntary muscle contractions. It also supports immune function, neuromuscular health, glucose metabolism, cellular growth, and regulation of inflammation.[157,158,170]

Certain foods naturally provide vitamin D, while others are fortified, and it is available in supplement form. In addition, the body can produce vitamin D when the skin is exposed to sunlight.

Deficiency can result from limited exposure to sunlight, low dietary intake, malabsorption, or impaired kidney function. It may lead to weakened bones or bone deformities, manifesting as osteomalacia in adults and as rickets in children.

Toxicity typically results from excessive supplementation, not from sun exposure or food. It can cause hypercalcemia, elevated serum 25(OH)D, and hypercalciuria. In severe cases, complications may include soft tissue calcification, cardiac arrhythmias, renal failure, or even death. Long-term high calcium intake (e.g., 2,100 mg/day) and moderate vitamin D intake (around 19 mcg/day) may increase the risk of kidney stones. Corticosteroids like prednisone can impair calcium absorption and interfere with vitamin D metabolism, potentially worsening bone loss or osteoporosis.[170]

Sources: fatty fish, fish liver oils, fortified milk, fortified cereals, and fortified margarine. Small amounts are also found in beef liver, cheese, egg yolks, and certain mushrooms.[160,170]

RDA (ages 14–70): men 15 mcg, women 15 mcg; (ages 70+) men 20 mcg, women 20 mcg
UL (ages 19+): 100 mcg[170]

Vitamin E

Vitamin E is the umbrella term for a group of fat-soluble compounds with distinctive antioxidant activities. Of the eight naturally occurring forms, only alpha-tocopherol meets human nutritional needs.

Vitamin E functions as an antioxidant and is essential for immune function, cell signaling, and gene expression. It helps halt the production of reactive oxygen species (ROS) during lipid oxidation, supports vascular health by reducing platelet aggregation and dilating blood vessels, and may help protect vitamin A and certain fats from oxidative damage. Alpha-tocopherol also inhibits protein kinase C (PKC), a group of enzymes involved in immune cells, platelets, and muscle cells. The inhibition of PKC is one of the ways it helps reduce inflammation, lower clot risk, and potentially protect cardiovascular health. Vitamin E may also contribute to cognitive protection and reduced Alzheimer's risk.[157,158,171]

Deficiency is rare but may occur in people with fat-malabsorption disorders or premature infants with very low birth weight. Symptoms can include ataxia, peripheral neuropathy, skeletal muscle weakness, retinopathy, and impaired immunity.

Consumption of foods abundant in vitamin E poses no risk for toxicity, but high-dose supplementation does. Excess alpha-tocopherol can interfere with blood clotting and increase bleeding risk. Animal studies suggest it may inhibit platelet aggregation and prolong clotting time.[171]

Sources: nuts, seeds, green leafy vegetables, fortified cereals, wheat germ, wheat germ oil, and polyunsaturated vegetable oils.[160,171]

RDA (ages 14+): men 15 mg, women 15 mg
UL (ages 14–18): 800 mg; (ages 19+) 1000 mg[171]

Vitamin K

Essential for blood clotting, bone metabolism, and cardiovascular health, vitamin K supports the production of proteins involved in various physiological functions. Inadequate levels can increase the risk of bleeding, bruising, fractures, and arterial calcification. It may also reduce the effectiveness of anticoagulants like warfarin, so consistent intake is important for those on blood thinners.[157,158,172]

Vitamin K is the collective term for a group of fat-soluble compounds with a common structure, primarily phylloquinone (vitamin K1) and menaquinones (vitamin K2). Phylloquinone, the main dietary form, is found in green leafy vegetables. Menaquinones (MK-4 through MK-13), mainly of bacterial origin, are found in fermented and animal-based foods and synthesized by gut bacteria. The only exception, MK-4, is produced in the body from phylloquinone.[172]

The bioavailability of phylloquinone from food is relatively low but improves when consumed together with fat. Supplements and oils offer higher absorption rates. Since adverse effects are rare, no official UL has been established for vitamin K.[172]

Sources: natto, fermented foods, soybean oil, canola oil, and green vegetables.[160,172]

RDA (ages 19+): men 120 mcg, women 90 mcg
UL: not established[172]

ESSENTIAL NUTRIENT

Choline

Although often grouped with the B-complex vitamins due to their similar functions, choline is an essential nutrient, not technically a vitamin. It is vital for healthy cell membranes, lipid metabolism, gene expression, and early brain development. Choline is also required to make acetylcholine, a neurotransmitter involved in memory, mood, and muscle control.[158,173]

While the liver produces some choline, endogenous synthesis is insufficient to meet human needs, so additional intake through food is necessary. Premenopausal women may require less from the diet because estrogen enhances choline synthesis.

Deficiency is rare but may occur during pregnancy, potentially leading to liver and muscle damage and contributing to nonalcoholic fatty liver disease. Excess intake can cause low blood pressure, vomiting, liver toxicity, excessive sweating, and a fishy body odor.

Sources: meat, beef liver, eggs, fish, dairy products, cruciferous vegetables, legumes, nuts, seeds, and whole grains.

RDA (ages 19+): men 550 mg, women 425 mg
UL (ages 19+): 3500 mg[173]

> **KEY TAKEAWAY**
>
> Vitamins are organic compounds needed for proper body function. Water-soluble vitamins must be consumed frequently, while fat-soluble ones can accumulate and reach toxic levels. Both deficiency and over-supplementation can cause problems, so food should remain the primary source, with testing recommended before supplementing.

CHAPTER 60

Minerals

Minerals, like vitamins, are vital for good health. They are inorganic elements present in rocks, soil, and water. Plants absorb them as they grow, and animals get them by eating plants or drinking mineral-rich water.

Essential minerals are classified into major (macro) and trace (micro) minerals or elements. The term "major" refers to the quantity the body needs, not its level of importance.

Macro (major) minerals:	calcium, chloride, magnesium, potassium, phosphorus, and sodium
Micro (trace) minerals:	chromium, copper, fluoride, iodine, iron, manganese, molybdenum, selenium, and zinc

MACRO (MAJOR) MINERALS

Calcium

Calcium is essential for the structure of teeth and bones. It also helps support movement by keeping tissues flexible, strong, and firm. In its free form within tissues, extracellular fluid, and the circulatory system, calcium helps control blood vessel contraction and dilation, blood clotting, muscle and nerve functions, and hormone release.

Vitamin D is required for calcium absorption in the gut and for maintaining adequate levels in the blood. About 98 percent of the body's calcium is stored in bones, which serve as a reservoir to help maintain calcium homeostasis. If dietary intake is insufficient, the body draws calcium from these reserves.

Deficiency can result in osteoporosis (fragile bones) and osteomalacia (inadequate mineralization and bone softening). Although more often caused by vitamin D deficiency, calcium deficiency can also lead to rickets in children.

In both osteomalacia and rickets, vitamin D and calcium needs appear to be interrelated: the lower the serum vitamin D levels, the higher the calcium requirement to prevent these conditions.

Hypocalcemia (abnormally low calcium levels in the blood) is usually caused by magnesium or vitamin D deficiency, impaired parathyroid hormone production, certain medical conditions, or the use of proton pump inhibitors, cisplatin, or bisphosphonates. It can also occur when bone resorption of calcium is impaired.

Mild or chronic hypocalcemia can be asymptomatic. When symptoms do occur, they often include neuromuscular irritability. Severe cases may lead to neurological complications, kidney damage, kidney failure, congestive heart failure, brain calcification, paresthesia, and, in rare cases, coma. Those at risk for deficiency include postmenopausal women and individuals who avoid dairy products.

Excessive calcium intake can lead to hypercalcemia (elevated blood calcium) and hypercalciuria (elevated urinary calcium). Both conditions can cause poor muscle tone, constipation, weight loss, nausea, fatigue, hypophosphatemia, heart arrhythmias, kidney problems, polyuria, and an increased risk of cardiovascular death. Calcium can also interact with medications such as quinolone antibiotics, lithium, levothyroxine, and dolutegravir.

Sources: dairy products such as yogurt, milk, mozzarella, and cottage cheese, firm tofu, sardines, salmon, fortified juices and cereals, spinach, kale, broccoli, soybeans, turnip greens, bok choy, pinto beans, among others.

Recommended Dietary Allowance (ages 19–50): men 1,000 mg, women 1,000 mg
RDA (ages 51–70): men 1,000 mg, women 1,200 mg
RDA (ages 70+): men 1,200 mg, women 1,200 mg
UL (ages 19–50): 2,500 mg
UL (ages 51+): men 2,000 mg, women 2,000 mg[174]

Chloride

Chloride is an electrolyte that helps regulate pH balance, blood pressure, and fluid levels in the body. Chloride is also essential for producing hydrochloric acid in the stomach, which supports protein digestion, mineral absorption, and activation of intrinsic factor needed for vitamin B12 uptake.

Chloride deficiency is rare, as nearly all foods containing sodium also contain chloride. However, excessive loss through vomiting, prolonged diarrhea, or heavy sweating can lead to a life-threatening condition known as alkalosis. Symptoms may include dehydration, loss of appetite, muscle weakness, lethargy, and irritability.

Chloride toxicity from dietary intakes is uncommon in healthy individuals but may occur with severe dehydration, kidney dysfunction or disease, or excessive salt consumption. Symptoms may include muscle weakness, fatigue, and high blood pressure.

Sources: table salt, seafood, seaweed, and high-sodium foods like cheese, potato chips, sausages, soy sauce, and ketchup.

Adequate Intake (AI) (ages 14–50): men 2.3 g, women 2.3 g
AI (ages 51–70): men 2 g, women 2 g
AI (ages 71+): men 1.8 g, women 1.8 g
UL (ages 14+): 3.6 g[175-177]

Magnesium

As a critical cofactor in over three hundred enzymatic reactions, magnesium plays a central role in regulating blood pressure and blood glucose, nerve function and impulse conduction, muscle function and contraction, protein synthesis, and maintaining a normal heart rhythm. It also supports cellular energy production and the synthesis of glutathione, DNA, RNA, and contributes to the structural development of bone.

More than half of the body's magnesium is stored in bones, while the rest is found in soft tissues. Less than 1 percent circulates in the blood, where levels are tightly regulated, primarily by the kidneys.

Magnesium deficiency is rare because the kidneys limit urinary excretion. However, chronically low intakes, long-term alcohol abuse, certain medications, and medical conditions can still cause deficiency. Early symptoms may include weakness, fatigue, nausea, vomiting, and loss of appetite. As it progresses, symptoms can include cramps, tingling, numbness, personality changes, seizures, coronary spasms, and abnormal heart rhythms. Severe deficiency can disrupt mineral balance, leading to hypokalemia or hypocalcemia (low serum potassium and calcium levels). Those at risk include older adults, individuals with type 2 diabetes or gastrointestinal diseases, and people with alcohol dependence.

Excess magnesium from food usually isn't harmful in healthy individuals because it's excreted in urine. However, large supplement doses can cause diarrhea, cramps, and nausea. Extremely high doses (>5,000 mg/d) from antacids and laxatives may be fatal due to hypermagnesemia. Those with kidney failure are at higher risk since they can't eliminate excess magnesium effectively.

Sources: pumpkin seeds, chia seeds, almonds, spinach, peanuts, cashews, soy milk, black beans, edamame, potato, rice, yogurt, fortified cereals, banana, salmon, halibut, raisins, whole wheat bread, avocado, chicken, and beef, among others.

RDA (ages 19–30): men 400 mg, women 310 mg
RDA (ages 31–50): men 420 mg, women 320 mg
RDA (ages 51+): men 420 mg, women 320 mg
UL (ages 19+): 350 mg (UL applies to supplements, not dietary magnesium)[178]

Phosphorus

Phosphorus is a component of DNA, RNA, cell membrane structure, and adenosine triphosphate (ATP)—the body's primary form of cellular energy. It is involved in building and maintaining bones and teeth, activating enzymes, regulating gene transcription, storing energy within cells, and maintaining proper pH levels in the blood.

Calcium and phosphorus are closely interrelated because their metabolism is regulated by the same hormones, such as parathyroid hormone (PTH) and vitamin D. Together, they form hydroxyapatite—the mineral compound that gives bones and tooth enamel structure and strength. The kidneys, intestines, and bones tightly regulate phosphorus levels to preserve the body's stores when dietary intake or absorption is insufficient.

Deficiency is rare and typically results from medical conditions like diabetic ketoacidosis, kidney tubule defects, or hyperparathyroidism. Symptoms may include anemia, anorexia, muscle weakness, bone pain, osteomalacia, rickets, paresthesias, confusion, ataxia, and increased infection risk.

Harmful effects from high phosphorus intakes are considered rare. Research findings are mixed: some studies link intakes of 1,000 mg or more to adverse impacts on kidneys, bones, and the cardiovascular system, while others show no increased disease risk.

Sources: dairy products, poultry, meat, eggs, fish, nuts, vegetables, legumes, and grains.

RDA (ages 12–18): men 1,250 mg, women 1,250 mg
RDA (ages 19+): men 700 mg, women 700 mg
UL (ages 9–70): 4,000 mg
UL (ages 71+): 3,000 mg[179]

Potassium

Helps maintain proper fluid volume within cells and supports electrochemical gradients across cell membranes, thereby ensuring normal cell function. Most potassium in the body is stored inside cells, with intracellular concentrations about thirty times higher than in the extracellular space. The sodium-potassium pump maintains this steep difference in potassium concentration across the cell membrane and is essential for cellular tonicity, muscle contraction, nerve transmission, and kidney function. Potassium and sodium are functionally interconnected, even though they have opposing effects.

Insufficient potassium intake raises risks of kidney stones, high blood pressure, urinary calcium loss, bone turnover, and salt sensitivity. Severe deficiency causes hypokalemia, initially leading to muscle weakness, fatigue, constipation, and malaise, and worsening symptoms like polyuria, glucose intolerance, poor respiration, paralysis, and arrhythmias. In kidney disease, it may cause brain dysfunction. As potassium is vital for muscle contraction and heartbeat, severe hypokalemia can be life-threatening.

Inadequate intake rarely causes hypokalemia on its own, but it can result from diarrhea, vomiting, dialysis, heavy sweating, refeeding syndrome, diuretics, or laxatives. Magnesium deficiency worsens hypokalemia by increasing urinary potassium loss and lowering intracellular levels, raising arrhythmia risk. Hypokalemia is more likely in people on certain medications, or with conditions such as inflammatory bowel disease or pica.

High dietary potassium intake does not pose a toxicity risk in healthy individuals with normal kidney function. No UL has been established due to insufficient evidence that high intakes cause hyperkalemia in healthy adults.

Sources: apricots, squash, lentils, raisins, prunes, potato, soybeans, kidney beans, orange juice, banana, milk, spinach, chicken breast, yogurt, salmon, beef, molasses, tomato, broccoli, cantaloupe, turkey breast, asparagus, apple, cashew, flaxseed, coffee, eggs, cheese, and others.

AI (ages 19+): men 3400 mg, women 2600 mg
UL: not established[180]

Sodium

Sodium functions as an electrolyte and helps maintain fluid balance and blood pressure, while also supporting muscle and nerve function. Like chloride and potassium, sodium forms specific channels in the cell membranes that regulate how much fluid enters and exits, allowing for proper nutrient transport and cellular activity.

Sodium deficiency is rare but can occur due to kidney dysfunction, prolonged vomiting or diarrhea, excessive sweating, or fluid overload that the kidneys cannot eliminate. Symptoms may include headaches, nausea, vomiting, lethargy, confusion, altered mental states, seizures, and coma.

Hypernatremia, or elevated serum levels, can result from dehydration, fever, infections, or diuretic use. Symptoms include weakness, nausea, loss of appetite, vomiting, excessive thirst, kidney damage, confusion, and fluid accumulation in the lungs. In severe cases, it may cause brain swelling, which can be life-threatening.

Sources: salt, soy sauce, processed foods, ham, bacon, pickles, parmesan, and others.

AI (ages 14+): men 1,500 mg, women 1,500 mg
CDRR (ages 14+): reduce intake if >2,300 mg/day = chronic-disease risk reduction target, not a UL.
UL: not established[181-183]

MICRO (TRACE) MINERALS/ELEMENTS

Chromium

Chromium may play a role in the metabolism of proteins, carbohydrates, and fats by enhancing insulin activity. It may also have antioxidant properties, though the exact mechanisms are not fully understood.

Deficiency has not been reported in healthy individuals, but levels can be reduced by diets high in simple sugars, strenuous exercise, infections, pregnancy, and lactation.[184]

RDAs have not been set, as the European Food Safety Authority (EFSA) concluded chromium is not essential—its absence does not cause symptoms that supplementation can reverse.[185] The FNB set AIs based on typical intakes in healthy people. No UL has been established due to limited evidence of harm, but caution is advised. Case reports suggest high-dose supplements may cause anemia, weight loss, thrombocytopenia, kidney and liver issues, dermatitis, and hypoglycemia.

Sources: grape juice, ham, brewer's yeast, orange juice, beef, lettuce, turkey breast, tomato juice, apples, green beans, bananas, and others.

AI (ages 19–50): men 35 mcg, women 25 mcg
AI (ages 51+): men 30 mcg, women 20 mcg
UL: not established[184,185]

Copper

Acts as a coenzyme in several enzyme systems involved in energy production, connective tissue formation, neurotransmitter synthesis, iron metabolism, and neuropeptide activation. It also contributes to immune function, blood vessel formation, brain development, neurohormone homeostasis, gene expression, and pigmentation.

Deficiency is uncommon but may develop due to malabsorption disorders like Menkes or celiac disease. Excessive zinc intake can also reduce copper absorption and lead to deficiency. Symptoms may include anemia, bone defects, osteoporosis, connective tissue abnormalities, loss of coordination, increased infection risk, hypopigmentation, and abnormal lipid metabolism.

Chronic exposure to high copper levels may result in gastrointestinal symptoms and liver damage. Although toxicity is uncommon in healthy individuals, it may result from drinking contaminated water due to copper pipes, fixtures, or plumbing systems.

Sources: liver, shellfish, oysters, shiitake mushrooms, potatoes, whole grains, nuts, seeds, beans, tofu, avocado, figs, prunes, cocoa, black pepper, and others.

RDA (ages 19+): men 900 mcg, women 900 mcg
UL: 10,000 mcg[186]

Fluoride

Crucial for both bone development and maintaining tooth health by preventing and potentially reversing cavities. Trace amounts of this mineral are naturally found in water, soil, and plants, while the major sources are fluoridated drinking water, foods made with it, and certain dental care products containing fluoride.

Although fluoride deficiency is rare, it can lead to weakened bones, particularly in children.

Excessive exposure to fluoride during early childhood can cause dental fluorosis. Ingesting high amounts may cause stomach pain, nausea, vomiting, diarrhea, and, although rarely, even death. Fluoride toxicity typically occurs only at very high doses. Still, long-term overexposure has been associated with skeletal fluorosis, a condition that involves joint pain, muscle degeneration, osteoporosis, and neurological issues.

Sources: fluoridated water, foods prepared with fluoridated water, tea, and small amounts in coffee, seafood.

AI (ages 19+): men 4 mg, women 3 mg
UL (ages 9+): 10 mg[187]

Iodine

Plays a vital role in the production of thyroid hormones, which control protein synthesis, enzyme activity, metabolism, skeletal development, and the growth of the central nervous system. Thyroid hormones also affect body temperature, muscle and nerve function, and reproduction.

Iodine deficiency causes growth and developmental issues, especially during pregnancy and infancy, leading to irreversible damage like growth retardation, CNS impairment, or miscarriage. Hypothyroidism with goiter can happen below 10–20 mcg/day. Mild deficiency in children may lower intelligence and is linked to ADHD. At-risk groups include pregnant women, those avoiding dairy, seafood, eggs, iodized salt, iodine-deficient areas, vitamin A or iron deficiencies, and consumption of goitrogenic foods such as soy, cabbage, broccoli, or cassava.

Excessive iodine intake can cause symptoms like iodine deficiency, including elevated TSH, hypothyroidism, and goiter. It may also lead to thyroiditis and thyroid cancer. Acute poisoning is rare, typically only caused by extremely high doses. Iodine levels in soil vary, affecting iodine content in crops. Salt iodization programs have significantly reduced deficiency worldwide.

Sources: iodized salt, seaweed, cod, shrimp, dairy products, enriched bread, pasta, cereals, eggs, and others.

RDA (ages 19+): men 150 mcg, women 150 mcg
UL: 1,100 mcg[188,189]

Iron

Iron is essential for oxygen transport because it is a key component of two important proteins: hemoglobin and myoglobin. Hemoglobin, found in red blood cells, carries oxygen from the lungs to the rest of the body. Myoglobin, located in muscles, helps store oxygen and releases it when muscles need it. Both proteins depend on iron to effectively bind and transport oxygen. Iron is also vital for neurological development, growth, hormone production, and cell function.

Dietary iron exists as heme from animals, which has a higher bioavailability, and nonheme from plants. Combining vitamin C, meat, and seafood in a mixed diet boosts nonheme absorption to 14–18 percent, whereas vegetarian diets absorb about 5–12 percent. Polyphenols, phytates, and calcium can inhibit absorption, but a varied diet generally balances these effects.

Iron deficiency is common among young children, pregnant women, and women of childbearing age. It progresses from mild deficiency (low ferritin and iron stores) to iron deficiency anemia, which is characterized by fatigue, cognitive issues, gastrointestinal disturbances, impaired immunity, and temperature regulation.

High dietary iron intakes are unlikely to cause harm in healthy adults. Still, high-dose supplementation may cause adverse effects like constipation, nausea, and abdominal pain, as well as reduced absorption and plasma concentrations of zinc. Taking iron supplements with meals can mitigate some of these effects. Doses of 130 mg have been shown to cause gastric lesions, and iron overdose (60 mg/kg) can result in convulsions, coma, and death. Between 1983 and 2000, iron overdose claimed the lives of forty-three children, prompting the introduction of safer packaging regulations.

People with hemochromatosis (iron overload) should avoid iron and vitamin

C supplements. For individuals with MCAS, iron supplementation should be used cautiously as it may trigger intense activation of mast cells.

Sources: red meat, poultry, seafood, eggs, fruits, green vegetables, legumes, fortified bread, and grain products.

RDA (ages 19–50): men 8 mg, women 18 mg
RDA (ages 51+): men 8 mg, women 8 mg
UL (ages 19+): 45 mg[190]

Manganese

Acts as a vital cofactor for several enzymes that aid in the metabolism of amino acids, glucose, carbohydrates, and cholesterol. It also plays a crucial role in combating reactive oxygen species, promoting reproductive health, facilitating bone formation, and supporting immune function.

Deficiency of manganese is highly uncommon, and as such, its symptoms are not clearly defined. However, some studies suggest that a lack of manganese might cause issues like growth retardation, alterations in bone health, hair loss, skin rashes, and exacerbated PMS symptoms.

While high dietary manganese intake poses no risk of toxicity, people exposed to high levels in work environments or drinking water may experience toxicity. Symptoms include muscle spasms, tremors, tinnitus, hearing loss, balance problems, insomnia, mood changes, and memory issues. Manganese toxicity can resemble Parkinson's disease.

Individuals with iron deficiency may be more vulnerable to manganese toxicity because low iron levels can increase manganese absorption. Additionally, those with chronic liver disease are at an elevated risk, as their ability to eliminate manganese through bile is impaired.

Sources: fish, grain products, vegetables, tea, seafood, nuts, rice, pineapple, soy, legumes, and others.

RDA: (ages 19+): men 2.3 mg, women 1.8 mg
UL: 11 mg[184,191]

Molybdenum

Functions as an integral component of molybdopterin, a cofactor of several enzymes responsible for the breakdown of heterocyclic compounds like pyrimidines and purines, and sulfur-containing amino acids, some of which can be toxic if not properly metabolized.

Deficiency is rare and has only been observed in cases of molybdenum cofactor deficiency, a rare genetic disorder.

Molybdenum toxicity is rare, as the body quickly excretes it in urine. Metal-workers, miners, and residents in molybdenum-rich areas may be at risk. A study in Armenia linked excessive molybdenum intake to joint pain, high uric acid, and gout-like symptoms.

Sources: legumes, particularly black-eyed peas and lima beans, nuts, whole grains, beef liver, dairy products, bananas, spinach, corn, rice, and more.

RDA (ages 19+): men 45 mcg, women 45 mcg
UL: 2,000 mcg[192,193]

Selenium

Plays a crucial role in reducing oxidative stress, protecting the body from infection, and supporting reproduction, DNA synthesis, and thyroid hormone metabolism.

Selenium deficiency does not pose a significant risk by itself. Still, combined with additional stresses like viral infections, it can contribute to conditions such as Kashin-Beck disease or male infertility. It may also exacerbate iodine deficiency.

Excessive intake can cause a metallic taste in the mouth, breath that smells like garlic, brittle or thinning hair and nails, fatigue, mottled teeth, skin rashes, nervous system issues, irritability, and digestive problems such as nausea and diarrhea. Acute toxicity may lead to serious symptoms like neurological and gastrointestinal problems, heart attack, ARDS, hair loss, tremors, light-headedness, kidney failure, muscle tenderness, and in extreme cases, death. Because of their high selenium content, regular consumption of Brazil nuts can pose a risk of toxicity.

Sources: Brazil nuts, organ meats, seafood, meat, dairy products, nuts, grains, eggs, and some plants (depending on the selenium content of the soil).

RDA (ages 14+): men 55 mcg, women 55 mcg
UL (ages 14+): 400 mcg[194]

Zinc

Zinc is essential for the function of hundreds of enzymes. It supports immune health, wound healing, protein and DNA synthesis, cell signaling, and cell division. Zinc is crucial for healthy growth and development during pregnancy and early years.

Deficiency symptoms vary by age, including diarrhea in infants, slow growth and infections in children, appetite loss, fertility problems, and pregnancy issues in adults. It can impair smell, taste, wound healing, cognition, and mood. Pregnant women, vegetarians, vegans, those with gastrointestinal issues, and bariatric surgery patients are at higher risk.

Excess zinc may lead to nausea, vomiting, dizziness, headaches, appetite loss, and GI symptoms. Long-term high-dose supplementation or use of zinc-containing denture adhesive creams can reduce the absorption of copper, potentially leading to neurological symptoms and anemia. Very high doses of zinc supplements (e.g., 142 mg/d) can also interfere with magnesium absorption.

Animal-based foods are the richest sources of zinc in the diet. While whole grains, legumes, and nuts also provide zinc, their bioavailability is lower due to phytates that bind minerals in the gut and hinder absorption.

Sources: oysters, beef, seafood, fortified cereals, pumpkin seeds, poultry, dairy products, eggs, and others.

RDA (ages 19+): men 11 mg, women 8 mg
UL: 40 mg[195]

> **KEY TAKEAWAY**
>
> Minerals, like vitamins, are vital for good health. They are inorganic elements in rocks, soil, and water absorbed by plants and passed on to animals and humans through food and water. Minerals are classified as major or trace, depending on how much the body requires.

CHAPTER 61

Proteins

Proteins are essential macronutrients that we must obtain in relatively large amounts through our diets. They play a role in nearly all cellular processes and support the function, regulation, and structure of our body's organs and tissues. Protein is found in every part and tissue of the body, including bone, muscle, skin, and hair.

Structure

Proteins are large molecules with a complex structure composed of many amino acids linked in long chains, similar to how beads are strung together to make a necklace. Although more than five hundred amino acids exist in nature, only twenty function as building blocks of proteins in the human body. A protein's specific shape and function are determined by the order of its amino acids, also known as the primary structure of a protein. The DNA sequence of a gene determines the sequence of amino acids.

Function

Proteins have a wide range of functions. They act as antibodies that help protect the body from foreign pathogens, such as bacteria and viruses. They carry out enzymatic reactions needed for chemical reactions in the cells and act as messengers to help coordinate biological functions between different organs, tissues, and cells. Additionally, proteins help maintain the shape of cells, provide structure in the cells and tissues, and assist in transporting and storing small molecules and atoms throughout the body and inside the cells.

Amino acids

Because the body does not store amino acids, we must regularly replenish them through the diet. The body can produce some from scratch and others by modifying existing ones, but nine of the twenty protein-building amino acids must be obtained through food, as the body cannot make them. These essential amino acids include histidine, isoleucine, leucine, lysine, methionine, phenylalanine, threonine, tryptophan, and valine.

Intake recommendations

Sedentary adults are generally advised to obtain at least 0.8 grams of protein per kilogram of body weight daily. However, protein requirements increase with age to help prevent sarcopenia (age-related muscle loss). Older adults typically need around 1.0–1.2g of protein per kilogram of body weight. Additionally, physically active individuals may have higher protein needs that will vary depending on their activity level.

According to the National Academy of Medicine, protein intake should make up 10 percent to 35 percent of daily calories. A Harvard study, which followed over 130,000 men and women over thirty-two years, found that the percentage of total caloric intake from protein did not affect overall mortality, but that the source of protein was significant.[196-198]

Deficiency

In developed countries, protein deficiency is rare but remains prevalent in underdeveloped areas. An estimated one billion people worldwide have chronically inadequate protein intakes. Protein-energy malnutrition (a lack of protein and total calories) is responsible for about six million deaths per year.

Insufficient protein can cause weakness, fatigue, fainting, headaches, muscle wasting, reduced oxygen transport, anemia, and impaired nutrient absorption. In children, it may stunt growth and delay development. Deficiency is also linked to reduced protein synthesis and increased protein breakdown in muscle and other tissues, impaired antioxidant responses, and reduced levels of growth hormone, insulin, and thyroid hormones, in addition to reduced levels of amino acids and IGF-I in blood plasma.

Additionally, protein deficiency may cause impaired immune responses, a high frequency of infections, increased mortality and morbidity from infectious diseases, and tissue fluid retention. Inadequate protein intake has also been linked to cardiovascular issues, reproductive issues, mood disorders, insomnia, skeletal and dental health problems, and poor skin and hair health.

During pregnancy, it can negatively affect the child's development and long-term health.[198]

Sources of Protein

Now it's clear we need protein for various reasons, but the source matters too. Each food that provides protein also contains other substances like sodium, fats, fiber, and more. Depending on these factors, some proteins are much healthier than others.

For example, 100 grams of sirloin steak provides 27 grams of protein, but also about 6 grams of saturated fat. Ham steak offers 18 grams of protein, but comes with roughly 1500 mg of sodium. In contrast, salmon is low in saturated fat and rich in omega-3 fatty acids, while lentils provide plenty of fiber and virtually no fat or sodium.

That's why it's best to get most of our protein from sources like legumes, nuts, fish, and poultry, while limiting red meats and cheeses and avoiding processed meats, bacon, and cold cuts altogether.[197]

PROTEIN & HISTAMINE

The problem for MCAS patients is that many proteins are high in histamine. Fish is a healthy source of protein because it is low in saturated fats and often rich in omega-3 fatty acids. However, to ensure safety in terms of histamine, it must be fresh-caught or frozen immediately after catch.

Legumes, like soybeans, beans, and lentils, are all high in histamine. Egg whites, though not high in histamine themselves, are known to trigger histamine release. Most nuts are high in histamine. Pork is also high in histamine and must be avoided. And then, many people are allergic to dairy, and some even react to red meats. However, we cannot possibly forgo eating protein to avoid histamine, because protein is crucial for good health.

Exploring alternatives

You could try protein powders, such as hydrolyzed whey protein, rice protein, hemp seed protein, flaxseed protein, or chia seed protein. Hemp and pumpkin seeds are rich in protein and low in histamine. Hemp seed protein is usually easy to digest and is one of the few plant foods with a complete amino acid profile.

Like always, you'll have to try and see what works for you. When I was searching for a protein powder I could tolerate, I contacted different manufacturers and asked them for samples. There's no sense in buying a whole bucket to try one spoonful and then not be able to use the rest.

Eating meat is likely the easiest way to obtain enough protein, but many health experts warn against consuming too much red meat. Organic skinless chicken is a safe low-histamine option. Some low-histamine vegetables contain relatively high amounts of protein, but it's practically impossible to meet the protein requirement from vegetables alone. For example, 100 grams of broccoli contain 2.8 grams of protein, meaning you would have to eat about 2.5 kg to get to 70 grams.

To get enough protein, aim to combine different low-histamine sources throughout the day. For breakfast, you might try oats with hempseed milk and blackberries, a chia seed pudding with blueberries, or a smoothie made with protein powder, flaxseed, and your favorite fruits or vegetables. If you prefer something savory, an omelet with turkey, eggs, cheese, broccoli, and sweet bell peppers can be a satisfying choice. For lunch or dinner, consider chicken with quinoa and broccoli, paired with a side salad topped with pumpkin seeds. The key is to include different protein sources in each meal. A chart of low-histamine proteins follows.

KEY TAKEAWAY

Proteins are essential for nearly all body functions, and a deficiency leads to widespread problems. They are made of amino acids, nine of which must come from food. Adults need about 0.8–1.2 g per kilogram of body weight, with higher needs in older or physically active individuals. Safer low-histamine proteins include fresh poultry, beef, lamb, and egg yolks, alongside seeds like pumpkin, chia, flax, and certain dairy products like young cheese and whey. Combining tolerated sources throughout the day helps meet requirements. Protein powders may be useful if tolerated.

LOW-HISTAMINE PROTEIN

Items in list provide approximate grams of protein per 100 g serving. Values compiled from Nutritionix[199] and the Swiss Interest Group Histamine Intolerance (SIGHI).[125]

Meat and Eggs

Turkey breast	30.0
Chicken breast	31.0
Beef steak	26.0
Lamb, ground	25.0
Lamb, tenderloin	31.0
Duck	19.0
Ostrich	22.1
Quail	19.2
Trout (freshwater)	27.0 (freshly caught)
Egg yolk (1 large)	2.7
Egg yolk (100g)	16.0

Seeds

Hempseed	31.7
Pumpkinseed	19.0
Flaxseed	18.0
Chia seed	17.0

Nuts

Almond	21.0 (small amounts)
Pistachio	21.0
Tiger nut	20.0
Brazil nut	14.0
Macadamia	7.9

Grains

Oats	13.0
Quinoa	4.4
Amaranth	3.8
Millet	3.5
Chestnut	3.2
Sweet corn	3.4

Asparagus	2.4
Broccoli	2.4
Watercress	2.3 [200]
Sweet potato	2.0
Mung bean sprouts	2.0 [201]

Dairy

Whey	78.0
Gouda (young)	25.0
Mozzarella	22.0
Farmer's cheese	18.0
Cottage cheese	11.0
Curd cheese	11.0
Ricotta	11.0
Cream cheese	6.2
Mascarpone	4.7
Heavy cream	2.8
Quark	10.0
Yogurt*	5.3
Goat milk	3.6
Sheep milk	3.5
Whole milk	3.2

* Tolerance varies by strain.

CHAPTER 62

Fats

Fats, also known as lipids, include fatty acids, monoglycerides, diglycerides, triglycerides, phospholipids, and sterols. Most dietary fat consists of triglycerides (triacylglycerol); the other main component is cholesterol.[202] Fat is an essential macronutrient that we must obtain through our diets in relatively large amounts. With nine calories per gram, fat is highly energy-dense, providing more than twice the energy of protein or carbohydrates (4 kcal/g).

In the body, fat provides energy and aids in transporting and absorbing fat-soluble vitamins and certain minerals. It is essential for constructing cell membranes and the protective layer around nerves called myelin sheaths.[203] Fat also acts as a precursor for cell signaling molecules and eicosanoids, playing important roles in inflammation, wound healing, and blood clotting.[204,205] Body fat cushions vital organs and insulates the body against extreme temperatures.

There is no established Recommended Dietary Allowance (RDA) for dietary fat, but the acceptable macronutrient distribution range (AMDR) is 25 to 30 percent of total calories. The 2015–2020 Dietary Guidelines for Americans recommend avoiding trans fats entirely and limiting saturated fat to 10 percent of daily calories, preferably replacing it with monounsaturated and polyunsaturated fats.[205]

MAIN TYPES OF FAT

Triglycerides

Triglycerides are made from three fatty acid molecules and a glycerol molecule. To absorb them, the body must first break them down through hydrolysis (splitting them into simpler compounds) into free fatty acids, mono- and diglycerides, and glycerol.

Once absorbed by intestinal cells, these parts are reassembled into triglycerides and packaged into chylomicrons with cholesterol, phospholipids, and proteins. Chylomicrons enter the lymphatic system and are transported throughout the body to supply peripheral tissues.[202,206]

Fatty acids

Fatty acids serve as cellular fuel and support many vital functions, including lipid and hormone synthesis, protein modification, cell signaling, and energy storage. They are the main component of lipids and consist of hydrocarbon chains with a carboxylic acid group at one end and a methyl group at the other.

Unsaturated fatty acids contain one or more double bonds, unlike saturated fats which have no double bonds. Saturation reflects how filled the chain is with hydrogen. Fully hydrogenated chains are saturated; variable chain length and saturation influence properties like fluidity and melting point.[207] Saturated fats are solid at room temperature, whereas unsaturated fats are liquid. Unsaturated fats are beneficial, reducing inflammation, improving cholesterol, and stabilizing heart rhythms.[208]

Fatty acids are classified by chain length, the presence of double bonds, and the position of the first double bond (counted from the methyl end). If the first double bond is at the third carbon atom, it is an omega-3 fatty acid. If the first double bond starts at the sixth carbon atom, it is an omega-6 fatty acid. Short-chain fatty acids have up to six carbon atoms, medium-chain have seven to twelve,[209] and long-chain have twelve to eighteen.[202]

Short- and medium-chain fatty acids are absorbed similarly to glucose and amino acids, while long-chain fatty acids follow the process explained above.[202] The omega-6 fatty acid linoleic acid (LA) and the omega-3 fatty acid alpha-linolenic acid (ALA) are considered essential fatty acids because the body cannot synthesize them and must obtain them through the diet.[210]

Cholesterol

Cholesterol helps form cell membranes, serves as a precursor for bile acids, and is required for synthesizing vitamin D and steroid hormones, including sex hormones, mineralocorticoids, and glucocorticoids.[211]

All cells in the body can synthesize cholesterol to a limited degree, but cholesterol synthesis occurs mainly in the liver.[211] Individuals who consume a regular diet usually also obtain a significant amount from food.

While cholesterol is essential for good health, excess levels in the bloodstream can be seriously harmful. It can build up in blood vessels, calcify, and eventually restrict blood flow, raising the risk of strokes and heart attacks. The body has a compensatory system that regulates how much cholesterol the liver synthesizes: the more you consume, the less the liver produces.[212]

Cholesterol is a 27-carbon molecule with four hydrocarbon rings, a tail, and a hydroxyl group.[211] Being water-insoluble, it binds to lipoproteins to travel in blood.[212] Low-density lipoproteins (LDLs) carry cholesterol from the liver to tissues, while high-density lipoproteins (HDLs) return excess cholesterol to the liver for conversion into bile acids for excretion. An easy way to remember this: LDL should be kept low ('L' for low), and HDL can be kept high ('H' for high).

Phospholipids

Unlike triglycerides, phospholipids are typically composed of one or two fatty acids, a phosphate group, and two alcohols.[213] They form the lipid bilayer, a two-layer structure that makes up cell membranes. This protective barrier shields cells from environmental stressors and supports many essential cellular processes.[214] As a key component of cell membranes, phospholipids are found in nearly all foods. High-quality sources include soybeans, eggs, milk, dairy products, and some vegetables.[215]

DIETARY FATS & SOURCES

Monounsaturated fat

Monounsaturated fat is found in avocados, canola oil, olive oil, peanut oil, most nuts, high-oleic safflower, and sunflower oils.[203]

Polyunsaturated fat (including the essential omega-3 and omega-6 fatty acids)

Polyunsaturated fat is needed for the structure and function of cell membranes, healthy vision, nervous system function, lipid mediator synthesis, and gene expression regulation.[210,216,217]

The body can synthesize arachidonic acid (AA) from linoleic acid (LA). It can also convert eicosapentaenoic acid (EPA) and docosahexaenoic acid (DHA) from alpha-linolenic acid (ALA)—but not in sufficient amounts. Therefore, EPA and DHA should be obtained through the diet.

For adults aged nineteen to seventy, the adequate intake (AI) of linoleic acid is 17 grams per day for men and 12 grams for women. For alpha-linolenic acid, the AI is 1.6 grams per day for men and 1.1 grams for women. Pregnant and breastfeeding women may require higher amounts.

- **Omega-3 fatty acids**
  Alpha-linolenic acid (ALA), eicosapentaenoic acid (EPA), and docosahexaenoic acid (DHA) are the most studied omega-3s. They support heart health by lowering heart rate, blood pressure, and improving blood vessel function. Higher doses may reduce triglycerides and inflammation, aiding in preventing atherosclerosis.[216] ALA is found in plants like flaxseed, chia seeds, walnuts, canola, soy, and mustard oil. EPA and DHA occur mainly in seafood such as salmon, herring, sardines, oysters, trout, sea bass, and shrimp.[217]
- **Omega-6 fatty acids**
  Linoleic acid (LA) and arachidonic acid (AA) are the most essential omega-6s. LA is mainly found in plant foods, such as safflower oil, sunflower seeds and oil, pine nuts, corn oil, soybean oil, pecans, Brazil nuts, and sesame oil. AA is found in animal foods like meat, poultry, and eggs. Supplements high in omega-6 fatty acids include black currant seed oil, evening primrose oil, and borage seed oil.[210]

Saturated fat

Saturated fat is mainly found in animal foods like fatty beef, lamb, pork, poultry with skin, lard, butter, cream, cheese, and other dairy products. It is also present in coconut, palm oil, and dark chocolate.[218,219]

Trans fats

Trans fats raise "bad" LDL cholesterol, lower "good" HDL cholesterol, and increase the risk of type 2 diabetes, heart disease, and stroke.[220] Industrially produced trans fats are made by adding hydrogen to vegetable oils to make them more solid. Since 2023, they have been officially banned in the U.S. because they offer no health benefits, and even small amounts are harmful.[203,221]

Some animal products, like meat and dairy, contain small amounts of naturally occurring trans fats. However, it's unclear whether these have a similarly harmful effect on cholesterol levels as industrially produced trans fats.

Trans fats are found in packaged and commercially fried foods like fast food, doughnuts, cakes, pie crusts, biscuits, frozen pizza, cookies, crackers, stick margarine, and other spreads.[220]

FATS & MCAS

Choosing the right fats can help lower inflammation and support a more stable immune response, better hormone balance, and improved nervous system function—all areas that can be disrupted in mast cell-related conditions. As always, be mindful of individual triggers and high-histamine sources.

> ### KEY TAKEAWAY
>
> Fat provides energy, supports absorption of fat-soluble nutrients, builds cell membranes and nerve coverings, and serves as a precursor for hormones and signaling molecules. Body fat cushions organs and regulates temperature. The healthiest fats are monounsaturated and polyunsaturated, while saturated fats should be limited, and trans fats should be avoided entirely.

CHAPTER 63

Carbohydrates

Carbohydrates (carbs) are essential macronutrients that we need to obtain in relatively large amounts through our diets. They come in the form of sugars, starches, and fibers. Together with fat and protein, they are one of the body's three main energy sources.

Types of carbohydrates

What matters most is the type of carbohydrates you eat. Prioritize complex carbohydrates and limit simple ones. Healthy sources include minimally processed whole grains, vegetables, whole fruits, and beans. Less healthy sources include highly processed foods like white bread, pastries, soda, candy, and fruit juice.

FUNCTIONS & REQUIREMENTS

Functions

Our muscles and nervous system rely on carbohydrates for energy. Carbs also help regulate blood glucose and insulin levels, support lipid metabolism, and promote fermentation in the gut. Adequate carbohydrate intake helps preserve lean muscle, as the body may break down protein for energy when carbs and fats are insufficient.[222,223] Remarkably, the brain alone uses about 20 percent of the body's glucose-derived energy.[224]

Deficiency

Carbohydrate deficiency can negatively impact the central nervous system, leading to dizziness and reduced physical and mental energy. It may also prompt the body to use protein for energy, which is not ideal, as protein is needed to build muscle. Low-carb intake may also cause constipation and digestive issues due to reduced fiber intake.[223]

Recommended intakes

For adults and children above age one, the Institute of Medicine (IOM) recommends that carbs make up 45 to 65 percent of total calories, or about 130 g of carbohydrates per day to ensure the brain gets enough glucose. However, intake should be adjusted based on individual needs.[225]

STRUCTURE

Carbohydrates are composed of carbon, hydrogen, and oxygen. Based on their chemical structure, they are classified as simple or complex.

Simple carbs contain one or two sugar molecules and are quickly digested and absorbed, providing the body with a quick source of energy, but they can cause unhealthy blood sugar spikes.

Complex carbohydrates consist of three or more sugar units and take longer to digest but provide longer-lasting energy without the downside of sugar highs.

During digestion, carbohydrates are broken down into glucose, which then enters the bloodstream and is shuttled throughout the body for energy. Up to 2,000 calories of extra glucose can be stored in the liver and muscles in the form of glycogen until more energy is needed. When glycogen stores are full, carbs are stored as fat.[222,223]

Sugar molecules are called saccharides. A single sugar is a monosaccharide. Two linked sugars form a disaccharide, three or more form oligosaccharides, and many monosaccharides linked together are called polysaccharides.

CARBOHYDRATE CLASSIFICATION

Simple Carbohydrates: Monosaccharides & Disaccharides

Simple carbohydrates have a simple chemical structure with only one or two sugar molecules linked together.

Monosaccharides

Examples include glucose (dextrose), galactose, fructose, and mannose.

- Glucose is found in candy, desserts, honey, syrups, and sodas. Fruits and vegetables are natural food sources of glucose.
- Fructose is the sugar found in fruit.
- Galactose is found in lactose, the sugar in milk and dairy products.[222,223]

Disaccharides

Examples include sucrose, lactose, lactulose, maltose, trehalose, and cellobiose.

- Sucrose (glucose + fructose) is table sugar, found in sugarcane or sugar beet, maple syrup, molasses, and fruit.
- Lactose (glucose + galactose) is the sugar in milk and milk products.
- Maltose (glucose + glucose) is found in malt beverages like beer, as well as in kamut, spelt, sweet potatoes, and high-maltose syrup. Maltose can also be made from corn.[226]

Complex Carbohydrates: Oligosaccharides & Polysaccharides

Complex carbohydrates have a more complex chemical structure of three or more simple sugars linked together.

Oligosaccharides

Apart from maltotriose, oligosaccharides are generally indigestible. They are fermented by the gut flora into absorbable nutrients and serve as soluble fiber to ease defecation. Some also function as prebiotics, promoting a healthy microbiome, which may benefit the lining of the large intestine.[227]

Examples include raffinose, oligofructose, and maltotriose.

- Raffinose (glucose, galactose + fructose) is found in asparagus, beans, broccoli, Brussels sprouts, cabbage, cottonseed, sugar beet molasses, sweet potatoes, and whole grains.[228]
- Oligofructose (3–10 sugar units) is found in many foods, including bananas, chicory, onion, and wheat.[229,230]
- Maltotriose (3 glucose units) is produced in the mouth and small intestine during starch digestion. It is found in brown rice syrup and liquid glucose and is sometimes used in baked goods to help retain moisture.[231]

Polysaccharides

Polysaccharides contain ten to several thousand monosaccharides linked together in long chains. Some polysaccharides can be digested, while others are indigestible but support regular bowel movements and feed healthy gut bacteria.

Examples include glycogen, cellulose, inulin, and starch.

- Glycogen is the main storage form of glucose in humans.
- Cellulose is what plant cell walls are primarily made of. It's indigestible but important as dietary fiber, promoting satiety, healthy bowel movements, and a healthy microbiome, and may lower the risk of diabetes and coronary heart disease.[222,223]
- Inulin is a polysaccharide of the fructan type (fructose molecules with a glucose molecule on the end) found in over 36,000 plants. The richest source is chicory root.[232–234]
- Starch (amylopectin + amylose) is the primary form in which plants store carbohydrates, and it's the main source of carbohydrates in the human diet. Some starches are digested in the small intestine, but cell wall polysaccharides and resistant starch are not. These act as dietary fiber and are fermented by the gut flora into short-chain fatty acids.[235] Starch is found in corn, cereals, grains, flour, rice, chickpeas, and root vegetables.[222,223,235]

THE GLYCEMIC INDEX & GLYCEMIC LOAD

The glycemic index (GI) tells us how quickly a carbohydrate turns into sugar after consumption.[236] Originally designed for diabetics, it serves as a basic guide for food selection.[237] Using a scale from 0 to 100 (100 representing pure sugar), it ranks carbohydrates based on how strongly they affect blood sugar levels. High-GI foods cause sharp blood sugar spikes, and excess intake is linked to an increased risk of weight gain, type 2 diabetes, and heart disease.

Generally speaking, the more fat and fiber a food contains, the lower its GI; the more processed it is, the higher its GI.[236] However, a low GI does not necessarily indicate high nutritional value, and high-GI foods may still provide benefits like greater satiety or lower energy density. Therefore, rather than placing too much emphasis on GI, it's better to focus on overall diet quality to reduce chronic disease risk.[236–238]

The glycemic load (GL) helps estimate how much a specific food raises an individual's blood glucose. It considers both the GI and the amount of digestible carbohydrates in a serving.

The GL is calculated by multiplying a food's GI by its carbohydrate content in grams, then dividing by 100. A GL of 20 or above is high, under 10 is low, and 11–19 is considered moderate. Because the GL takes portion size into account, a food ranking high on the GI scale may still have a low glycemic load, making it a better choice for blood sugar management, according to Harvard Medical School.[238,239]

CARBOHYDRATES & DIETARY APPROACHES

While experts generally agree that carbohydrates are essential to a balanced diet, some dietary approaches consider them nonessential. Ketogenic and carnivore diets, for example, suggest the body can adapt to using fats and proteins as primary energy sources. Proponents argue that carbohydrates are not required, since the liver can produce sufficient glucose from amino acids.

> ### KEY TAKEAWAY
>
> Carbohydrates provide energy, regulate blood sugar, support fat metabolism, and aid digestion. Deficiency can cause fatigue, muscle breakdown, and digestive issues, while excess intake may contribute to obesity, diabetes, and heart disease. The healthiest sources are complex carbs from vegetables, fruits, legumes, and whole grains, while processed foods, sugary drinks, and refined flours should be minimized.

CHAPTER 64

Coffee, Yes or No?

While some say coffee is okay on a low-histamine diet, others say it's high in histamine and should be avoided. Some claim it's a histamine liberator, others disagree. Coffee is known to inhibit DAO, which may contribute to digestive problems or issues from excess histamine. It's also a stimulant, and excessive stimulation can worsen mast cell–related symptoms. Therefore, even for those who tolerate it, moderation is key.

Reports from self-help groups show that some can handle coffee fine, while others can't. As with most MCAS-related dietary concerns, you need to experiment to see what works.

I am a coffee lover, but much to my regret, I started reacting to it. Stubborn as I am sometimes, I didn't just give up on it, but tried to find a way to keep having it. Sure, I could have cut it out altogether, but I just really wanted to keep something I could enjoy in my life. So, despite some painful reactions, I kept trying to find a way to have my coffee and still be fine afterward. First, I needed to know which coffee beans I could tolerate, and then I experimented with different brewing techniques. Finally, I came up with the following insights:

MAKING COFFEE WORK FOR YOU

Quality

Buy sustainably farmed beans. These are usually treated with fewer pesticides, fungicides, and insecticides, to which we might react.

Roasting degree

Dark roasts may be better, as roasting can lower the acidity of coffee beans.[240]

Storage

Store the beans in an airtight container in a cool, dark place, away from moisture and heat.

Freshness

Grind the beans fresh for each cup. Whole beans keep fresh longer than ground coffee, which makes a big difference.

Brewing methods

Cold-brew coffee is said to be the least acidic, but I like to prepare my coffee with a French press or barista coffee machine. Both methods have short brewing times, reducing the coffee's acidity. Stovetop espresso machines or mocha pots could also be an option, but they are sometimes made from potentially toxic materials and can accumulate mold and bacteria if not cleaned properly.

Avoid coffee vending machines

Automatic coffee machines are often not cleaned properly. They continuously heat water, and the brewed coffee then drips down through tubes that may accumulate bacteria and mold. Since you don't have any control over the cleanliness of such machines, I'd say it's best to skip the coffee if a vending machine is your only option.

> **KEY TAKEAWAY**
>
> Coffee tolerance varies in MCAS: some manage it well, while others react. It may block DAO, act as a histamine liberator, and overstimulate the system, so moderation is key. Quality and preparation matter too: buy sustainably farmed beans, store them in an airtight container in the dark, grind fresh, and consider darker roasts to reduce acidity. Cold brew is the least acidic, though French press or a barista-style espresso machine may also work well.

CHAPTER 65

Menu Ideas

The menu suggestions below are low in histamine, gluten-free, and dairy-free.

Dishes with meat

- Thinly sliced chicken breast sautéed with white onion and bell pepper, served with a side of jasmine rice
- Oven-baked chicken breast with mashed potatoes and baked zucchini with a seasoned almond flour crust
- Rosemary-seasoned lamb chops sprinkled with Himalayan crystal salt, served alongside golden-brown oven-baked potato wedges
- Beef steak served with steamed broccoli and a quinoa pilaf cooked with onion and carrot
- Homemade hamburger patties with oven-baked broccoli and roasted potatoes
- Turkey steak with asparagus and a side of diced potatoes with homemade mayo

Vegetarian dishes

- Hash browns served with hard-boiled egg yolks and a side of carrot salad dressed with homemade apple-chive-mayo
- Stir-fry with white onions, carrots, bok choy, and rice noodles, garnished with watercress and pumpkin seed oil
- Roasted pumpkin served with quinoa mixed with raisins and almonds, accompanied by an iceberg salad with cucumber, apple, and hulled hemp seeds
- Crispy sweet potato fries with homemade mayo, served alongside steamed broccoli or a fresh side salad topped with aromatic herbs
- Millet, zucchini, and fennel gratin baked in a creamy coconut sauce and topped with fresh savory

Salads

- Iceberg lettuce salad with red bell pepper and cucumber, topped with almond flour, oregano, a pinch of salt, and a drizzle of olive oil
- Carrot salad with homemade dressing made with mayonnaise, salt, chives, and the juice of about a quarter of an apple
- Diced bell pepper (red/yellow) and cucumber, mixed with fresh cilantro and the white part of spring onions, seasoned with Himalayan crystal salt and a drizzle of olive oil
- Quinoa and pomegranate salad with fresh herbs

Desserts

- Caramelized apples topped with coconut cream and maple syrup
- Coconut-chia pudding with fresh blueberries and nectarines sprinkled with brown sugar and cardamom
- Fruit salad with apricots, cherries, apples, and raisins
- Fried sticky rice served with a fresh mango sauce (mango is often well-tolerated, but not always) or topped with crushed macadamia nuts, coconut cream, maple syrup, and a sprinkle of goji berries
- Fresh grapes or fruit of your choice
- Homemade vegan caramels

Breakfast

- Smoothie with hemp milk, protein powder, blueberries, gluten-free oats, and dates
- Homemade granola with gluten-free oats, almond, pumpkin seeds, maple syrup, and raisins
- Fried egg yolks with bell pepper, bok choy, broccoli, and a side of potatoes
- Rice cakes with almond butter and apple

Juices (freshly juiced)

- Apple, celery, fennel
- Apple, cucumber, mint
- Apple, beetroot, carrot, ginger
- Carrot, ginger
- Yellow pepper (unexpectedly tasty!)
- ...or any of these ingredients by themselves.

Useful Go-Tos

Experts and clinicians

- Dr. Lawrence Afrin, New York, NY, USA (aimcenterpm.com)
- Dr. Tania Dempsey, New York, NY, USA (drtaniadempsey.com)
- Dr. Anne Maitland, Eastchester, NY, USA (drannemaitland.net)
- Dr. T.C. Theoharides, Boston, MA, USA (drtheoharides.com, mastcellmaster.com)
- Dr. Jill R. Schofield, Denver, CO, USA (centerformultisystemdisease.com)
- Dr. Matthew J. Hamilton, Boston, MA, USA (HMS, BWH, AIM)
- Dr. Mariana Castells, Boston, MA, USA (HMS, BWH, AIM)
- Dr. Cem Akin, Ann Arbor, MI, USA (University of Michigan, AIM)
- Dr. Gerhard J. Molderings, Bonn, Germany (humangenetics-bonn.de, mcsciences.com)
- Dr. Theo Gulen, Stockholm, Sweden (Karolinska Institutet)
- Dr. Peter Valent, Vienna, Austria (MedUni Vienna, ECNM, AIM)

Organizations and patient support

- tmsforacure.org – The Mastocytosis Society, USA
- mastocytosis-mcas.org – Global Resource for Mast Cell Diseases
- mastocytosis.org.au – Australia
- mastocytosis.ca – Canada
- mastcellaction.org – United Kingdom
- ukmasto.org – United Kingdom
- mcas-hope.de – Germany

Practical resources, education, and patient support

- mastcell360.com
- mastattack.org
- supertmastcell.org
- eds.clinic
- ehlers-danlos.com

Books in English

- *Never Bet Against Occam: Mast Cell Activation Disease and the Modern Epidemics of Chronic Illness and Medical Complexity*
  by Dr. Lawrence B. Afrin
- *Mast Cells United: A Holistic Approach to Mast Cell Activation Syndrome*
  by Amber Walker
- *The Trifecta Passport: Tools for Mast Cell Activation Syndrome, Postural Orthostatic Tachycardia Syndrome and Ehlers-Danlos Syndrome*
  by Amber Walker
- *My Crazy Life: A Humorous Guide to Understanding Mast Cell Disorders*
  by Daniel & Pamela Hodge

Books in German

- *Die systemische Mastzellerkrankung: MCAS und SM: Symptome einordnen, die Diagnose finden und die besten Therapien nutzen. Die wichtigsten Fragen und Antworten*
  by Prof. med. Gerhard J. Molderings and Prof. Dr. med. Martin Mücke
- *MCAS Mastzell-Aktivierungs-Syndrom: Die überaktive Mastzelle beruhigen – das praktische Mutmach-Buch einer Betroffenen*
  by Nina Chen
- *MCAS Die Verborgene Krankheit: Mastzell- aktivierungssyndrom – Symptome erkennen, behandeln und damit leben*
  by Jeanette Grametzki and Dr. med. Katja Aschenbrenner

Support groups on Facebook (not inclusive)

- The Mastocytosis Society
- Mastocytosis and Mast Cell Disorders - An Integrative Approach
- My Crazy Life with Mast Cell Disorder
- Mastocytosis and Mast Cell Disorders - A Holistic and Integrative Approach
- Mastocytosis Awareness and Support Group
- Mastocytosis Awareness
- Mast Cell Activation Disorders Forum
- Masto Moms
- Masto Kids
- Mastozytose (German)
- Mast Movement

Safe Home Checklist

CHECK, REMOVE, AND REPLACE

Scented products

▸ avoid completely

- ☐ Candles
- ☐ Incense
- ☐ Air fresheners
- ☐ Body care
- ☐ Perfume
- ☐ Toilet paper
- ☐ Sanitary pads
- ☐ Garbage bags
- ☐ Cleaning products
- ☐ Laundry detergents
- ☐ Dryer sheets

Textiles

▸ avoid direct skin contact with PPD, formaldehyde resins, and synthetics

- ☐ Clothing
- ☐ Bedding
- ☐ Blankets
- ☐ Pillows
- ☐ Mattress
- ☐ Sofas
- ☐ Carpets
- ☐ Upholstery

Furniture

► avoid flame-retardants, toxic glues, and toxic finishes

- ☐ Bedframe
- ☐ Night table
- ☐ Wardrobe
- ☐ Chairs
- ☐ Cupboards, etc.

Building materials

► avoid VOCs and formaldehyde (plywood, MDF, and particleboard)

- ☐ Flooring
- ☐ Walls

Heating

► avoid gas, fan, quartz tube infrared, electric convection, and oil-filled heaters

- ☐ Safer options: central heating, geothermal, radiant tile heaters, and hydronic radiators

BEDROOM SETUP

- ☐ Mellow lighting
- ☐ Calming colors
- ☐ Tolerated blanket covers
- ☐ Natural material blankets and pillows
- ☐ Dust-mite-proof casing
- ☐ Toxicity-free mattress
- ☐ Scent-free environment
- ☐ Blackout curtains or outside shutters
- ☐ Keep temperature around 61–65°F
- ☐ Air out room before sleep
- ☐ Avoid formaldehyde-based furniture
- ☐ No electrical appliances (reduce EMF)
- ☐ Turn off Wi-Fi before sleep

KITCHEN SETUP

► avoid BPA, PFOA, PTFE

- ☐ Scent-free dishwashing liquid
- ☐ Scent-free dishwasher tabs
- ☐ Range hood (ideally ducted, venting outside) or portable options like the AirHood
- ☐ Non-toxic cookware
- ☐ Non-toxic utensils
- ☐ BPA-free plastics or glass storage solutions

HELPFUL HABITS

- ☐ Change clothing daily
- ☐ Change bedding often
- ☐ Clean frequently
- ☐ Air out rooms regularly
- ☐ Declutter your home
- ☐ Dry laundry outside in fresh air

UPGRADE WHEN POSSIBLE

- ☐ Microfiber cleaning rags
- ☐ Vacuum with HEPA filter
- ☐ Steam vacuum
- ☐ Air filter
- ☐ The AirHood
- ☐ Water filter
- ☐ Dishwasher
- ☐ Washing machine
- ☐ Food processor

Trigger Management Kit

Keep these essentials with you whenever you leave the house to help avoid triggers, quickly soothe reactions, and stay prepared if you need to eat. Use travel-sized containers to keep things light, and store the items—clothing aside—in a designated MCAS pouch so you can easily grab it and go.

Medications

- ☐ Emergency set: EpiPen, antihistamines, corticosteroids, medical emergency card
- ☐ Mast cell stabilizers
- ☐ Personal medications (day pack)

Trigger Reduction

- ☐ Mask or scarf
- ☐ Earplugs or noise-cancelling headphones
- ☐ Sunglasses
- ☐ Baseball cap or hat (light-sensitivity, sun protection)
- ☐ Hoodie (extra protection from wind and light)

Trigger Management

- ☐ Avène thermal water spray (to quickly calm skin reactions)
- ☐ Eyedrops

Eating Away from Home

- ☐ Tolerated salt (no iodine)
- ☐ List of tolerated foods
- ☐ Hand soap
- ☐ Microfiber travel towel

Optional

- ☐ Backup shirt and socks
- ☐ Sun protection (long sleeves or parasol)
- ☐ Pocket warmer

Foods Rich in Quercetin List

This list provides quercetin content in foods alongside their histamine compatibility. It is based on the information in Chapter 52, "Foods Rich in Quercetin," and the SIGHI Food Compatibility List (Swiss Interest Group Histamine Intolerance). Items not included in SIGHI were cross-checked for accuracy using InTolerApp, Histamino.com, and Casa de Sante.[125,241-243]

The Histamine Compatibility | Notes column reflects typical tolerability for individuals sensitive to histamine or mast cell stimulators.

Food	Quercetin mg per 100g/ml	Histamine Compatibility | Notes
Capers	233.84	insufficient data
Capers, canned	172.55	incompatible / high histamine due to pickling
Lovage leaves	170	insufficient data / likely safe
Elderberry juice concentrate*	108.16	insufficient data / fruit safe / juice concentrate variable
Dock	86.2	insufficient data
Radish leaves	70.37	insufficient data / likely safe
Wild rocket	66.19	incompatible / histamine liberator
Dill	55.15	tolerated in small amounts / mild liberator / high salicylate
Cilantro	52.9	safe in small amounts
Banana peppers	50.63	insufficient data / may stimulate mast cells due to capsaicin
Fennel leaves	48.8	insufficient data / likely safe
Juniper berries	46.61	insufficient data / likely safe
Mexican oregano	42	insufficient data / likely safe
Yellow onion, cooked	41.9	moderate / histamine liberator
Red onions	39.21	moderate / histamine liberator
Carob flour	38.78	incompatible / potential histamine liberator

Food	Quercetin mg per 100g/ml	Histamine Compatibility | Notes
Radicchio	31.51	contradictory data / likely safe / moderate
Red leaf lettuce	30.6	likely safe
Spring onions (red bulb)	30.6	safe / mild liberator for some
Watercress	29.99	safe
Hartwort leaves	29.3	insufficient data
Ancho peppers	27.6	problematic / mast cell stimulator due to capsaicin
Elderberries	26.77	insufficient data / likely safe / variable
Hawthorn leaves**	24.1	insufficient data / likely safe
Asparagus, cooked	23.6	safe
Kale	22.58	insufficient data / likely safe
Okra	20.97	insufficient data / likely safe
Bee pollen	20.95	insufficient data / variable
Cocoa powder	20	high histamine / histamine liberator / other amines
Apples, skin only	19.36	safe
Chia seeds	18.42	safe
Moringa	16.65	insufficient data / likely safe
Saskatoons	16.64	insufficient data
Annual sow thistle	16	insufficient data
Serrano peppers	15.98	problematic / mast cell stimulator due to capsaicin
Buckwheat	15.38	incompatible / potential histamine liberator / other amines
Hot green chili pepper	14.7	problematic / mast cell stimulator due to capsaicin
Cranberries	14	safe
Goji berries, dried	13.6	safe if unsulfured
Red spring onion leaves	12.6	insufficient data / likely safe
Black diamond plums	12.45	insufficient data / likely moderate / mild histamine liberator

Food	Quercetin mg per 100g/ml	Histamine Compatibility | Notes
Romaine lettuce (source 1)	12	safe
Yellow onion, cooked (summer)	11	moderate / mild histamine liberator
Scallions	10.68	likely safe / mild histamine liberator
Red leaf lettuce (winter)	10.3	likely safe
Tarragon	10	insufficient data / likely moderate
Green chili pepper, cooked	9.9	problematic / mast cell stimulator due to capsaicin
Sweet potato leaves, cooked	9.84	insufficient data / likely safe
Mustard greens	8.8	insufficient data / likely safe
Arugula	7.92	likely safe
Blueberries	7.67	safe
Sea buckthorn	7.58	safe
Red Swiss chard	7.5	moderate / potential histamine liberator
Lingonberries	7.4	safe if not overripe
Oregano	7.3	safe
Red kidney beans, boiled	6.82	low in histamine / potential histamine liberator
Chicory greens	6.49	likely safe / problematic for some due to inulin content
Long yellow peppers (hot)	6.45	problematic / mast cell stimulator due to capsaicin
Figs	5.47	moderate / mild histamine liberator

Food	Quercetin mg per 100g/ml	Histamine Compatibility | Notes
Yardlong bean, cooked	5.3	insufficient data
White sweet onion	5.19	safe
Jalapeño peppers	5.07	problematic / mast cell stimulator due to capsaicin
Turmeric, steamed	4.92	safe
Chives	4.77	moderate / safe in small amounts
Acerola	4.74	safe
Brussels sprouts, cooked	4.33	moderate / safe for most / mild liberator
Green leaf lettuce	4.16	safe
Tomato products, no salt added	4.12	high histamine / histamine liberator
Apples, all varieties, w/skin	4.01	safe
Spinach	3.97	contradictory data / incompatible / fresh may be compatible
Tart or sour cherry juice	3.88	safe / variable / potential histamine liberator
Blackberries	3.58	safe
Celery	3.5	safe
Cherry tomatoe	3.3	potentially compatible if not overripe
Broccoli	3.26	safe
Bay leaves	3.19	likely safe
Concord grapes	3.11	likely safe in moderation / may contain other amines
Bilberries	3.04	insufficient data / likely safe
Snap green peas	2.73	insufficient data / moderate / safe for some
Butterhead lettuce	2.73	safe

Food	Quercetin mg per 100g/ml	Histamine Compatibility | Notes
Green tea, brewed	2.69	incompatible / moderate / DAO blocker (fermentation)
Collard greens	2.57	insufficient data / likely safe
Black grapes	2.54	likely safe in moderation / may contain other amines
Cayenne peppers	2.48	problematic / mast cell stimulator due to capsaicin
Broccoli rabe	2.25	safe
Green bell peppers	2.21	compatible / mild liberator for some
White Swiss chard	2.2	moderate / potential histamine liberator
Romaine lettuce (source 2)	2.2	safe
Black tea, brewed	2.19	incompatible / high histamine / DAO blocker
Japanese green tea, brewed	2.1	incompatible / moderate / DAO blocker (fermentation)
Applesauce, canned	2	likely safe / potential histamine liberator due to preservation
Garlic	1.74	moderate / well tolerated in small amounts and cooked
Apricots	1.63	safe
Pistachio nuts	1.46	safe for most
Red potatoes with skin, baked	1.43	insufficient data / likely safe / skin might be problematic
Iceberg lettuce	1.42	safe
Oolong tea, brewed	1.3	insufficient data / variable / problematic due to fermentation
Cherries	1.2	safe

Food	Quercetin mg per 100g/ml	Histamine Compatibility | Notes
Strawberries	1.11	high histamine / histamine liberator / biogenic amines
Apples, all, fruit without skin	1.05	safe
Broccoli rabe cooked	1.05	safe
Red raspberries	1.05	incompatible
Red grapes	1.04	likely safe in moderation / may contain other amines
Red wine	1.0	high histamine / liberator / biogenic amines / DAO blocker

* Elderberry juice may provoke flare-ups in autoimmune diseases.
** Hawthorn leaves are not recommended for low blood pressure.[125]

Anti-Inflammatory Foods List

This list provides anti-inflammatory foods alongside their histamine compatibility. It is based on the foods mentioned in Chapter 53, "Anti-Inflammatory Foods," and the SIGHI Food Compatibility List (Swiss Interest Group Histamine Intolerance).[125] Items not included in SIGHI were cross-checked for accuracy using InTolerApp, Histamino.com, and Casa De Sante.[241–243]

The Histamine Compatibility / Notes column reflects typical tolerability for individuals sensitive to histamine or mast cell stimulators.

Fruits	Histamine Compatibility | Notes
Acai berries	insufficient data / likely moderate
Apricots	safe
Avocado	incompatible / high histamine / histamine liberator
Banana	high histamine / biogenic amines / occasionally tolerated when underripe
Blackberries	safe
Blueberries	safe
Cranberries	safe
Grapefruit	incompatible / high histamine / histamine liberator / biogenic amines
Grapes	likely safe in moderation / may contain other amines
Lemon	incompatible / high histamine / histamine liberator / biogenic amines
Lime	incompatible / high histamine / histamine liberator / biogenic amines
Mango	moderate / debated; often tolerated
Mandarins	incompatible / high histamine
Mulberry	insufficient data
Oranges	incompatible / high histamine / histamine liberator / biogenic amines

Papaya	incompatible / high histamine / histamine liberator / biogenic amines
Peach	safe
Pear	conflicting data / likely moderate / other biogenic amines
Pink guava	contradictory data / likely incompatible
Pomegranate	safe
Rhubarb	controversial / moderate / often well tolerated / contains oxalic acid
Rose hip	moderate / histamine liberator
Sour/tart cherries	safe
Strawberries	incompatible / high histamine / histamine liberator / biogenic amines
Tangerine	insufficient data / likely incompatible
Watermelon	moderate / potential histamine liberator

Vegetables & Leafy Greens	**Histamine Compatibility | Notes**
Asparagus	safe
Bell peppers (sweet)	safe
Broccoli	safe
Brussels sprouts	moderate / histamine liberator
Cabbage (unpickled)	safe
Carrots	safe
Cauliflower	safe
Chard	moderate / potential histamine liberator
Collard greens	insufficient data / likely safe
Green beans	moderate / variable / well tolerated in some cases
Kale	insufficient data / likely safe
Lettuce	safe
Mustard greens	insufficient data / likely safe
Okra	insufficient data / likely safe
Olives	often incompatible due to fermentation with intolerated ingredients
Pumpkin	safe
Pepper (hot)	problematic / mast cell stimulator due to capsaicin

Radish	safe
Spinach	contradictory data / incompatible / fresh may be compatible
Sweet potato	safe
Turnip	contradictory data / safe / moderate

Herbs, Spices & Flavorings	**Histamine Compatibility | Notes**
Angelica root	insufficient data / likely compatible
Basil (sweet basil)	safe
Bay leaves	safe
Cardamom	safe
Chili peppers	problematic / mast cell stimulator due to capsaicin
Ginger	moderate / small amounts are often well tolerated
Honey	usually safe / contains benzoic acid
Ironwort	insufficient data
Lemongrass	insufficient data / likely safe
Mint	safe / high in salicylates
Moringa leaves	insufficient data / likely safe
Oregano	safe
Parsley	safe
Rosemary	safe
Sage	safe
Thyme	safe
Turmeric	safe

Legumes, Beans & Pulses	**Histamine Compatibility | Notes**
Black beans	insufficient data / likely incompatible / histamine liberator
Black soybeans	incompatible / histamine liberator / DAO blocker
Chickpeas	incompatible
Fava beans	incompatible / high histamine
Field peas	safe / moderate / small portions are often well tolerated

Lentils	contradictory data / moderate / incompatible
Peas (snap, green)	insufficient data / moderate / safe for some
Soybeans	incompatible / histamine liberator / DAO blocker

Nuts & Seeds	**Histamine Compatibility | Notes**
Black sesame	moderate
Chia seeds	safe
Flaxseeds	safe
Peanuts	incompatible / high histamine
Pistachios	safe
Sesame seeds	moderate
Walnuts	incompatible / histamine liberator / other biogenic amines

Protein Sources	**Histamine Compatibility | Notes**
Fatty fish	freshly caught or frozen immediately = safe / otherwise high histamine
Chicken (skinless)	safe

Other Foods	**Histamine Compatibility | Notes**
Brown seaweed	incompatible / histamine liberator / extremely rich in iodine
Macroalgae	incompatible / histamine liberator / extremely rich in iodine
Microalgae	incompatible / histamine liberator / extremely rich in iodine
Cacao / cocoa	incompatible / histamine liberator / biogenic amines
Coffee	moderate / potential mast cell stimulator
Japanese knotweed	insufficient data
Salvia species	insufficient data
Sea buckthorn	safe

Tea (green)	incompatible / moderate / DAO blocker (fermentation)
Tea (black)	incompatible / high histamine / DAO blocker
Tea (oolong)	insufficient data / variable / problematic due to fermentation
Wine	high histamine / liberator / biogenic amines / DAO blocker

References

1. Afrin LB, Ackerley MB, Bluestein LS, et al. Diagnosis of mast cell activation syndrome: a global "consensus-2." Diagnosis (Berl). 2020;8(2):137-152. doi:10.1515/dx-2020-0005
2. Krystel-Whittemore M, Dileepan KN, Wood JG. Mast cells: a multi-functional master cell. Front Immunol. 2016;6:620. doi:10.3389/fimmu.2015.00620
3. da Silva EZ, Jamur MC, Oliver C. Mast cell function: a new vision of an old cell. J Histochem Cytochem. 2014;62(10):698-738. doi:10.1369/0022155414545334
4. Molderings GJ, Mücke M. Die systemische Mastzellerkrankung: MCAS und SM: Symptome einordnen, die Diagnose finden und die besten Therapien nutzen. Die wichtigsten Fragen und Antworten. Stuttgart, Germany: TRIAS Verlag; 2023
5. Gulen T. Using the right criteria for MCAS. Curr Allergy Asthma Rep. 2024;24(2):39-51. doi:10.1007/s11882-024-01126-0
6. Afrin LB, Self S, Menk J, Lazarchick J. Characterization of mast cell activation syndrome. Am J Med Sci. 2017;353(3):207-215. doi:10.1016/j.amjms.2016.12.013
7. Valent P, Akin C, Arock M, et al. Definitions, criteria and global classification of mast cell disorders with special reference to mast cell activation syndromes: a consensus proposal. Int Arch Allergy Immunol. 2012;157(3):215-225. doi:10.1159/000328760
8. Valent P, Akin C. Doctor, I think I am suffering from MCAS: differential diagnosis and separating facts from fiction. J Allergy Clin Immunol Pract. 2019;7(4):1109-1114. doi:10.1016/j.jaip.2018.11.045
9. Shea-Donohue T, Stiltz J, Zhao A, Notari L. Mast cells. Curr Gastroenterol Rep. 2010;12(5):349-357. doi:10.1007/s11894-010-0132-1
10. Fong M, Crane JS. Histology, mast cells. StatPearls [Internet]. Treasure Island (FL): StatPearls Publishing; 2023. Accessed August 2023
11. Breedveld A, Groot Kormelink T, van Egmond M, de Jong EC. Granulocytes as modulators of dendritic cell function. J Leukoc

Biol. 2017;102(4):1003-1016. doi:10.1189/jlb.4MR0217-048RR

12. Baran J, Sobiepanek A, Mazurkiewicz-Pisarek A, et al. Mast cells as a target—a comprehensive review of recent therapeutic approaches. Cells. 2023;12(8):1187. doi:10.3390/cells12081187
13. Abraham SN, St John AL. Mast cell-orchestrated immunity to pathogens. Nat Rev Immunol. 2010;10(6):440-452. doi:10.1038/nri2782
14. Arun S, Storan A, Myers B. Mast cell activation syndrome and the link with long COVID. Br J Hosp Med (Lond). 2022;83(7):1-10. doi:10.12968/hmed.2022.0123
15. Jackson CW, Pratt CM, Rupprecht CP, Pattanaik D, Krishnaswamy G. Mastocytosis and mast cell activation disorders: clearing the air. Int J Mol Sci. 2021;22(20):11270 doi:10.3390/ijms222011270
16. Klimas L. Mast cell diseases. MastAttack website. Accessed March 2024. https://www.mastattack.org/mast-cell-diseases
17. Molderings GJ, Zienkiewicz T, Homann J, Menzen M, Afrin LB. Risk of solid cancer in patients with mast cell activation syndrome: results from Germany and USA. F1000Res. 2017;6:1889. doi:10.12688/f1000research.12730.1
18. Valent P, Akin C, Hartmann K, et al. Updated diagnostic criteria and classification of mast cell disorders: a consensus proposal. Hemasphere. 2021;5(11):e646. doi:10.1097/HS9.0000000000000646
19. Brockow K, Bent RK, Schneider S, et al. Challenges in the diagnosis of cutaneous mastocytosis. Diagnostics (Basel). 2024;14(2):161. doi:10.3390/diagnostics14020161
20. Pardanani A. Systemic mastocytosis in adults: 2023 update on diagnosis, risk stratification and management. Am J Hematol. 2023;98(7):1097-1116. doi:10.1002/ajh.26962
21. Gülen T, Akin C, Bonadonna P, et al. Selecting the right criteria and proper classification to diagnose mast cell activation syndromes: a critical review. J Allergy Clin Immunol Pract. 2021;9(11):3918-3928. doi:10.1016/j.jaip.2021.06.011
22. US National Cancer Institute. Mast cell sarcoma. SEER Hematopoietic and Lymphoid Tumor Database website. Updated February 7, 2020. Accessed July 30, 2025. https://seer.cancer.gov/seertools/hemelymph/51f6cf5ae3e27c3994bd54c2/
23. von Bubnoff D, Koch D, Stocker H, Ludwig RJ, Wortmann F, von

Bubnoff N. The clinical features of hereditary alpha-tryptasemia—implications for interdisciplinary practice. Dtsch Arztebl Int. 2024;121(8):258-264. doi:10.3238/arztebl.m2023.0287

24. The EDS Clinic. Mast cell activation is linked to a wide range of other conditions. The EDS Clinic website. Published December 2024. Accessed December 29, 2024 https://www.eds.clinic/articles/mast-cell-activation-is-linked-to-a-wide-range-of-other-conditions.
25. Theoharides TC, Valent P, Akin C. Mast cells, mastocytosis, and related disorders. N Engl J Med. 2015;373(2):163-172. doi:10.1056/NEJMra1409760
26. Özdemir Ö, Kasımoğlu G, Bak A, Sütlüoğlu H, Savaşan S. Mast cell activation syndrome: an up-to-date review of literature. World J Clin Pediatr. 2024;13(2):92813. doi:10.5409/wjcp.v13.i2.92813
27. Molderings GJ, Afrin LB. A survey of the currently known mast cell mediators with potential relevance for therapy of mast cell-induced symptoms. Naunyn Schmiedebergs Arch Pharmacol. 2023;396(11):2881-2891. doi:10.1007/s00210-023-02545-y
28. Picard M, Giavina-Bianchi P, Mezzano V, Castells M. Expanding spectrum of mast cell activation disorders: monoclonal and idiopathic mast cell activation syndromes. Clin Ther. 2013;35(5):548-562. doi:10.1016/j.clinthera.2013.04.001
29. Molderings GJ, Haenisch B, Brettner S, et al. Pharmacological treatment options for mast cell activation disease. Naunyn Schmiedebergs Arch Pharmacol. 2016;389(7):671-694. doi:10.1007/s00210-016-1247-1
30. Schofield JR, Afrin LB. Recognition and management of medication excipient reactivity in patients with mast cell activation syndrome. Am J Med Sci. 2019;357(6):507-511. doi:10.1016/j.amjms.2019.03.005
31. Molderings GJ, Kolck UW, Scheurlen W, Homann J, Frieling T. Multiple novel alterations in KIT tyrosine kinase in patients with gastrointestinally pronounced systemic mast cell activation syndrome: a case series. Scand J Gastroenterol. 2014;49(3):323-335. doi:10.3109/00365521.2013.867468
32. Encyclopaedia Britannica. Histamine. Encyclopaedia Britannica website. Updated February 23, 2024. Accessed February 27, 2024. https://www.britannica.com/science/histamine

33. Patel RH, Mohiuddin SS. Biochemistry, histamine. StatPearls [Internet]. Treasure Island (FL): StatPearls Publishing; 2023. Accessed February 2024.
34. Swiss Interest Group Histamine Intolerance (SIGHI). Histaminosis and histamine metabolism. SIGHI website. Updated March 18, 2023. Accessed February 27, 2024. https://www.histaminintoleranz.ch/en/histaminosis_histaminemetabolism.html
35. Branco ACCC, Yoshikawa FSY, Pietrobon AJ, Sato MN. Role of histamine in modulating the immune response and inflammation. Mediators Inflamm. 2018;2018:9524075. doi:10.1155/2018/9524075
36. Tiligada E, Ennis M. Histamine pharmacology: from Sir Henry Dale to the 21st century. Br J Pharmacol. 2020;177(3):469-489. doi:10.1111/bph.14524
37. Schirmer B, Neumann D. The function of the histamine H4 receptor in inflammatory and inflammation-associated diseases of the gut. Int J Mol Sci. 2021;22(11):6116. doi:10.3390/ijms22116116
38. Heidari A, Tongsook C, Najafipour R, et al. Mutations in the histamine N-methyltransferase gene, HNMT, are associated with nonsyndromic autosomal recessive intellectual disability. Hum Mol Genet. 2015;24(20):5697-5710. doi:10.1093/hmg/ddv286
39. Pearlman DS. Antihistamines: pharmacology and clinical use. Drugs. 1976;12(4):258-273. doi:10.2165/00003495-197612040-00002
40. Simons FE, Simons KJ. H1 antihistamines: current status and future directions. World Allergy Organ J. 2008;1(9):145-155. doi:10.1186/1939-4551-1-9-145
41. Parsons ME, Ganellin CR. Histamine and its receptors. Br J Pharmacol. 2006;147(Suppl 1):S127-S135. doi:10.1038/sj.bjp.0706440
42. Rusjan P, Sabioni P, Di Ciano P, et al. Exploring occupancy of the histamine H3 receptor by pitolisant in humans using PET. Br J Pharmacol. 2020;177(15):3464-3472. doi:10.1111/bph.15067
43. Zampeli E, Tiligada E. The role of histamine H4 receptor in immune and inflammatory disorders. Br J Pharmacol. 2009;157(1):24-33. doi:10.1111/j.1476-5381.2009.00151.x

44. Tiligada E, Zampeli E, Sander K, Stark H. Histamine H3 and H4 receptors as novel drug targets. Expert Opin Investig Drugs. 2009;18(10):1519-1531. doi:10.1517/14728220903188438
45. Criado PR, Criado RF, Maruta CW, Machado Filho CD. Histamine, histamine receptors and antihistamines: new concepts. An Bras Dermatol. 2010;85(2):195-210. doi:10.1590/S0365-05962010000200010
46. Handley DA, Magnetti A, Higgins AJ. Therapeutic advantages of third generation antihistamines. Expert Opin Investig Drugs. 1998;7(7):1045-1054. doi:10.1517/13543784.7.7.1045
47. Mayo Clinic. Allergy medications: know your options. Mayo Clinic website. Updated March 5, 2022. Accessed February 27, 2024. https://www.mayoclinic.org/diseases-conditions/allergies/in-depth/allergy-medications/art-20047403
48. Finn DF, Walsh JJ. Twenty-first century mast cell stabilizers. Br J Pharmacol. 2013;170(1):23-37. doi:10.1111/bph.12138
49. Billie Shellist. 15 natural anti-histamines and mast cell stabilizers. Functional Diagnostic Healing website. Accessed October 2019. https://www.functionaldiagnostichealing.com
50. Minutello K, Gupta V. Cromolyn sodium. StatPearls [Internet]. Treasure Island (FL): StatPearls Publishing; 2024. Accessed November 2024. https://www.ncbi.nlm.nih.gov/books/NBK557473/.
51. Weng Z, Zhang B, Asadi S, et al. Quercetin is more effective than cromolyn in blocking human mast cell cytokine release and inhibits contact dermatitis and photosensitivity in humans. PLoS One. 2012;7(3):e33805. doi:10.1371/journal.pone.0033805
52. Hamilton MJ. Nonclonal mast cell activation syndrome: a growing body of evidence. Immunol Allergy Clin North Am. 2018;38(3):469-481. doi:10.1016/j.iac.2018.04.002
53. Sokol KC, Amar NK, Starkey J, Grant JA. Ketotifen in the management of chronic urticaria: resurrection of an old drug. Ann Allergy Asthma Immunol. 2013;111(6):433-436. doi:10.1016/j.anai.2013.10.003
54. Ang DC, Hilligoss J, Stump T. Mast cell stabilizer (ketotifen) in fibromyalgia: phase 1 randomized controlled clinical trial. Clin J Pain. 2015;31(9):836-842. doi:10.1097/AJP.0000000000000169
55. Shaik Y, Caraffa A, Ronconi G, Lessiani G, Conti P. Impact of

polyphenols on mast cells with special emphasis on the effect of quercetin and luteolin. Cent Eur J Immunol. 2018;43(4):476-481. doi:10.5114/ceji.2018.81347
56. Lin Y, Shi R, Wang X, Shen HM. Luteolin, a flavonoid with potential for cancer prevention and therapy. Curr Cancer Drug Targets. 2008;8(7):634-646. doi:10.2174/156800908786241050
57. Theoharides TC. Ways to address perinatal mast cell activation and focal brain inflammation, including response to SARS-CoV-2, in autism spectrum disorder. J Pers Med. 2021;11(9):860. doi:10.3390/jpm11090860
58. Kritas SK, Saggini A, Varvara G, et al. Luteolin inhibits mast cell-mediated allergic inflammation. J Biol Regul Homeost Agents. 2013;27(4):955-959
59. Liao H, Ye J, Gao L, Liu Y. The main bioactive compounds of Scutellaria baicalensis Georgi. for alleviation of inflammatory cytokines: a comprehensive review. Biomed Pharmacother. 2021;133:110917. doi:10.1016/j.biopha.2020.110917
60. Wang ZL, Wang S, Kuang Y, Hu ZM, Qiao X, Ye M. A comprehensive review on phytochemistry, pharmacology, and flavonoid biosynthesis of Scutellaria baicalensis. Pharm Biol. 2018;56(1):465-484. doi:10.1080/13880209.2018.1492620
61. Nijkamp FP, Sitsen JM. Leukotrienes, allergy and inflammation. Pharm Weekbl Sci. 1982;4(6):165-171. doi:10.1007/BF01959134
62. Schapowal A; Petasites Study Group. Randomised controlled trial of butterbur and cetirizine for treating seasonal allergic rhinitis. BMJ. 2002;324(7330):144-146. doi:10.1136/bmj.324.7330.144
63. Kälin P. The common butterbur (Petasites hybridus)—portrait of a medicinal herb. Forsch Komplementarmed Klass Naturheilkd. 2003;10(Suppl 1):41-44. doi:10.1159/000071691
64. Siddiqui MZ. Boswellia serrata, a potential antiinflammatory agent: an overview. Indian J Pharm Sci. 2011;73(3):255-261. doi:10.4103/0250-474X.93507
65. Sultana A, Rahman KU, Padmaja AR, Rahman SU. Boswellia serrata Roxb. A traditional herb with versatile pharmacological activity—a review. Int J Pharm Sci Res. 2013;4(6):2106-2117. doi:10.13040/IJPSR.0975-8232.4(6).2106-17

66. McKenna M, McDougall JJ. Cannabinoid control of neurogenic inflammation. Br J Pharmacol. 2020;177(19):4386-4399. doi:10.1111/bph.15208
67. Timoszuk M, Bielawska K, Skrzydlewska E. Evening primrose (Oenothera biennis) biological activity dependent on chemical composition. Antioxidants (Basel). 2018;7(8):108. doi:10.3390/antiox7080108
68. Fecker R, Buda V, Alexa E, et al. Phytochemical and biological screening of Oenothera biennis L. hydroalcoholic extract. Biomolecules. 2020;10(6):818. doi:10.3390/biom10060818
69. Sharifi M, Nourani N, Sanaie S, et al. The effect of Oenothera biennis (evening primrose) oil on inflammatory diseases: a systematic review of clinical trials. BMC Complement Med Ther. 2024;24(1):89. doi:10.1186/s12906-024-04378-5
70. Pareek A, Suthar M, Rathore GS, Bansal V. Feverfew (Tanacetum parthenium L.): a systematic review. Pharmacogn Rev. 2011;5(9):103-110. doi:10.4103/0973-7847.79105
71. Hasan MR, Alotaibi BS, Althafar ZM, et al. An update on the therapeutic anticancer potential of Ocimum sanctum L.: "elixir of life." Molecules. 2023;28(3):1193. doi:10.3390/molecules28031193
72. Cohen MM. Tulsi - Ocimum sanctum: a herb for all reasons. J Ayurveda Integr Med. 2014;5(4):251-259. doi:10.4103/0975-9476.146554
73. Han S, Sun L, He F, Che H. Anti-allergic activity of glycyrrhizic acid on IgE-mediated allergic reaction by regulation of allergy-related immune cells. Sci Rep. 2017;7(1):7222. doi:10.1038/s41598-017-07833-1
74. Yang R, Yuan BC, Ma YS, Zhou S, Liu Y. The anti-inflammatory activity of licorice, a widely used Chinese herb. Pharm Biol. 2017;55(1):5-18. doi:10.1080/13880209.2016.1225775
75. Sharma V, Katiyar A, Agrawal RC. Glycyrrhiza glabra: chemistry and pharmacological activity. In: Sweeteners. 2017;87-100. doi:10.1007/978-3-319-27027-2_21
76. Flora K, Hahn M, Rosen H, Benner K. Milk thistle (Silybum marianum) for the therapy of liver disease. Am J Gastroenterol. 1998;93(2):139-143. doi:10.1111/j.1572-0241.1998.00139

77. Bhusal KK, Magar SK, Thapa R, et al. Nutritional and pharmacological importance of stinging nettle (Urtica dioica L.): a review. Heliyon. 2022;8(6):e09717. doi:10.1016/j.heliyon.2022.e09717
78. Devkota HP, Paudel KR, Khanal S, et al. Stinging nettle (Urtica dioica L.): nutritional composition, bioactive compounds, and food functional properties. Molecules. 2022;27(16):5219. doi:10.3390/molecules27165219
79. Roschek B Jr, Fink RC, McMichael M, Alberte RS. Nettle extract (Urtica dioica) affects key receptors and enzymes associated with allergic rhinitis. Phytother Res. 2009;23(7):920-926. doi:10.1002/ptr.2763
80. Sharma SC, Sharma S, Gulati OP. Pycnogenol inhibits the release of histamine from mast cells. Phytother Res. 2003;17(1):66-69. doi:10.1002/ptr.1240
81. Adam G, Robu S, Flutur MM, et al. Applications of Perilla frutescens extracts in clinical practice. Antioxidants (Basel). 2023;12(3):727. doi:10.3390/antiox12030727
82. Carr AC, Maggini S. Vitamin C and immune function. Nutrients. 2017;9(11):1211. doi:10.3390/nu9111211
83. Yazdani Shaik BD, Conti P. Relationship between vitamin C, mast cells and inflammation. J Nutr Food Sci. 2016;6:456. doi:10.4172/2155-9600.1000456
84. Kempuraj D, Mentor S, Thangavel R, et al. Mast cells in stress, pain, blood-brain barrier, neuroinflammation, and Alzheimer's disease. Front Cell Neurosci. 2019;13:54. doi:10.3389/fncel.2019.00054
85. Kempuraj D, Selvakumar GP, Thangavel R, et al. Mast cell activation in brain injury, stress, and post-traumatic stress disorder and Alzheimer's disease pathogenesis. Front Neurosci. 2017;11:703. doi:10.3389/fnins.2017.00703
86. Morales-Gutierrez J, Díaz-Cortés S, Montoya-Giraldo MA, Zuluaga AF. Toxicity induced by multiple high doses of vitamin B12 during pernicious anemia treatment: a case report. Clin Toxicol (Phila). 2020;58(2):129-131. doi:10.1080/15563650.2019.1606432
87. Meyer HE, Willett WC, Fung TT, et al. Association of high intakes of vitamins B6 and B12 from food and supplements with risk of hip fracture among postmenopausal women in the Nurses' Health

Study. JAMA Netw Open. 2019;2(5):e193591. doi:10.1001/jamanetworkopen.2019.3591

88. Breit S, Kupferberg A, Rogler G, Hasler G. Vagus nerve as modulator of the brain-gut axis in psychiatric and inflammatory disorders. Front Psychiatry. 2018;9:44. doi:10.3389/fpsyt.2018.00044
89. Irwin MR, Olmstead R, Carroll JE. Sleep disturbance, sleep duration, and inflammation: a systematic review and meta-analysis of cohort studies and experimental sleep deprivation. Biol Psychiatry. 2016;80(1):40-52. doi:10.1016/j.biopsych.2015.05.014
90. Elliot AJ. Color and psychological functioning: a review of theoretical and empirical work. Front Psychol. 2015;6:368. doi:10.3389/fpsyg.2015.00368
91. Miraj S, Rafieian-Kopaei M, Kiani S. Melissa officinalis L: a review study with an antioxidant prospective. J Evid Based Complement Altern Med. 2017;22(3):385-394. doi:10.1177/2156587216663433
92. Koulivand PH, Khaleghi Ghadiri M, Gorji A. Lavender and the nervous system. Evid Based Complement Alternat Med. 2013;2013:681304. doi:10.1155/2013/681304
93. Knufinke M, Fittkau-Koch L, Møst EIS, Kompier MAJ, Nieuwenhuys A. Restricting short-wavelength light in the evening to improve sleep in recreational athletes: a pilot study. Eur J Sport Sci. 2019;19(6):728-735. doi:10.1080/17461391.2018.1544278
94. Barsam T, Monazzam MR, Haghdoost AA, Ghotbi MR, Dehghan SF. Effect of extremely low frequency electromagnetic field exposure on sleep quality in high voltage substations. Iranian J Environ Health Sci Eng. 2012;9(1):15. doi:10.1186/1735-2746-9-15
95. No Radiation for You. No Radiation for You. No Radiation for You website. Accessed September 2025. https://www.norad4u.com
96. Strøm-Tejsen P, Zukowska D, Wargocki P, Wyon DP. The effects of bedroom air quality on sleep and next-day performance. Indoor Air. 2016;26(5):679-686. doi:10.1111/ina.12254
97. Pache M, Kräuchi K, Cajochen C, et al. Cold feet and prolonged sleep-onset latency in vasospastic syndrome. Lancet. 2001;358(9276):125-126. doi:10.1016/S0140-6736(01)05344-2

98. Sleep Foundation. Napping. Sleep Foundation website. Accessed September 2025. https://www.sleepfoundation.org/sleep-hygiene/napping
99. Medic G, Wille M, Hemels ME. Short- and long-term health consequences of sleep disruption. Nat Sci Sleep. 2017;9:151-161. doi:10.2147/NSS.S134864
100. Masters A, Pandi-Perumal SR, Seixas A, et al. Melatonin, the hormone of darkness: from sleep promotion to Ebola treatment. Brain Disord Ther. 2014;4(1):1000151. doi:10.4172/2168-975X.1000151
101. Costello RB, Lentino CV, Boyd CC, et al. The effectiveness of melatonin for promoting healthy sleep: a rapid evidence assessment of the literature. Nutr J. 2014;13:106. doi:10.1186/1475-2891-13-106
102. Gröber U, Schmidt J, Kisters K. Magnesium in prevention and therapy. Nutrients. 2015;7(9):8199-8226. doi:10.3390/nu7095388
103. Abbasi B, Kimiagar M, Sadeghniiat K, et al. The effect of magnesium supplementation on primary insomnia in elderly: a double-blind placebo-controlled clinical trial. J Res Med Sci. 2012;17(12):1161-1169.
104. Chandrashekhar VM, Halagali KS, Nidavani RB, et al. Anti-allergic activity of German chamomile (Matricaria recutita L.) in mast cell mediated allergy model. J Ethnopharmacol. 2011;137(1):336-340. doi:10.1016/j.jep.2011.05.029
105. Srivastava JK, Shankar E, Gupta S. Chamomile: a herbal medicine of the past with bright future. Mol Med Rep. 2010;3(6):895-901. doi:10.3892/mmr.2010.377
106. National Center for Complementary and Integrative Health. Chamomile. NCCIH website. Accessed September 2025. https://www.nccih.nih.gov/health/chamomile
107. Franco L, Sánchez C, Bravo R, Rodriguez A, Barriga C, Juánez JC. The sedative effects of hops (Humulus lupulus), a component of beer, on the activity/rest rhythm. Acta Physiol Hung. 2012;99(2):133-139. doi:10.1556/APhysiol.99.2012.2.6
108. Bent S, Padula A, Moore D, Patterson M, Mehling W. Valerian for sleep: a systematic review and meta-analysis. Am J Med. 2006;119(12):1005-1012. doi:10.1016/j.amjmed.2006.02.026

109. Mount Sinai Health Library. Valerian. Mount Sinai Health Library website. Accessed 2020. https://www.mountsinai.org/health-library/herb/valerian.

110. Miroddi M, Calapai G, Navarra M, Minciullo PL, Gangemi S. Passiflora incarnata L.: ethnopharmacology, clinical application, safety and evaluation of clinical trials. J Ethnopharmacol. 2013;150(3):791-804. doi:10.1016/j.jep.2013.09.047

111. Toda K, Hitoe S, Takeda S, Shimizu N, Shimoda H. Passionflower extract induces high-amplitude rhythms without phase shifts in the expression of several circadian clock genes in vitro and in vivo. Int J Biomed Sci. 2017;13(2):84-92.

112. Mount Sinai Health Library. Passionflower. Mount Sinai Health Library website. Accessed 2020. https://www.mountsinai.org/health-library/herb/passionflower

113. Frank S, Gonzalez K, Lee-Ang L, Young MC, Tamez M, Mattei J. Diet and sleep physiology: public health and clinical implications. Front Neurol. 2017;8:393. doi:10.3389/fneur.2017.00393

114. Peuhkuri K, Sihvola N, Korpela R. Dietary factors and fluctuating levels of melatonin. Food Nutr Res. 2012;56:17252. doi:10.3402/fnr.v56i0.17252

115. St-Onge MP, Mikic A, Pietrolungo CE. Effects of diet on sleep quality. Adv Nutr. 2016;7(5):938-949. doi:10.3945/an.116.012336

116. Zeng Y, Yang J, Du J, et al. Strategies of functional foods promote sleep in human being. Curr Signal Transduct Ther. 2014;9(3):148-155. doi:10.2174/1574362410666150205165504

117. Doherty R, Madigan S, Warrington G, Ellis J. Sleep and nutrition interactions: implications for athletes. Nutrients. 2019;11(4):822. doi:10.3390/nu11040822

118. Whitbread D. Top 10 foods highest in tryptophan. MyFoodData website. Accessed September 2025. https://www.myfooddata.com/articles/high-tryptophan-foods.php

119. Ryberg K, Goossens A, Isaksson M, et al. Is contact allergy to disperse dyes and related substances associated with textile dermatitis? Br J Dermatol. 2009;160(1):107-115. doi:10.1111/j.1365-2133.2008.08953.x

120. Lundius EG, Sanchez-Alavez M, Ghochani Y, Klaus J, Tabarean IV. Histamine influences body temperature by acting at H1 and H3

receptors on distinct populations of preoptic neurons. J Neurosci. 2010;30(12):4369-4381. doi:10.1523/JNEUROSCI.0378-10.2010

121. Guo EL, Katta R. Diet and hair loss: effects of nutrient deficiency and supplement use. Dermatol Pract Concept. 2017;7(1):1-10. doi:10.5826/dpc.0701a01

122. Mayo Clinic Staff. Hair loss. Mayo Clinic website. Published January 19, 2024. Accessed March 12, 2024. https://www.mayoclinic.org/diseases-conditions/hair-loss/symptoms-causes/syc-20372926

123. Garza LA, Liu Y, Yang Z, et al. Prostaglandin D2 inhibits hair growth and is elevated in bald scalp of men with androgenetic alopecia. Sci Transl Med. 2012;4(126):126ra34. doi:10.1126/scitranslmed.3003122

124. Nesterenko S. Histaminintoleranz, die unentdeckte Krankheit. 2nd ed. Weinheim, Germany: Rainer Bloch Verlag; 2017.

125. Swiss Interest Group Histamine Intolerance (SIGHI). Food compatibility list: histamine. SIGHI website. Updated April 1, 2023. Accessed March 12, 2024. https://mastzellaktivierung.info/en/downloads.html#lm_en

126. Suzzi G, Torriani S. Editorial: biogenic amines in foods. Front Microbiol. 2015;6:472. doi:10.3389/fmicb.2015.00472

127. Özogul Y, Özogul F. Biogenic amines formation, toxicity, regulations in food. In: Saad B, Tofalo R, eds. Biogenic Amines in Food: Analysis, Occurrence and Toxicity. Cambridge, UK: Royal Society of Chemistry; 2020:1-17. doi:10.1039/9781788017527-00001

128. Ruiz-Capillas C, Herrero AM. Impact of biogenic amines on food quality and safety. Foods. 2019;8(2):62. doi:10.3390/foods8020062

129. Li Y, Yao J, Han C, et al. Quercetin, inflammation and immunity. Nutrients. 2016;8(3):167. doi:10.3390/nu8030167

130. Drugs.com. Quercetin. Drugs.com website. Updated December 19, 2022. Accessed December 13, 2023. https://www.drugs.com/npp/quercetin.html

131. Quercetin.com. Dietary sources of quercetin. Quercetin.com website. Accessed March 12, 2024. https://quercetin.com/overview/dietary-sources-of-quercetin

132. Superfoodly. 100 quercetin foods: best natural sources ranked. Superfoodly website. Published August 14, 2020. Accessed December 13, 2023. https://www.superfoodly.com/quercetin-foods/
133. Smalley WE, Ray WA, Daugherty JR, Griffin MR. Nonsteroidal anti-inflammatory drugs and the incidence of hospitalizations for peptic ulcer disease in elderly persons. Am J Epidemiol. 1995;141(6):539-545. doi:10.1093/oxfordjournals.aje.a117469
134. Sinha M, Gautam L, Shukla PK, Kaur P, Sharma S, Singh TP. Current perspectives in NSAID-induced gastropathy. Mediators Inflamm. 2013;2013:258209. doi:10.1155/2013/258209
135. Dugowson CE, Gnanashanmugam P. Nonsteroidal anti-inflammatory drugs. Phys Med Rehabil Clin N Am. 2006;17(2):347-354. doi:10.1016/j.pmr.2005.12.012
136. Fosbøl EL, Gislason GH, Jacobsen S, et al. Risk of myocardial infarction and death associated with the use of nonsteroidal anti-inflammatory drugs (NSAIDs) among healthy individuals: a nationwide cohort study. Clin Pharmacol Ther. 2009;85(2):190-197. doi:10.1038/clpt.2008.204
137. Meek IL, van de Laar MAFJ, Vonkeman HE. Non-steroidal anti-inflammatory drugs: an overview of cardiovascular risks. Pharmaceuticals (Basel). 2010;3(7):2146-2162. doi:10.3390/ph3072146
138. Gupta C, Prakash D. Phytonutrients as therapeutic agents. J Complement Integr Med. 2014;11(3):151-169. doi:10.1515/jcim-2013-0021
139. Kumar A, P N, Kumar M, et al. Major phytochemicals: recent advances in health benefits and extraction method. Molecules. 2023;28(2):887. Published January 16, 2023. doi:10.3390/molecules28020887
140. Kiokias S, Oreopoulou V. A review of the health protective effects of phenolic acids against a range of severe pathologic conditions (including coronavirus-based infections). Molecules. 2021;26(17):5405. doi:10.3390/molecules26175405
141. Al-Khayri JM, Mascarenhas R, Harish HM, et al. Stilbenes, a versatile class of natural metabolites for inflammation—an overview. Molecules. 2023;28(9):3786. Published April 28, 2023. doi:10.3390/molecules28093786

142. Zamora-Ros R, Andres-Lacueva C, Lamuela-Raventós RM, et al. Concentrations of resveratrol and derivatives in foods and estimation of dietary intake in a Spanish population: European Prospective Investigation into Cancer and Nutrition (EPIC)-Spain cohort. Br J Nutr. 2008;100(1):188-196. doi:10.1017/S0007114507882997
143. Jang WY, Kim MY, Cho JY. Antioxidant, anti-inflammatory, anti-menopausal, and anti-cancer effects of lignans and their metabolites. Int J Mol Sci. 2022;23(24):15482. Published December 7, 2022. doi:10.3390/ijms232415482
144. Ojo MA. Tannins in foods: nutritional implications and processing effects of hydrothermal techniques on underutilized hard-to-cook legume seeds—a review. Prev Nutr Food Sci. 2022;27(1):14-19. doi:10.3746/pnf.2022.27.1.14
145. Magrone T, Magrone M, Russo MA, Jirillo E. Recent advances on the anti-inflammatory and antioxidant properties of red grape polyphenols: in vitro and in vivo studies. Antioxidants (Basel). 2019;9(1):35. doi:10.3390/antiox9010035
146. Ajanaku CO, Ademosun OT, Atohengbe PO, et al. Functional bioactive compounds in ginger, turmeric, and garlic. Front Nutr. 2022;9:1012023. Published December 8, 2022. doi:10.3389/fnut.2022.1012023
147. Suzuki Y, Miyoshi N, Isemura M. Health-promoting effects of green tea. Proc Jpn Acad Ser B Phys Biol Sci. 2012;88(3):88-101. doi:10.2183/pjab.88.88
148. Krinsky NI, Johnson EJ. Carotenoid actions and their relation to health and disease. Mol Aspects Med. 2005;26(6):459-516. doi:10.1016/j.mam.2005.10.001
149. Crupi P, Faienza MF, Naeem MY, Corbo F, Clodoveo ML, Muraglia M. Overview of the potential beneficial effects of carotenoids on consumer health and well-being. Antioxidants (Basel). 2023;12(5):1069. Published May 10, 2023. doi:10.3390/antiox12051069
150. Gutiérrez-Del-Río I, López-Ibáñez S, Magadán-Corpas P, et al. Terpenoids and polyphenols as natural antioxidant agents in food preservation. Antioxidants (Basel). 2021;10(8):1264. Published August 8, 2021. doi:10.3390/antiox10081264
151. Verkerk R, Schreiner M, Krumbein A, et al. Glucosinolates in

Brassica vegetables: the influence of the food supply chain on intake, bioavailability and human health. Mol Nutr Food Res. 2009;53(Suppl 2):S219. doi:10.1002/mnfr.200800065

152. Chang A, Rosani A, Quick J. Capsaicin. In: StatPearls [Internet]. Treasure Island (FL): StatPearls Publishing; 2025 Jan–. Updated May 23, 2023. Available from: https://www.ncbi.nlm.nih.gov/books/NBK459168/

153. Chen M, Xu L, Van Horn L, Manson JE, Tucker KL, Du X, Feng N, Rong S, Zhong VW. Association of 8-hour time-restricted eating with all-cause and cause-specific mortality. Poster presentation. American Heart Association. Published March 2024. Accessed August 2024. https://s3.amazonaws.com/cms.ipressroom.com/67/files/20242/8-h+TRE+and+mortality+AHA+poster_031924.pdf

154. British Heart Foundation. Intermittent fasting: what does the evidence say? Heart Matters Magazine. Published March 22, 2024. Accessed August 24, 2024. https://www.bhf.org.uk/informationsupport/heart-matters-magazine/news/behind-the-headlines/intermittent-fasting

155. British Nutrition Foundation. The science of protein. British Nutrition Foundation website. Accessed December 2023. https://www.nutrition.org.uk/nutritional-information/protein/?level=Health%20professional

156. Mayo Clinic Staff. Carbohydrates: How carbs fit into a healthy diet. Mayo Clinic website. Published March 22, 2022. Accessed December 15, 2023. https://www.mayoclinic.org/healthy-lifestyle/nutrition-and-healthy-eating/in-depth/carbohydrates/art-20045705

157. HealthLink BC. Vitamins: their function and sources. HealthLink BC website. Updated March 1, 2023. Accessed January 30, 2024. https://www.healthlinkbc.ca/health-topics/ta3868

158. Harvard Health Publishing. Listing of vitamins. Harvard Health Publishing website. Published August 31, 2020. Accessed January 30, 2024. https://www.health.harvard.edu/staying-healthy/listing_of_vitamins

159. National Institutes of Health, Office of Dietary Supplements. Vitamin C: Fact Sheet for Health Professionals. ODS, NIH website. Updated March 26, 2021. Accessed January 29, 2024. https://ods.

od.nih.gov/factsheets/VitaminC-HealthProfessional
160. Self Nutrition Data. Self Nutrition Data. Self Nutrition Data website. Archived at: https://web.archive.org/web/20180707024905/http://nutritiondata.self.com/.Accessed November 20,2019.
161. National Institutes of Health, Office of Dietary Supplements. Thiamin: Fact Sheet for Health Professionals. ODS, NIH website. Updated Feb 9, 2023. Accessed January 29, 2024 https://ods.od.nih.gov/factsheets/Thiamin-HealthProfessional
162. National Institutes of Health, Office of Dietary Supplements. Riboflavin: Fact Sheet for Health Professionals. ODS, NIH website. Updated May 11, 2022. Accessed January 29, 2024. https://ods.od.nih.gov/factsheets/Riboflavin-HealthProfessional
163. National Institutes of Health, Office of Dietary Supplements. Niacin: Fact Sheet for Health Professionals. ODS, NIH website. Updated Nov 18, 2022. Accessed January 28, 2024. https://ods.od.nih.gov/factsheets/Niacin-HealthProfessional
164. National Institutes of Health, Office of Dietary Supplements. Pantothenic acid: Fact Sheet for Health Professionals. ODS, NIH website. Updated March 26, 2021. Accessed January 28, 2024. https://ods.od.nih.gov/factsheets/PantothenicAcid-HealthProfessional
165. National Institutes of Health, Office of Dietary Supplements. Vitamin B6: Fact Sheet for Health Professionals. ODS, NIH website. Updated June 16, 2023. Accessed January 28, 2024. https://ods.od.nih.gov/factsheets/VitaminB6-HealthProfessional
166. National Institutes of Health, Office of Dietary Supplements. Biotin: Fact Sheet for Health Professionals. ODS, NIH website. Updated January 10, 2022. Accessed January 28, 2024. https://ods.od.nih.gov/factsheets/Biotin-HealthProfessional
167. National Institutes of Health, Office of Dietary Supplements. Folate: Fact Sheet for Health Professionals. ODS, NIH website. Updated November 30, 2022. Accessed January 27, 2024. https://ods.od.nih.gov/factsheets/Folate-HealthProfessional
168. National Institutes of Health, Office of Dietary Supplements. Vitamin B12: Fact Sheet for Health Professionals. ODS, NIH website. Updated December 15, 2023. Accessed January 27, 2024.

https://ods.od.nih.gov/factsheets/VitaminB12-HealthProfessional
169. National Institutes of Health, Office of Dietary Supplements. Vitamin A: Fact Sheet for Health Professionals. ODS, NIH website. Updated December 15, 2023. Accessed January 27, 2024. https://ods.od.nih.gov/factsheets/VitaminA-HealthProfessional
170. National Institutes of Health, Office of Dietary Supplements. Vitamin D: Fact Sheet for Health Professionals. ODS, NIH website. Updated September 18, 2023. Accessed January 25, 2024. https://ods.od.nih.gov/factsheets/VitaminD-HealthProfessional
171. National Institutes of Health, Office of Dietary Supplements. Vitamin E: Fact Sheet for Health Professionals. ODS, NIH website. Updated March 26, 2021. Accessed January 25, 2024. https://ods.od.nih.gov/factsheets/VitaminE-HealthProfessional
172. National Institutes of Health, Office of Dietary Supplements. Vitamin K: Fact Sheet for Health Professionals. ODS, NIH website. Updated March 29, 2021. Accessed January 25, 2024. https://ods.od.nih.gov/factsheets/VitaminK-HealthProfessional
173. National Institutes of Health, Office of Dietary Supplements. Choline: Fact Sheet for Health Professionals. ODS, NIH website. Updated June 2, 2022. Accessed January 25, 2024. https://ods.od.nih.gov/factsheets/Choline-HealthProfessional
174. National Institutes of Health, Office of Dietary Supplements. Calcium: Fact Sheet for Health Professionals. ODS, NIH website. Updated June 2, 2022. Accessed February 27, 2024. https://ods.od.nih.gov/factsheets/Calcium-HealthProfessional
175. Meletis CD. Chloride: The forgotten essential mineral. Return2Health website. Published September 15, 2009. Accessed March 10, 2024. https://return2health.com.au/articles/chloride-the-forgotten-essential-mineral
176. Harvard T.H. Chan School of Public Health. Chloride. The Nutrition Source. Harvard T.H. Chan School of Public Health website. Last reviewed March 2023. Accessed March 10, 2024. https://www.hsph.harvard.edu/nutritionsource/chloride
177. University of Florida Health. Chloride in diet. Conditions and Treatments. Last reviewed March 11, 2021. Accessed March 10, 2024. https://ufhealth.org/conditions-and-treatments/chloride-in-diet
178. National Institutes of Health, Office of Dietary Supplements.

Magnesium: Fact Sheet for Health Professionals. ODS, NIH website. Updated June 2, 2022. Accessed February 26, 2024. https://ods.od.nih.gov/factsheets/Magnesium-HealthProfessional

179. National Institutes of Health, Office of Dietary Supplements. Phosphorus: Fact Sheet for Health Professionals. ODS, NIH website. Updated March 4, 2023. Accessed February 24, 2024. https://ods.od.nih.gov/factsheets/Phosphorus-HealthProfessional
180. National Institutes of Health, Office of Dietary Supplements. Potassium: Fact Sheet for Health Professionals. ODS, NIH website. Updated June 2, 2022. Accessed February 24, 2024. https://ods.od.nih.gov/factsheets/Potassium-HealthProfessional
181. European Food Information Council. Sodium: foods, functions, how much do you need & more. EUFIC website. Updated January 11, 2021. Accessed March 12, 2024. https://www.eufic.org/en/vitamins-and-minerals/article/sodium-foods-functions-how-much-do-you-need-more
182. Harvard T.H. Chan School of Public Health. Salt and sodium. The Nutrition Source. Harvard T.H. Chan School of Public Health website. Last reviewed March 2023. Accessed March 12, 2024. https://www.hsph.harvard.edu/nutritionsource/salt-and-sodium
183. National Academies of Sciences, Engineering, and Medicine. Sodium and potassium dietary reference intake values updated in new report; introduces new category for sodium based on chronic disease risk reduction. News Release March 5, 2019. Accessed March 12, 2024. https://www.nationalacademies.org/news/2019/03/sodium-and-potassium-dietary-reference-intake-values-updated-in-new-report
184. Institute of Medicine (US) Panel on Micronutrients. Dietary reference intakes for vitamin A, vitamin K, arsenic, boron, chromium, copper, iodine, iron, manganese, molybdenum, nickel, silicon, vanadium, and zinc. Washington, DC: National Academies Press; 2001.
185. National Institutes of Health, Office of Dietary Supplements. Chromium: Fact Sheet for Health Professionals. ODS, NIH website. Updated June 2, 2022. Accessed February 23, 2024. https://ods.od.nih.gov/factsheets/Chromium-HealthProfessional
186. National Institutes of Health, Office of Dietary Supplements.

Copper: Fact Sheet for Health Professionals. ODS, NIH website. Updated October 18, 2022. Accessed February 24, 2024. https://ods.od.nih.gov/factsheets/Copper-HealthProfessional

187. Harvard T.H. Chan School of Public Health. Fluoride. The Nutrition Source. Last reviewed March 2023. Accessed February 22, 2024. https://www.hsph.harvard.edu/nutritionsource/fluoride

188. World Health Organization. Assessment of iodine deficiency disorders and monitoring their elimination: a guide for programme managers. 3rd ed. Geneva, Switzerland: World Health Organization; 2007. Accessed February 21, 2024. https://www.who.int/publications/i/item/9789241595827

189. National Institutes of Health, Office of Dietary Supplements. Iodine: Fact Sheet for Health Professionals. ODS, NIH website. Updated October 13, 2023. Accessed February 21, 2024. https://ods.od.nih.gov/factsheets/Iodine-HealthProfessional

190. National Institutes of Health, Office of Dietary Supplements. Iron: Fact Sheet for Health Professionals. ODS, NIH website. Updated June 15, 2023. Accessed February 24, 2024. https://ods.od.nih.gov/factsheets/Iron-HealthProfessional

191. National Institutes of Health, Office of Dietary Supplements. Manganese: Fact Sheet for Health Professionals. ODS, NIH website. Updated March 29, 2021. Accessed February 21, 2024. https://ods.od.nih.gov/factsheets/Manganese-HealthProfessional

192. National Institutes of Health, Office of Dietary Supplements. Molybdenum: Fact Sheet for Health Professionals. ODS, NIH website. Updated March 30, 2021. Accessed February 21, 2024. https://ods.od.nih.gov/factsheets/Molybdenum-HealthProfessional

193. National Library of Medicine. Molybdenum cofactor deficiency. MedlinePlus Genetics website. Updated March 1, 2014. Accessed February 21, 2024. https://medlineplus.gov/genetics/condition/molybdenum-cofactor-deficiency/#causes

194. National Institutes of Health, Office of Dietary Supplements. Selenium: Fact Sheet for Health Professionals. ODS, NIH website. Updated March 26, 2021. Accessed February 21, 2024. https://ods.od.nih.gov/factsheets/Selenium-HealthProfessional

195. National Institutes of Health, Office of Dietary Supplements. Zinc: Fact Sheet for Health Professionals. ODS, NIH website. Updated

September 28, 2022. Accessed February 26, 2024. https://ods.od.nih.gov/factsheets/Zinc-HealthProfessional
196. National Library of Medicine. What are proteins and what do they do? MedlinePlus Genetics website. Updated March 26, 2021. Accessed January 15, 2024. https://medlineplus.gov/genetics/understanding/howgeneswork/protein/
197. Harvard T.H. Chan School of Public Health. Protein. The Nutrition Source. Harvard T.H. Chan School of Public Health website. Accessed January 14, 2024. https://www.hsph.harvard.edu/nutritionsource/what-should-you-eat/protein/
198. Wu G. Dietary protein intake and human health. Food Funct. 2016;7(3):1251-1265. doi:10.1039/c5fo01530h
199. Nutritionix. Accessed January 2024. https://www.nutritionix.com
200. Goda Y, Hoshino K, Akiyama H, et al. Constituents in watercress: inhibitors of histamine release from RBL-2H3 cells induced by antigen stimulation. Biol Pharm Bull. 1999;22(12):1319-1326. doi:10.1248/bpb.22.1319
201. Li L, Li MH, Ren HK, Shi YJ, Dong YM. Anti-allergic effects and related active constituents of mung bean (Vignaradiatus Linn) sprouts. Food Sci Biotechnol. 2016;25(2):553-559. Published April 30, 2016. doi:10.1007/s10068-016-0077-8
202. Lichtenstein AH, Kennedy E, Barrier P, Danford D, Ernst ND, Grundy SM, et al. Dietary fat consumption and health. Nutr Rev. 1998;56(5):3-19. doi:10.1111/j.1753-4887.1998.tb01728.x
203. Harvard Health Publishing. The truth about fats: the good, the bad, and the in-between. December 12, 2019. Harvard Medical School website. Accessed February 14, 2024. https://www.health.harvard.edu/staying-healthy/the-truth-about-fats-bad-and-good
204. European Food Information Council (EUFIC). The functions of fats in the body. Updated February 13, 2015. Accessed February 14, 2024. https://www.eufic.org/en/whats-in-food/article/facts-on-fats-dietary-fats-and-health
205. Field CJ, Robinson L. Dietary fats. Adv Nutr. 2019;10(4):722-724. doi:10.1093/advances/nmz052
206. News-Medical. Triglycerides – what do they do? Updated June 18, 2023. Accessed February 14, 2024. https://www.news-medical.net/health/Triglycerides-What-do-they-do.aspx
207. Biology Dictionary. Fatty acids. Updated October 4, 2019.

Accessed February 13, 2024. https://biologydictionary.net/fatty-acids/

208. Harvard T.H. Chan School of Public Health. Types of fat. The Nutrition Source website. Accessed February 13, 2024. https://www.hsph.harvard.edu/nutritionsource/what-should-you-eat/fats-and-cholesterol/types-of-fat/

209. Schönfeld P, Wojtczak L. Short- and medium-chain fatty acids in energy metabolism: the cellular perspective. J Lipid Res. 2016;57(6):943-954. doi:10.1194/jlr.R067629

210. Oregon State University, Linus Pauling Institute. Essential fatty acids. Reviewed June 2019. Accessed February 12, 2024. https://lpi.oregonstate.edu/mic/other-nutrients/essential-fatty-acids

211. Craig M, Yarrarapu SNS, Dimri M. Biochemistry, cholesterol. In: StatPearls [Internet]. Treasure Island (FL): StatPearls Publishing; January 2024. Updated August 8, 2023. https://www.ncbi.nlm.nih.gov/books/NBK513326/

212. Encyclopaedia Britannica. Cholesterol. Encyclopaedia Britannica website. Updated January 30, 2024. Accessed February 12, 2024. https://www.britannica.com/science/cholesterol

213. Encyclopaedia Britannica. Phospholipid. Encyclopaedia Britannica website. Updated January 30, 2024. Accessed February 13, 2024. https://www.britannica.com/science/phospholipid

214. Dai Y, Tang H, Pang S. The crucial roles of phospholipids in aging and lifespan regulation. Front Physiol. 2021;12:775648. Published November 23, 2021. doi:10.3389/fphys.2021.775648

215. Wehrmüller K. Impact of Dietary Phospholipids on Human Health. Technical-scientific information. No. 524. ALP Science; 2008. ISBN 978-3-905667-63-9

216. Harvard T.H. Chan School of Public Health. Omega-3 fatty acids: an essential contribution. The Nutrition Source website. Accessed February 13, 2024. https://www.hsph.harvard.edu/nutritionsource/what-should-you-eat/fats-and-cholesterol/types-of-fat/omega-3-fats/

217. National Institutes of Health. Office of Dietary Supplements. Omega-3 fatty acids: Fact Sheet for Health Professionals. Updated February 15, 2023. Accessed February 13, 2024. https://ods.od.nih.gov/factsheets/Omega3FattyAcids-HealthProfessional

218. American Heart Association. Saturated fat. Accessed February 12,

2024. https://www.heart.org/en/healthy-living/healthy-eating/eat-smart/fats/saturated-fats

219. MyFoodData. Top 10 foods highest in saturated fat. Updated May 29, 2023. Accessed February 12, 2024. https://www.myfooddata.com/articles/foods-highest-in-saturated-fat.php
220. American Heart Association. Trans fats. Accessed February 13, 2024. https://www.heart.org/en/healthy-living/healthy-eating/eat-smart/fats/trans-fat
221. U.S. Food and Drug Administration. Trans fat. Accessed February 13, 2024. https://www.fda.gov/food/food-additives-petitions/trans-fat
222. Holesh JE, Aslam S, Martin A. Physiology, carbohydrates. In: StatPearls [Internet]. Treasure Island (FL): StatPearls Publishing; May 12, 2023. Accessed January 10, 2024. https://www.ncbi.nlm.nih.gov/books/NBK459280/
223. Szalay J. What are carbohydrates? Live Science. July 15, 2017. Updated July 20, 2022. Accessed January 10, 2024. https://www.livescience.com/51976-carbohydrates.html
224. Mergenthaler P, Lindauer U, Dienel GA, Meisel A. Sugar for the brain: the role of glucose in physiological and pathological brain function. Trends Neurosci. 2013;36(10):587-597. doi:10.1016/j.tins.2013.07.001
225. Slavin J, Carlson J. Carbohydrates. Adv Nutr. 2014;5(6):760-761. doi:10.3945/an.114.006163.
226. Nutrients Review. Disaccharides. Accessed January 9, 2024. https://www.nutrientsreview.com/carbs/disaccharides.html.
227. Nutrients Review. Oligosaccharides. Accessed January 9, 2024. https://www.nutrientsreview.com/carbs/oligosaccharides.html.
228. Nutrients Review. Raffinose, stachyose, and verbascose. Accessed January 10, 2024. https://www.nutrientsreview.com/carbs/soluble-fiber-raffinose-stachyose-verbascose.html.
229. Niness KR. Inulin and oligofructose: what are they? J Nutr. 1999;129(7Suppl):1402S-1406S. doi:10.1093/jn/129.7.1402S.
230. Milner JA. Functional foods and health promotion. J Nutr. 1999;129(7Suppl):1395S-1397S. doi:10.1093/jn/129.7.1395S.
231. Nutrients Review. Maltotriose. Accessed January 9, 2024. https://www.nutrientsreview.com/carbs/oligosaccharides-maltotriose.html.

232. Gupta N, Jangid AK, Pooja D, Kulhari H. Inulin: a novel and stretchy polysaccharide tool for biomedical and nutritional applications. Int J Biol Macromol. 2019;132:852-863. doi:10.1016/j.ijbiomac.2019.03.188.
233. Shoaib M, Shehzad A, Omar M, et al. Inulin: properties, health benefits and food applications. Carbohydr Polym. 2016;147:444-454. doi:10.1016/j.carbpol.2016.04.020.
234. Nutrients Review. Inulin. Accessed January 8, 2024. https://www.nutrientsreview.com/carbs/soluble-fiber-inulin.html.
235. Lovegrove A, Edwards CH, De Noni I, et al. Role of polysaccharides in food, digestion, and health. Crit Rev Food Sci Nutr. 2017;57(2):237-263. doi:10.1080/10408398.2014.939263.
236. Harvard Health Publishing. The lowdown on glycemic index and glycemic load. August 2, 2023. Accessed January 8, 2024. https://www.health.harvard.edu/diseases-and-conditions/the-lowdown-on-glycemic-index-and-glycemic-load.
237. Venn BJ, Green TJ. Glycemic index and glycemic load: measurement issues and their effect on diet–disease relationships. Eur J Clin Nutr. 2007;61 Suppl 1:S122-S131. doi:10.1038/sj.ejcn.1602942.
238. Harvard T.H. Chan School of Public Health. Carbohydrates and blood sugar. Accessed January 9, 2024. https://www.hsph.harvard.edu/nutritionsource/carbohydrates/carbohydrates-and-blood-sugar/
239. Vega-López S, Venn BJ, Slavin JL. Relevance of the glycemic index and glycemic load for body weight, diabetes, and cardiovascular disease. Nutrients. 2018;10(10):1361. doi:10.3390/nu10101361.
240. Pilipczuk T, Kusznierewicz B, Zielińska D, Bartoszek A. The influence of roasting and additional processing on the content of bioactive components in special purpose coffees. J Food Sci Technol. 2015;52(9):5736-5744. doi:10.1007/s13197-014-1646-6.
241. InTolerApp. Version 3.3.21 [iOS mobile app]. 2025. Accessed November 2025. https://apps.apple.com
242. Onyx A. Casa de Sante. Casa de Sante website. 2025. Accessed November 2025. https://casadesante.com
243. Histamino. Histamino website. 2025. Accessed November 2025. https://histamino.com

Acknowledgments

I want to take a moment to acknowledge all the people who supported me on this journey—those who stood by me in difficult times and everyone who helped bring this book to life.

First and foremost, I thank my partner and my friends for believing in me and sticking with me through the years when I was unavailable for anything but this project. It claimed so much of our time together, and I deeply appreciate your understanding of how important it was for me to write this book.

I'm grateful to Holly Emma for early editing and structural improvements, and to Patrick M. Parker for reminding me to paint pictures with my words. Thank you as well to everyone who helped with countless rounds of feedback and proofreading: Imogen Solloway, Melissa Gilly†, Dr. John van Limburg-Stirum, Dr. Protazy Rejmer, Dr. Simon Reichel, Sean Less, Ellie Fletcher, Molly Stauffer, and Charles C. Dahinden.

I'm especially indebted to my production team: Michael Tizzano for his input and an amazing collaboration in the final phase of editing; Trinity McFadden for her last-minute proofreading; Denise Gibbon for her careful legal review; Jennifer Federico Stimson for her patience, flexibility, and the beautiful cover; Arjan van Woensel for his fantastic typesetting; Will Allan for indexing, and Rodney Hatfield for helping the book find its audience. My gratitude also to Christina DeFranco of KN Literary Arts for a pivotal call that shaped the book's direction, and to Shana Hartman for sharing her insights on bringing books to the market.

Endless gratitude goes to my medical team for their steadfast support and guidance—Dr. John van Limburg-Stirum, Dr. Simon Reichel, Dr. Franziska Saissi, Dr. René Zenhäusern, Rebekka Kraemer, Dr. Karoline Zepter, and Cilgia Pfleiderer—and especially to Dr. Protazy Rejmer for his meticulous medical review, ingenuity, and forthright feedback and support. I'm equally grateful to the doctors who generously shared their feedback but prefer to remain unnamed.

Finally, I extend heartfelt appreciation to the self-help community—organizations, group leaders, and participants—for your engagement, support, and help in sharing this information.

Without all of you, the process of writing this book, and my life in general, would have been so much harder, and the outcome nowhere near as good!

Thank you with all my heart; you all mean so much to me!

About the Author

Joy A. Schweizer is a writer, patient advocate, and independent health researcher living with Mast Cell Activation Syndrome (MCAS), Ehlers-Danlos Syndrome (EDS), Hereditary Alpha Tryptasemia (HαT), and Immune Thrombocytopenia (ITP). After being told in her teens that she would likely never regain the use of her hands due to a disabling inflammatory condition, she embarked on a path of self-guided rehabilitation and deep research that defied medical expectations.

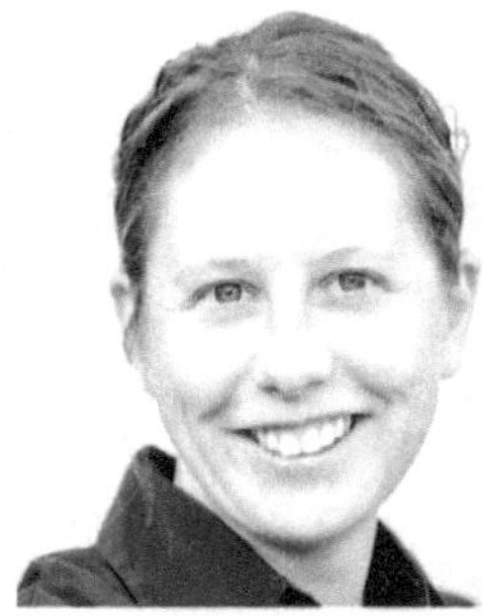

Unable to pursue a conventional career because of ongoing health challenges, Joy developed a uniquely diverse background spanning fields such as sales, food service, creative arts, and wellness. This breadth of experience, combined with years of patient-led inquiry and engagement with medical professionals and chronic illness communities, informs the grounded and compassionate approach she brings to her writing.

Her book, *Managing Mad Mast Cells,* was born from the insights she wished she had when she was first diagnosed. With it, she aims to bridge the gap between clinical knowledge and real-world experience—offering practical strategies, encouragement, and clarity for others navigating MCAS.

Joy lives in her mountain home in Switzerland. When she's not writing, she enjoys spending time in nature, painting, cooking, and making music.

A Note to Readers

If this book has been helpful to you, I'd truly appreciate it if you would take a moment to leave a review on Amazon. Your feedback not only supports my work but also helps others living with MCAS—or those seeking to understand it—discover this book.

For updates and downloadable resources please visit www.mcas-book.com.

Thank you for joining me on this journey!

Joy

Index

www.ingramcontent.com/pod-product-compliance
Lightning Source LLC
Chambersburg PA
CBHW031335230926
51848CB00002B/239

9783952627303